BRAIN CHEMISTRY AND MENTAL DISEASE

Proceedings of a Symposium on Brain Chemistry and Mental Disease held at the Texas Research Institute, Houston, Texas, November 18-20, 1970

Edited by
Beng T. Ho and William M. McIsaac
Texas Research Institute of Mental Sciences
Texas Medical Center
Houston, Texas

 PLENUM PRESS · NEW YORK–LONDON · 1971

The present volume, Volume 1 of the new series *Advances in Behavioral Biology,* simultaneously constitutes Volume 4 of *Advances in Mental Science,* a series of proceedings of annual symposia held since 1967 at the Texas Research Institute of Mental Sciences in Houston. The preceding volumes are *Congenital Mental Retardation, Drug Dependence,* and *Biological Aspects of Alcohol,* which were published by University of Texas Press.

Library of Congress Catalog Card Number 78-165398

SBN 306-37901-5

© 1971 Plenum Press, New York
A Division of Plenum Publishing Corporation
227 West 17th Street, New York, N.Y. 10011

United Kingdom edition published by Plenum Press, London
A Division of Plenum Publishing Company, Ltd.
Davis House (4th Floor), 8 Scrubs Lane, Harlesden, NW10 6SE, England

All rights reserved

No part of this publication may be reproduced in any form
without written permission from the publisher

Printed in the United States of America

PREFACE

This volume contains the proceedings of the fourth international symposium held in November 1970 at the Texas Research Institute of Mental Sciences in Houston. Leading psychiatrists, biochemists, and pharmacologists from the United States and Great Britain presented new material and reviewed current concepts concerning schizophrenia and the affective disorders, with particular reference to the neurochemical basis of the etiology and chemotherapy of these diseases.

Although the multiple mechanisms of mental disease are still not fully understood, substantial progress has definitely been made. The greatest contribution has come through the development of new therapeutic agents that not only provide invaluable help to the mentally ill but serve as chemical tools for studying the biological mechanisms associated with the disease state. Studies concerning the proposed catecholamine and indolealkylamine hypotheses for affective disorders and the possible formation of endogenous toxins in schizophrenia have stimulated significant new research.

This book presents new studies of schizophrenia and the affective disorders in one volume. It is our hope that it represents an effective integration of basic biochemical and pharmacological research with current clinical findings and that it will increase understanding of the etiology of mental disease and provide an impetus for the development of more effective therapeutic agents.

We thank Drs. Gordon Farrell, Samuel Gershon, A. Horita, Irwin Kopin, and Joseph Schildkraut for their help with the organization of the meeting and for chairing the corresponding sessions.

We are grateful to CIBA Pharmaceutical Company, Mead Johnson, New England Nuclear Corporation, Sandoz Pharmaceuticals, Schering Corporation, Smith Kline & French Laboratories, E. R. Squibb & Sons, and The Pauline Sterne Wolff Memorial Home for their generous financial support.

Our special thanks to the many staff members who contributed to the smooth running of the symposium, especially Suzanne Barnes, Chester Calhoun, Gail Cox, Ed Fritchie, Pat Gardner, Jack Palmer, Lillie Mae Phillips, Wallace Ragan, Dr. Mary K. Roach, Jere Schulze, Harry Turley, and Frank Womack. Our personal appreciation to Lore Feldman for her help in editing the manuscript, and to Gerry Musgrove for her assistance in typing it for publication.

Beng T. Ho

William M. McIsaac

CONTRIBUTORS

Lacoe B. Alltop, M.S.P.H.
    Biostatistician, North Carolina Department of Health, Chapel Hill, North Carolina

Fuad Antun, M.D.
    Research Fellow, Department of Psychiatry, University of Edinburgh, Edinburgh, Scotland

George R. Breese, Ph.D.
    Assistant Professor of Pharmacology and Psychiatry, The University of North Carolina School of Medicine, Chapel Hill, North Carolina

Bruce Buckingham
    Research Associate, Department of Psychiatry, School of Medicine, University of California, San Diego; La Jolla, California

William E. Bunney, Jr., M.D.
    Chief, Section on Psychiatry, Laboratory of Clinical Science, National Institute of Mental Health, Bethesda, Maryland

John D. Connor, Ph.D.
    Assistant Professor, Department of Pharmacology, The Milton Hershey Medical Center of The Pennsylvania State University College of Medicine, Hershey, Pennsylvania

Alec Coppen, M.D.
    Clinical Director, Medical Research Council Laboratories, Neuropsychiatric Research Unit, Clinical Investigation Ward, Greenbank, West Park Hospital, Epsom, Surrey, England

Erminio Costa, M.D.
    Chief, Laboratory of Preclinical Pharmacology, National Institute of Mental Health–St. Elizabeths Hospital, Washington, D. C.

Gerald Curzon, Ph.D., D.Sc.
    Reader in Biochemistry, Department of Chemical Pathology, Institute of Neurology, London, England

Paul R. Draskoczy, M.D.
    Pharmacologist, Neuropsychopharmacology Laboratory, Massachusetts Mental Health Center, and Lecturer in Pharmacology, Harvard Medical School, Boston, Massachusetts

David L. Dunner, M.D.
   Clinical Associate, Section on Psychiatry, Laboratory of Clinical Science, National Institute of Mental Health, Bethesda, Maryland. Dr. Dunner is now at the New York State Psychiatric Institute, New York, New York

Donald Eccleston, M.D.
   Assistant Director, Medical Research Council Brain Metabolism Unit, Department of Pharmacology, University of Edinburgh, Edinburgh, Scotland

Samuel Eiduson, Ph.D.
   Associate Professor, Departments of Psychiatry and Biological Chemistry, Neuropsychiatric and Brain Institutes, University of California, Los Angeles, California

Gordon L. Farrell, M.D.
   Assistant Director, Texas Research Institute of Mental Sciences; Professor of Mental Sciences, The University of Texas Graduate School of Biomedical Sciences, Houston, Texas. Dr. Farrell is now in private practice.

Elliot S. Gershon, M.D.
   Clinical Associate, Section on Psychiatry, Laboratory of Clinical Science, National Institute of Mental Health, Bethesda, Maryland. Dr. Gershon is now at Ezrath Nahim Mental Hospital, Jerusalem, Israel

Samuel Gershon, M.B.B.S., D.P.M.
   Professor of Psychiatry and Director, Neuropsychopharmacology Research Unit, New York University Medical Center School of Medicine, New York, New York

Frederick K. Goodwin, M.D.
   Unit Chief, Section on Psychiatry, Laboratory of Clinical Science, National Institute of Mental Health, Bethesda, Maryland

Edwin L. Grab, A.M.
   Assistant Chemist, Neuropsychopharmacology Laboratory, Massachusetts Mental Health Center, Boston, Massachusetts

George M. Henry, M.D.
   Clinical Associate, Section on Psychiatry, Laboratory of Clinical Science, National Institute of Mental Health, Bethesda, Maryland

Beng T. Ho, Ph.D.
   Assistant Director, Texas Research Institute of Mental Sciences; Professor of Mental Sciences, The University of Texas Graduate School of Biomedical Sciences, Houston, Texas

Leo E. Hollister, M.D.
   Associate Chief of Staff and Medical Investigator, Veterans Administration Hospital, Palo Alto, California; Associate Professor of Medicine, Stanford University School of Medicine, Stanford, California

Akira Horita, Ph.D.
   Professor, Department of Pharmacology, University of Washington School of Medicine, Seattle, Washington

CONTRIBUTORS

Seymour S. Kety, M.D.
   Director, Psychiatric Research Laboratories, Massachusetts General Hospital, and Professor of Psychiatry, Harvard Medical School, Boston, Massachusetts

Gerald L. Klerman, M.D.
   Professor of Psychiatry, Harvard Medical School–Massachusetts General Hospital, Boston, Massachusetts

Angelina Knox, M.D.
   Unit Director, Dorothea Dix Hospital, Raleigh, North Carolina

Irwin J. Kopin, M.D.
   Chief, Laboratory of Clinical Science, National Institute of Mental Health, Bethesda, Maryland

Morris A. Lipton, Ph.D., M.D.
   Professor and Chairman, Department of Psychiatry, The University of North Carolina School of Medicine, Chapel Hill, North Carolina

James W. Maas, M.D.
   Director of Research, Illinois State Psychiatric Institute, and Professor of Psychiatry, University of Illinois College of Medicine, Chicago, Illinois

Arnold J. Mandell, M.D.
   Professor and Chairman, Department of Psychiatry, School of Medicine, University of California, San Diego; La Jolla, California

Billy R. Martin, B.S.
   Chief Technician, Department of Psychiatry, The University of North Carolina School of Medicine, Chapel Hill, North Carolina

Dennis L. Murphy, M.D.
   Unit Chief, Section on Psychiatry, Laboratory of Clinical Science, National Institute of Mental Health, Bethesda, Maryland

José M. Musacchio, M.D.
   Associate Professor, Department of Pharmacology, New York University Medical Center School of Medicine, New York, New York

George Wilson McBee, B.A.
   Chief of Systems Analysis, Texas Research Institute of Mental Sciences, Houston, Texas

Thomas K. McClane, M.D.
   Lakeland, Florida

William M. McIsaac, M.D., Ph.D., D.Sc.
   Director, Texas Research Institute of Mental Sciences; Professor of Mental Sciences, The University of Texas Graduate School of Biomedical Sciences; Associate Professor of Biochemistry and Psychiatry, Baylor College of Medicine, Houston, Texas

M. K. Naimzada, M.D.
  Laboratory of Preclinical Pharmacology, National Institute of Mental Health—St. Elizabeths Hospital, Washington, D. C.

William L. Nyhan, M.D., Ph.D.
  Professor and Chairman, Department of Pediatrics, University of California School of Medicine, San Diego; La Jolla, California

Arthur J. Prange, Jr., M.D.
  Professor of Psychiatry and Director of Research Development, Department of Psychiatry, The University of North Carolina School of Medicine, Chapel Hill, North Carolina

Peter Reich, M.D.
  Senior Associate in Medicine and Assistant Professor of Psychiatry, Peter Bent Brigham Hospital, Harvard Medical School, Boston, Massachusetts

A. Revuelta, D.M.D.
  Laboratory of Preclinical Pharmacology, National Institute of Mental Health—St. Elizabeths Hospital, Washington, D. C.

Joseph J. Schildkraut, M.D.
  Director, Neuropsychopharmacology Laboratory, and Associate Professor of Psychiatry, Massachusetts Mental Health Center and Harvard Medical School, Boston, Massachusetts

David Segal, Ph.D.
  Assistant Research Psychobiologist, Department of Psychiatry, School of Medicine, University of California, San Diego; La Jolla, California

Charles R. Shaw, M.D.
  Professor of Biology, The University of Texas M. D. Anderson Hospital and Tumor Institute at Houston, Houston, Texas

Jean-Hung C. Shih, Ph.D.
  Assistant Resident Biological Chemist, Department of Psychiatry, Medical School, University of California, Los Angeles, California

Baron Shopsin, M.D.
  Research Psychiatrist, Neuropsychopharmacology Research Unit, Department of Psychiatry, New York University Medical Center School of Medicine, New York, New York

J. R. Smythies, M.D.
  Reader in Psychiatry, Department of Psychiatry, University of Edinburgh, Edinburgh, Scotland

Dorothy Taylor, M.S.
  Research Assistant, Texas Research Institute of Mental Sciences, Houston, Texas

Ian C. Wilson, M.B., D.P.M.
  Research Psychiatrist, North Carolina Department of Mental Health, Chapel Hill, North Carolina

CONTENTS

Preface v
Contributors vii

ENZYMES: IMPLICATIONS IN MENTAL DISEASE

Introduction 1
    A. Horita

Multiple Forms of Monoamine Oxidase in Developing Tissues:
The Implications for Mental Disorder 3
    Jean-Hung C. Shih and Samuel Eiduson

Regulation of Catecholamine Biosynthesis:
Tyrosine Hydroxylase and Dihydropteridine Reductase 21
    José M. Musacchio

Behavioral, Metabolic, and Enzymatic Studies of a
Brain Indoleethylamine N-Methylating System 37
    Arnold J. Mandell, Bruce Buckingham, and David Segal

Transmethylation Processes in Schizophrenia 61
    F. Antun, D. Eccleston, and J. R. Smythies

PSYCHOACTIVE AGENTS: BIOLOGICAL ACTIONS

Effects of Drugs on Catecholamine Synthesis 73
    Irwin J. Kopin

Pharmacological Implications of the Effects of Amphetamine
and Its Analogs on the Turnover Rate of Tissue
Catecholamines 83
    E. Costa, M. K. Naimzada, and A. Revuelta

Studies on the Mechanism of Action of 6-Methoxytetrahydro-Beta-
Carboline in Elevating Brain Serotonin 97
    Beng T. Ho, Dorothy Taylor, and William M. McIsaac

Comparison of the Effects of Electrical Stimulation
and Iontophoretic Dopamine on Neurons of the
Nigro-Neostriatal Pathway 113
    John D. Connor

BIOLOGICAL ASPECTS OF AFFECTIVE DISORDERS

Biogenic Amines and Affective Disorders 123
    Alec Coppen

Catecholamines and Affective Illness: Studies with
L-DOPA and Alpha-Methyl-Para-Tyrosine 135
    Elliot S. Gershon, William E. Bunney, Jr., Frederick K. Goodwin,
    Dennis L. Murphy, David L. Dunner, and George M. Henry

Relationships between Stress and Brain 5-Hydroxy-
tryptamine and their Possible Significance in
Affective Disorders 163
    G. Curzon

Interactions between Adrenocortical Steroid
Hormones, Electrolytes, and the Catecholamines 177
    James W. Maas

Thyroid-Imipramine Interaction: Clinical Results
and Basic Mechanism 197
    Arthur J. Prange, Jr., Ian C. Wilson, Angelina E. Knox,
    Thomas K. McClane, George R. Breese, Billy R. Martin,
    Lacoe B. Alltop, and Morris A. Lipton

Effects of Tricyclic Antidepressants on Norepinephrine Metabolism:
Basic and Clinical Studies 215
    Joseph J. Schildkraut, Paul R. Draskoczy, Elliot S. Gershon,
    Peter Reich, and Edwin L. Grab

BRAIN AMINES AND AFFECTIVE DISORDERS

Overall Review 237
    Seymour S. Kety

Panel Discussion 245

GENETIC AND METABOLIC FACTORS IN MENTAL DISORDERS

Heterogeneous Distributions of Schizophrenia 265
    George Wilson McBee

Frequency of Genetic Polymorphism: Implications for Mental Disease 275
    Charles R. Shaw

Purine Metabolism and Abnormal Behavior in Children 281
    William L. Nyhan

MODERN CONCEPTS OF CHEMOTHERAPY

Chemotherapy of Schizophrenia 303
    Leo E. Hollister

Chemotherapy of Manic-Depressive Disorder
    Baron Shopsin and Samuel Gershon

    I. Introduction 319
    II. Chemotherapy of Mania 320
    III. Prophylaxis Against Manic and Depressive Relapses 346
    IV. Behavioral Toxicity 354
    V. Psychoactive Drugs Versus Other Forms of Therapy 356
    VI. Psychoactive Drug Choice 356
    VII. General Conclusions and Principles of Drug Treatment 357
    VIII. Problems of Drug Evaluation in Mania: Research Design and Methodology 359
    IX. Mood Disorders in Children and Adolescents: Diagnostic Problems
        and Chemotherapy with Lithium 362

Chemotherapy of Depression 379
    Gerald L. Klerman

Index 403

INTRODUCTION

ENZYMES: IMPLICATIONS IN MENTAL DISEASE

A. Horita

School of Medicine, University of Washington

Seattle, Washington

In the title for this morning's session, the term "implications" is quite appropriate, for there is at present no known enzyme that is responsible for the genesis of mental illness. Thus, selecting topics and speakers for this session was rather difficult for Dr. Ho and me, because we did not want "just another" symposium on the biochemistry of mental disease. We decided that the topics for this session should represent not only those areas of interest today, but also those most likely to exert a significant impact on future progress in understanding the biochemistry of mental illness. We selected four areas of research that in our opinion have exciting possibilities. These include the advances in the areas of monoamine oxidase, tyrosine hydroxylase, and the enzymes involved in the transmethylation of the biogenic amines.

The probable role of monoamine oxidase in behavior modification is well known. Inhibition of this enzyme with various agents has shown striking psychopharmacological actions in both man and in animals. Now there is evidence that monoamine oxidase in brain is comprised of several forms--possibly isoenzymes--and this finding opens up new explorations that may further clarify the nature and function of this poorly understood enzyme in the central nervous system.

The second enzyme system to be discussed, tyrosine hydroxylase, is the rate-limiting step in the biosynthesis of norepinephrine. Historically, this was the last step to be discovered, and with it, the total picture of catecholamine metabolism was completed. Although the isolation and characterization of tyrosine hydroxylase of adrenal medulla was accomplished only six years ago, the importance of this enzyme in the overall regulation of the sympathetic nervous system, both central and peripheral, is becoming recognized rapidly. This was quite evident from the number of papers and the enthusiasm on this subject of this year's Federation and Pharmacological Society meetings. Much more is to be learned, not only about the biochemical properties of tyrosine hydroxylase, but also about the various influences that regulate its activity and synthesis in the intact animal.

Although they are important in the overall regulation of catecholamine metabolism, the two enzyme systems, monoamine oxidase and tyrosine hydroxylase, have yet to be seriously implicated in mental illness. They are essential for normal behavior, as is evident from inhibition studies. There is no evidence as yet, however, that an excess or deficiency of these enzymes is associated with any known form of psychopathology. But there is the hypothesis that abnormal transmethylation processes may be involved in the genesis of mental illness. The assumption is that abnormal transmethylation of either catecholamines or indoleamines can occur, resulting in the formation of psychotomimetic agents that resemble mescaline or bufotenine. The fact that such substances have been reported in the urine of schizophrenic patients makes the abnormal transmethylation hypothesis even more attractive. I should emphasize, however, that this hypothesis is not totally accepted, because many inconsistencies and negative results have also been found. The present status of the transmethylation system in mental illness constitutes a major part of this discussion.

Only time will tell whether our selection of topics was correct as a forecast for research trends in mental health. In any event, I believe that many of the investigations in these areas will continue to serve as stepping stones toward our ultimate goal, namely, understanding the biochemical basis of mental disease.

MULTIPLE FORMS OF MONOAMINE OXIDASE IN DEVELOPING TISSUES:

THE IMPLICATIONS FOR MENTAL DISORDER

Jean-Hung C. Shih and Samuel Eiduson

Neuropsychiatric and Brain Institutes
University of California at Los Angeles Medical School

Los Angeles, California

For a number of years our laboratory has been concerned with the developmental characteristics of the biogenic amines in the maturing brain (Eiduson 1966; Eberle and Eiduson 1968). More specifically, we believe as others do that a knowledge of how the biosynthesis, tissue levels, and catabolism of these amines are regulated during brain development may lead to a greater understanding of the biochemical and behavioral individuality exhibited by higher organisms and man himself. Little knowledge has been adduced about these regulatory mechanisms, especially during the formative period of development, although some workers have suggested end-product feed-back inhibition in the case of norepinephrine biosynthesis (Spector et al. 1967), or end-product feed-back repression of the enzyme involved in the first step of serotonin biosynthesis (Eiduson 1966). Thus we have been led to speculate about the possible mechanisms that may play a role in the regulation of these amines in different parts of the brain, and especially during development of the brain. These considerations, as well as our search and interpretation of the literature, have led us to consider the notion that there may exist multiple forms (isoenzymes) of monoamine oxidase (monoamine: O_2-oxidoreductase [deaminating] EC 1.4.3.4) that may play a significant role in the regulation of these important neurohumoral substances. We shall be using the terms "multiple forms" of an enzyme and "isoenzyme" interchangeably since it is difficult to give a very precise definition of the word "isoenzyme." We shall accept as definition for the time being, as was suggested by Latner and Skillen (1968), that "...most authorities believe that a broad definition such as 'different proteins with similar enzymatic activity' best suits the current state of our knowledge. It is customary, for the most part, to limit this definition to multiple enzymes obtained from one tissue of one individual animal or plant or possibly a small organ, or a culture of a unicellular organism." Accordingly, the properties of monoamine oxidase (MAO) and especially its activity in developing brain (and other tissues of the maturing organism), as well as in certain clinical disease entities, serve as the subject matter of this paper.

That an approach of this kind may be exceedingly useful is well demonstrated not only by our own and other investigators' work on MAO, but also by the already considerable evidence of the existence of multiple forms of other enzymes and especially those of lactic dehydrogenase (LDH). Studies with the isoenzymes of lactic dehydrogenase have shown that there exist not only species and organ specificities but, importantly, developmental changes in the appearance of multiple forms of this enzyme. Markert and Ursprung (1962) have shown, for example, that the patterns of LDH isoenzyme distribution in embryonic tissues of the mouse differ from those of the adult; that is, LDH-5, which is found principally in embryonic tissue, changes gradually to LDH-1 in adult tissues. These workers also point out that since these isoenzymes differ in kinetic properties, substrate concentration optima, etc., it is likely that they fulfill distinct metabolic roles in cellular metabolism; "LDH-5 is more abundant in tissues subject to relative anaerobiosis, and the isoenzymes at the other end of the spectrum are more abundant in highly oxygenated tissues." The work of Fine, Kaplan and Kuftinec (1963) has also demonstrated developmental changes; that is, the human embryonic liver contains the H-type LDH almost exclusively, while the adult has very little of this type. These workers also have observed a considerable difference in the type of LDH present in liver of various adult species, and they speculate that this variation in the multiple forms of LDH is not a random occurrence but is of functional importance in liver metabolism. These developmental changes have also been seen in mouse heart (Smith and Kissane 1963). More recently, the work of Schultz and Ruth (1968) and Wuntch, Chen and Vessell (1970) suggests the possibility that different isoenzymes may be subject to different kinds of regulation and that they, in turn, regulate different functions.

The suggestion by a number of investigators that there might be multiple forms of monoamine oxidase is based on indirect evidence derived from multiple substrate and inhibitor studies (Werle and Röwer 1952; Oswald and Strittmatter 1963; Hardegg and Heilbronn 1961; Fellman and Roth 1965; Gorkin *et al.* 1964). There are even some reports detailing the attempt to isolate the pure enzyme that also suggest the possibility of the existence of one or more multiple forms of MAO (Gorkin 1963; Youdim and Sourkes 1966; Youdim and Sandler 1967; Kim and D'Iorio 1968; Squires 1968; Ragland 1968; Gomes *et al.* 1969). Recently, Youdim, Collins, and Sandler (1969) reported that, using gel electrophoresis, they were able to obtain four bands from rat brain mitochondria that had MAO activity. These workers observed that these bands showed different substrate specificities and inhibitor sensitivities. Unfortunately, to our knowledge, there has been little information to date on the developmental nature and significance of these multiple forms of MAO or the role they play in the metabolism of the biogenic amines. Neither have there been any reports on the possible significance of these MAO isoenzymes for any disease state, except for the speculative remarks by Youdim, Collins and Sandler (1969) that, since some MAO inhibitors are used for alleviating depression, the multiple forms of MAO may possibly be involved in the biochemistry of depression.

Last year Dr. Jean Shih and I published our first results on the polyacrylamide gel patterns of monoamine oxidase derived from newborn and adult chick brain (Shih and Eiduson 1969). At that time we presented evidence for the existence of multiple forms of MAO and for the change that takes place during brain development. These studies have now been extended to demonstrate the existence of multiple forms of MAO in rat brain, heart, and liver and to show the developmental changes that take place in these tissues.

In brief, the technique was to obtain the tissues at zero degrees following decapitation of the rat and to homogenize them in cold buffer. The MAO was solubilized by either sonic oscillation or by homogenizing the tissue in the presence of a non-ionic detergent (Triton X-100). Following centrifugation, aliquots of the supernatant were applied to the gels and run for two hours in the cold. The staining technique for visualizing the MAO bands was essentially that of Glenner's, using nitro-blue tetrazolium dye and either tryptamine, benzylamine or serotonin as substrate for the enzyme.

Figure 1 shows the MAO patterns comparing brain, heart, and liver obtained for newborn and adult rats (Sprague-Dawley). In this figure, tryptamine was used as substrate for the enzyme. It is clear from the results that there were bands staining for MAO, with tryptamine as substrate, in the adult tissue that were not present in the newborn. In every case, at least twice as many MAO-staining bands appeared in the adult tissue as in that of the infant. In addition, it was apparent that the two infant bands migrated to a position similar to two such bands obtained from adult tissues. In almost every instance, the newborn tissues contained both the slowest and the fastest moving of the multiple forms of the adult MAO, while the adult tissues also had bands showing an intermediate speed. Since the MAO bands do not photograph nor project well, we have made diagrammatic sketches of the gels. Figure 2 is a diagram of Figure 1. The results obtained from adult and infant tissues, using 5-hydroxytryptamine as substrate for the MAO, are shown in Figure 3. Again, the MAO patterns derived from the

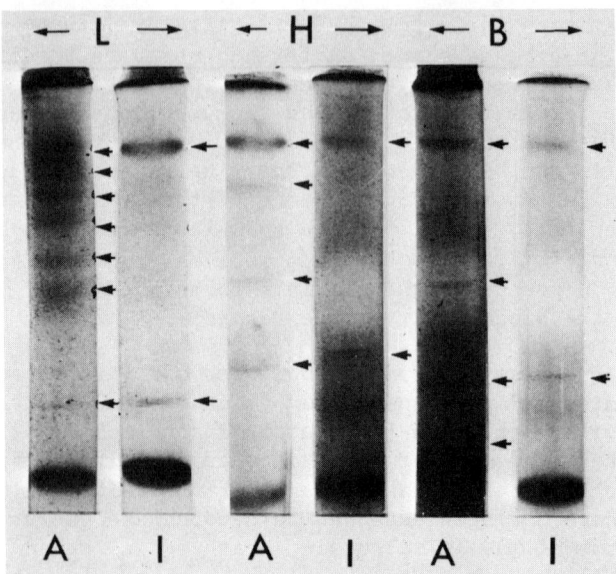

Figure 1. Gel-electrophoretic patterns of MAO from newborn (1) and adult (A) rat tissues: liver (L), heart (H), brain (B). The substrate employed was tryptamine.

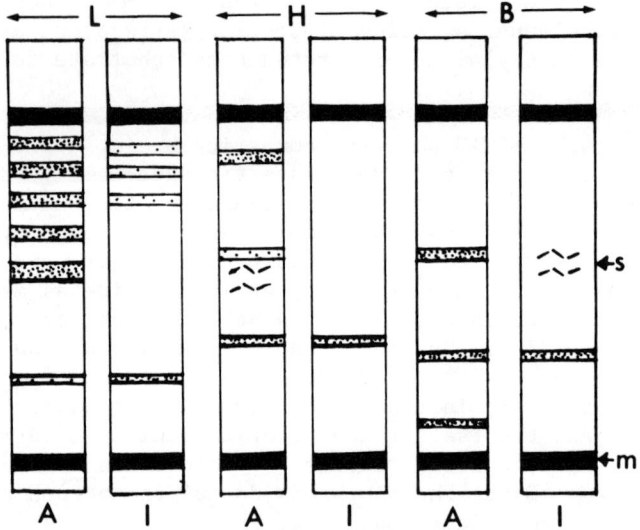

Figure 2. Diagrammatic representation of Figure 1. "s" defines a clean, colorless space in the gel; "m" refers to the position of the dye marker.

MAO IN DEVELOPING BRAIN

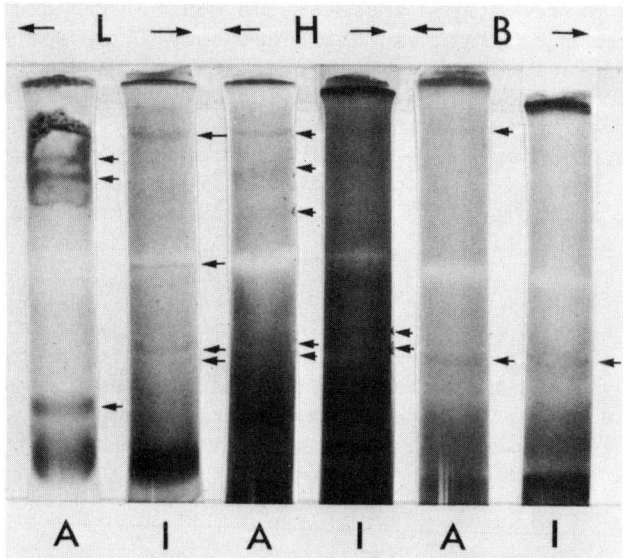

Figure 3. Same as Figure 1, except that 5-hydroxytryptamine was used as substrate for the MAO.

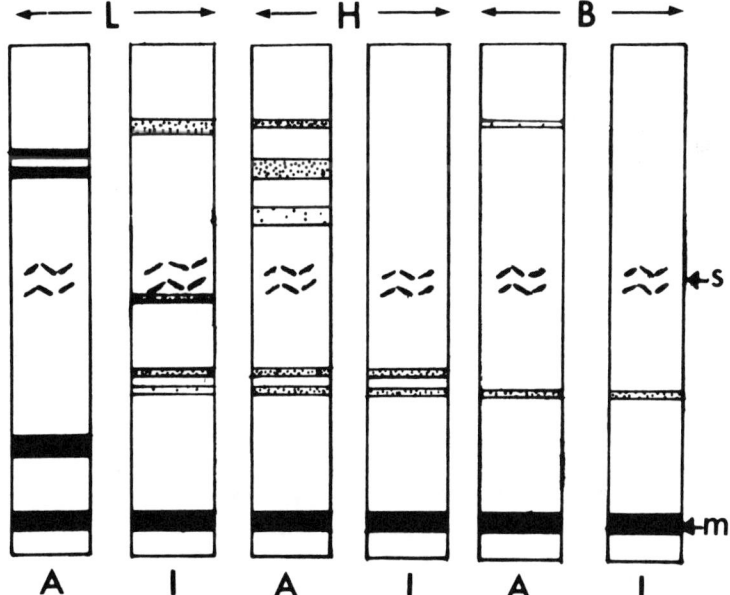

Figure 4. Diagrammatic representation of Figure 3.

infant tissues differed from those of the adult. The adult MAO patterns derived from brain and heart not only possessed the bands seen with the infant, but they showed additional bands. The infant liver tissue showed four bands of MAO activity while the adult liver tissue showed three distinct bands of activity. It is hazardous, of course, to compare the multiple forms of MAO across tissues, but it may be tentatively proposed that different tissues may possess different multiple forms of the enzyme. Figure 4 is the diagram of the previous figure.

In order to begin to assess whether these multiple forms of MAO have different substrate specificities beyond what we have already shown with our method, newborn tissues (brain, heart, and liver) were assayed for MAO active bands, using three different substrates for the enzyme: 5-hydroxytryptamine, benzylamine, and tryptamine. Figure 5 shows the results obtained from newborn brain in

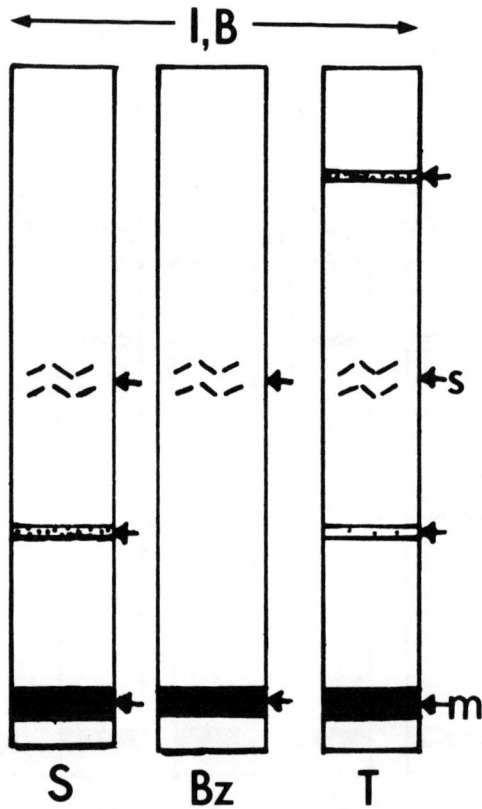

Figure 5. Diagram of MAO gel patterns obtained from newborn (one-day-old) rat brain. Substrates used were serotonin (S), benzylamine (Bz), tryptamine (T).

diagrammatic form. It was apparent that, when tryptamine was used as substrate for the enzyme, two bands possessing MAO activity appeared. When serotonin was used as substrate, only one of the bands appeared. Apparently the slower moving (upper) form of MAO had little or no affinity for the 5-hydroxytryptamine. Further, it seemed that with newborn brain MAO, benzylamine could not be used equally well as substrate.

One can clearly see the substrate specificity of the MAO derived from infant rat heart (Figure 6). The slower (upper) moving

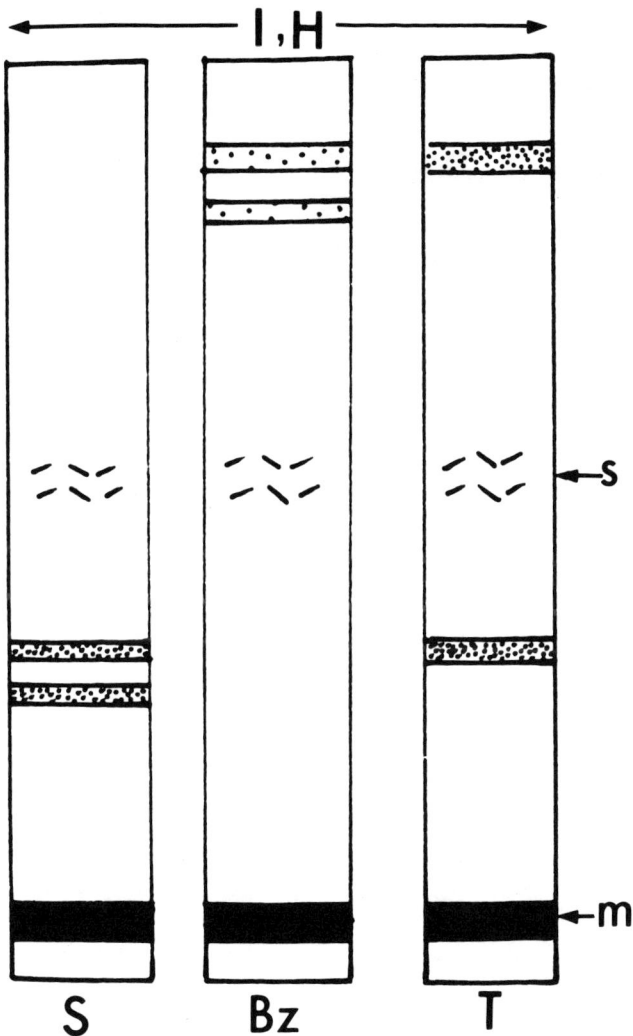

Figure 6. Same as Figure 5, except that MAO was derived from newborn rat heart.

band can use both tryptamine and benzylamine as substrate, but not serotonin. The faster (bottom) band can utilize both serotonin and tryptamine, but not benzylamine. There seems to be an additional slow-moving band of MAO that can only use benzylamine as substrate.

The results obtained from infant liver are shown in Figure 7.

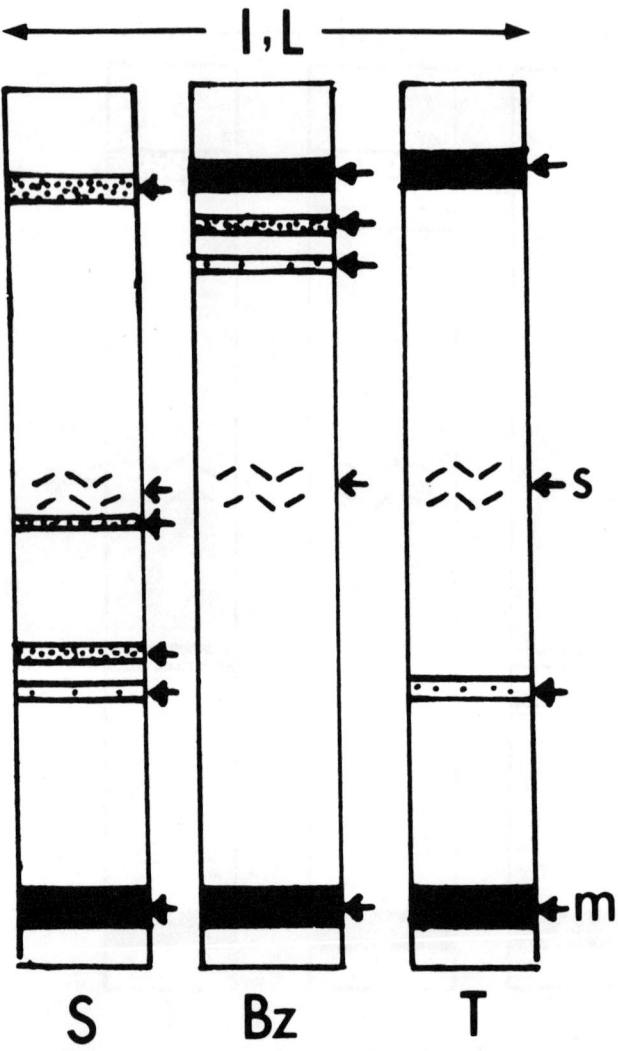

Figure 7. Diagram of MAO pattern derived from newborn rat liver. Symbols are the same as for Figure 5.

In this tissue, as seen previously, two MAO bands appeared when tryptamine was used as substrate for the enzyme. Significantly, the slower moving band stained much more heavily than the faster-moving band. In contrast to the infant brain, the MAO derived from infant liver with serotonin as substrate showed four MAO bands. Significantly too, unlike the activity observed with brain tissue, the slower moving forms of the enzyme could readily use serotonin as substrate. In addition, the infant liver possessed at least three MAO forms that could use benzylamine as substrate. The two slower moving forms of infant liver MAO could not be seen with either serotonin or tryptamine as substrate. On the other hand, the fast-moving band demonstrated an affinity for both serotonin and tryptamine, but not benzylamine.

Because the technique of gel-staining may lead to artifacts (Brooke and Engel 1966; Otsuka and Kobayashi 1964), we have employed radioactive substrate incubated with segments of the gel to check the authenticity of the stained bands that are presumed to be MAO. A comparison of brain MAO activity on the gels, as seen by the staining technique and as determined by assay with ^{14}C-labeled serotonin, is shown in Figure 8. The stained gel, with

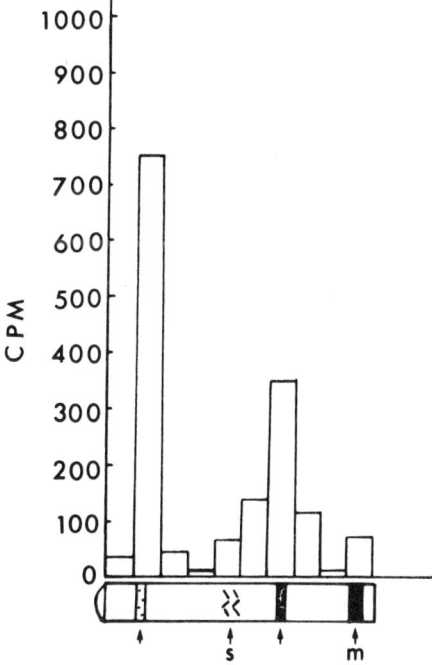

Figure 8. Comparison of MAO-stained gel to segments of a gel incubated with 5-hydroxytryptamine-2-^{14}C (see text for details). MAO was derived from adult rat brain.

serotonin as substrate, showed the bands as indicated in the figure. This was compared with the radioactivity exhibited by a duplicate gel run at the same time. It can clearly be seen that the bands, which stained for MAO activity, also exhibited MAO activity by conversion of the labeled substrate to product.

In Figure 9, the MAO derived from adult rat heart was run on the

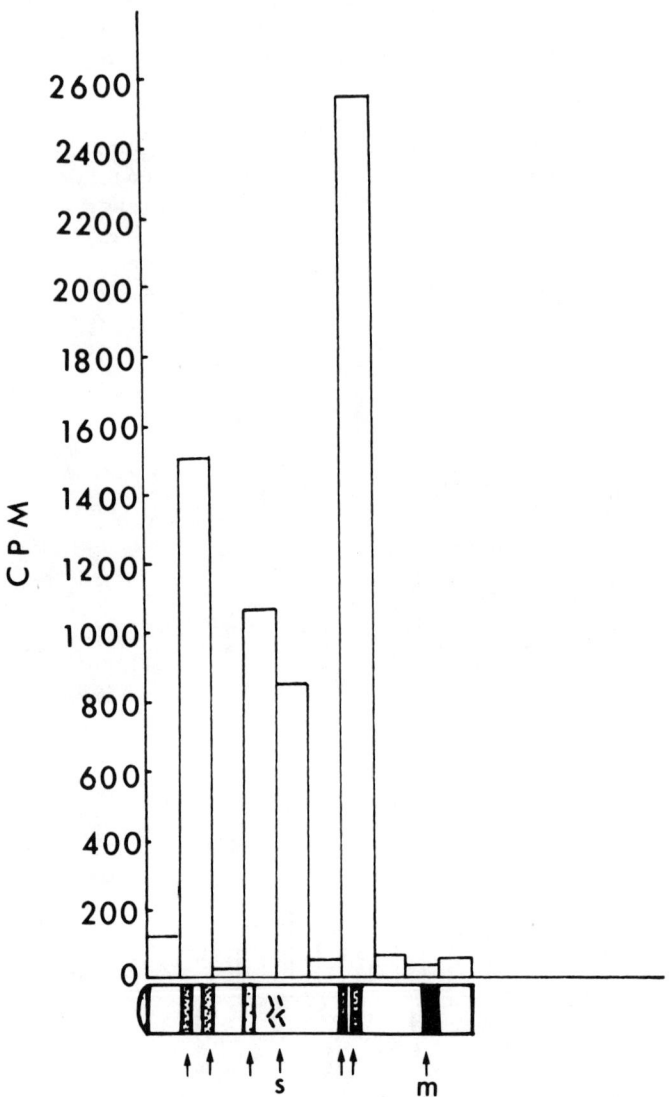

Figure 9. Same as Figure 8, except that MAO was derived from adult rat heart.

gel, and the same comparison was made between the two methods. The staining method indicated the presence of about five bands of MAO activity with serotonin as substrate. The labeling experiment indicated that MAO activity, as determined by counting the radioactive product, was essentially in the same position on the gel as were the stained bands. In addition, the very light band in the center of the gel, although it did not show a MAO stain, exhibited significant MAO activity when tested with labeled substrate.

Adult rat liver was analyzed for MAO activity as above, and the data obtained are shown in Figure 10. As seen in the previous

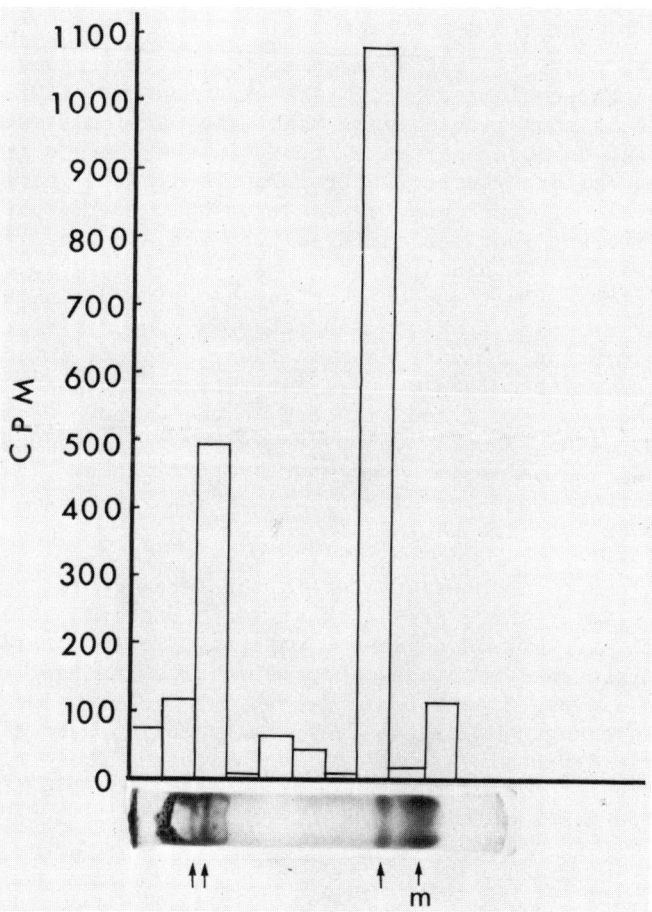

Figure 10. Same as Figure 8, except that MAO was derived from adult rat liver.

two figures, the label appeared in the same positions on the gel as did the three bands stained for activity. The liver, however, like the brain but unlike the heart, did not possess a defined, clear band in the center of the gel, and it also did not show any MAO activity in that region as determined by the labeling experiment.

It seems reasonable to assume from these data that there are indeed multiple forms of monoamine oxidase in brain and other tissues. It is clear that the total MAO pattern derived from infant tissue differs strikingly from that of the adult, thus signaling changes during development. There seems to be no question that these various forms have different affinities for the various substrates used. (We are currently finding that the different forms respond differently when incubated with a variety of MAO inhibitors.)

In view of all this, we naturally began to think and speculate about the role these multiple forms of MAO may play in human disease states. We considered, for example, that if there was any validity in the catecholamine hypothesis of affective disorders, then isoenzymes of monoamine oxidase might play an important role in regulating the turnover of the amines. Further, since it is well known that children suffering from Down's syndrome have low circulating levels of serotonin, we wondered whether the patterns of MAO were different in these children from normal. Unfortunately, we have no access to the brain of the human individual, so we must resort to indirect reflections of what may be going on in the brain by looking, for example, at blood MAO patterns. We would like to present some of our preliminary data on these. First, let me say that, since the dye technique we used for tissue MAO is not well suited for blood, we used a modification of the Graham (Graham and Karnovsky 1965) method whereby the hydrogen peroxide produced by MAO oxidation of the amine is acted upon by peroxidase. To the incubation media of the gel are added 3-amino-9-ethylcarbazol along with substrate to localize the MAO on the gel.

Figure 11 shows the MAO patterns in the serum of two normal individuals. Clearly there are at least two different patterns. For our preliminary work on depressed patients, we arbitrarily listed three different groupings. Depression 1 contained individuals who were diagnosed as chronic depressives; depression 2 were those listed as endogenous depressives; and number 3 were classified as neurotic depressives. As I have indicated, these classes were not rigorously defined for these preliminary observations and, thus, for our purposes at this time, the classes of 1, 2 or 3 can serve just as well.

The next three figures (Figures 12, 13, and 14) show the variations in MAO patterns derived from "depressed" patients' serum. It

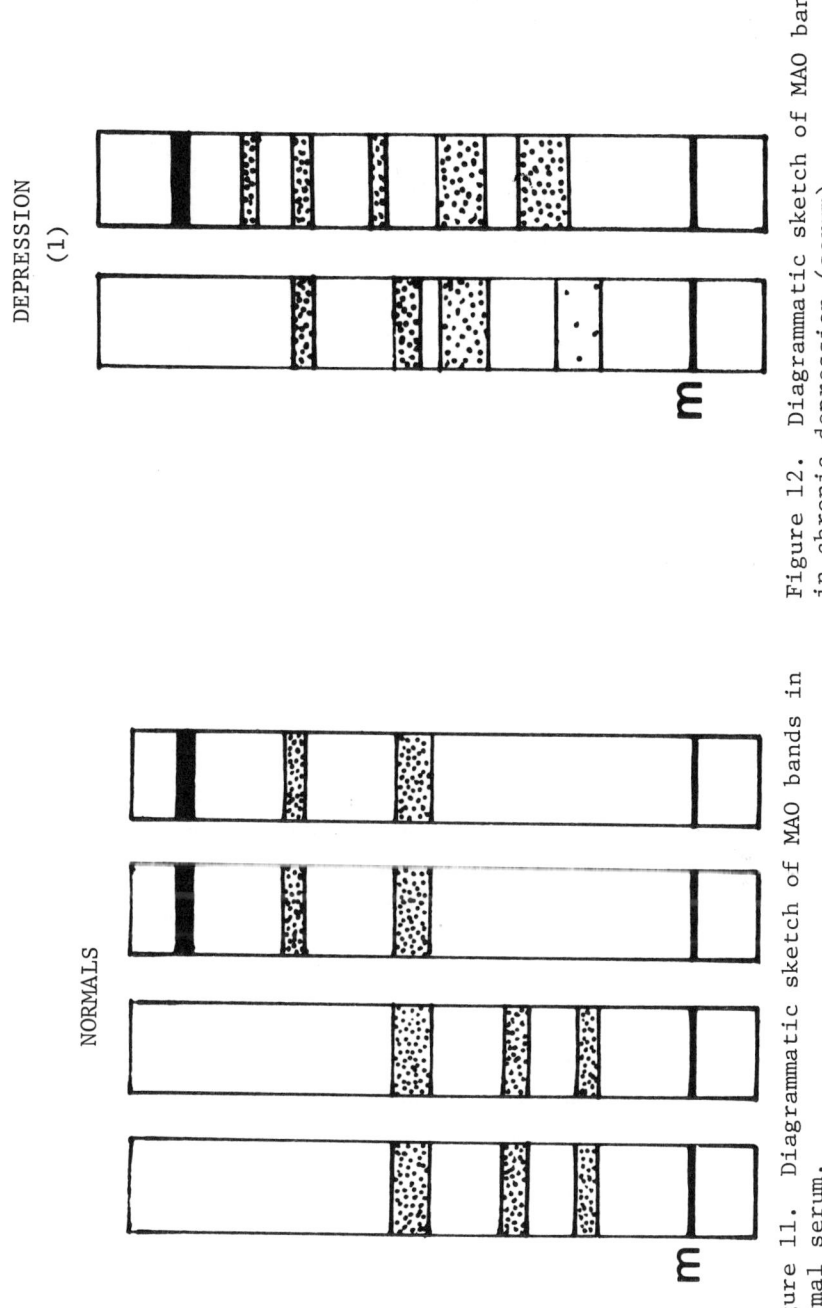

Figure 11. Diagrammatic sketch of MAO bands in normal serum.

Figure 12. Diagrammatic sketch of MAO bands in chronic depression (serum).

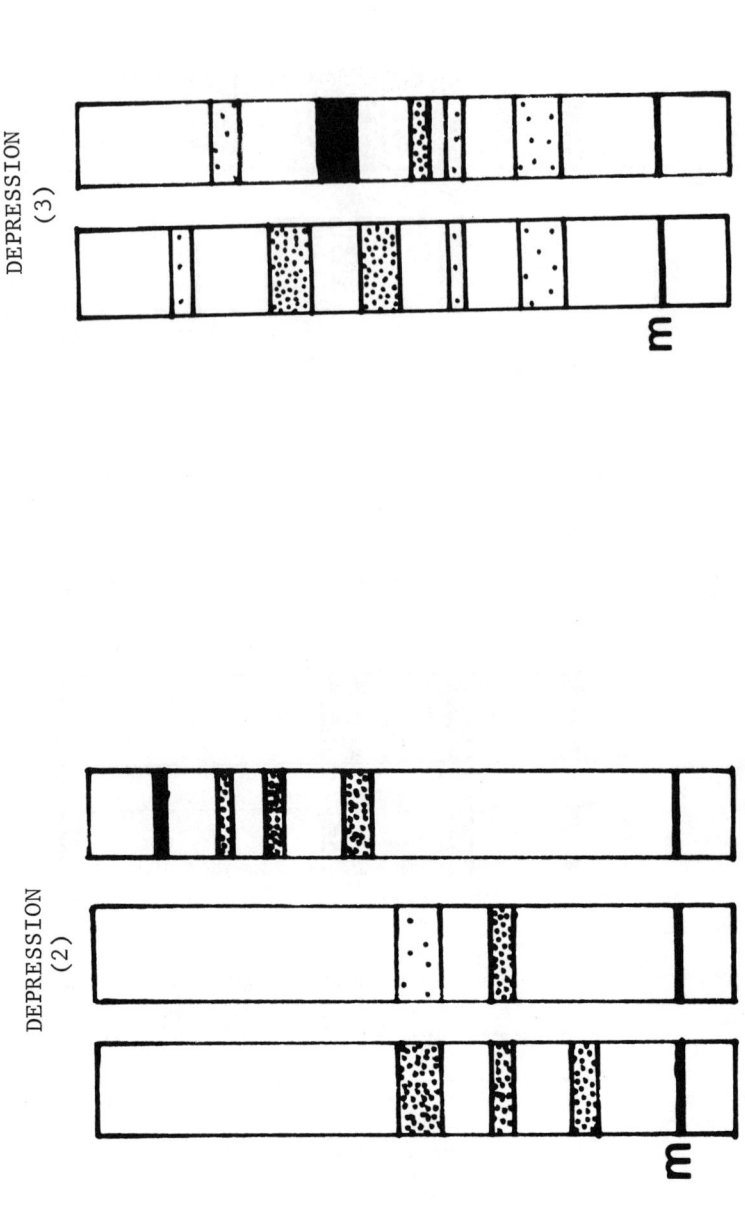

Figure 13. Diagrammatic sketch of MAO bands in endogenous depression (serum).

Figure 14. Diagrammatic sketch of MAO bands in neurotic depression (serum).

MAO IN DEVELOPING BRAIN 17

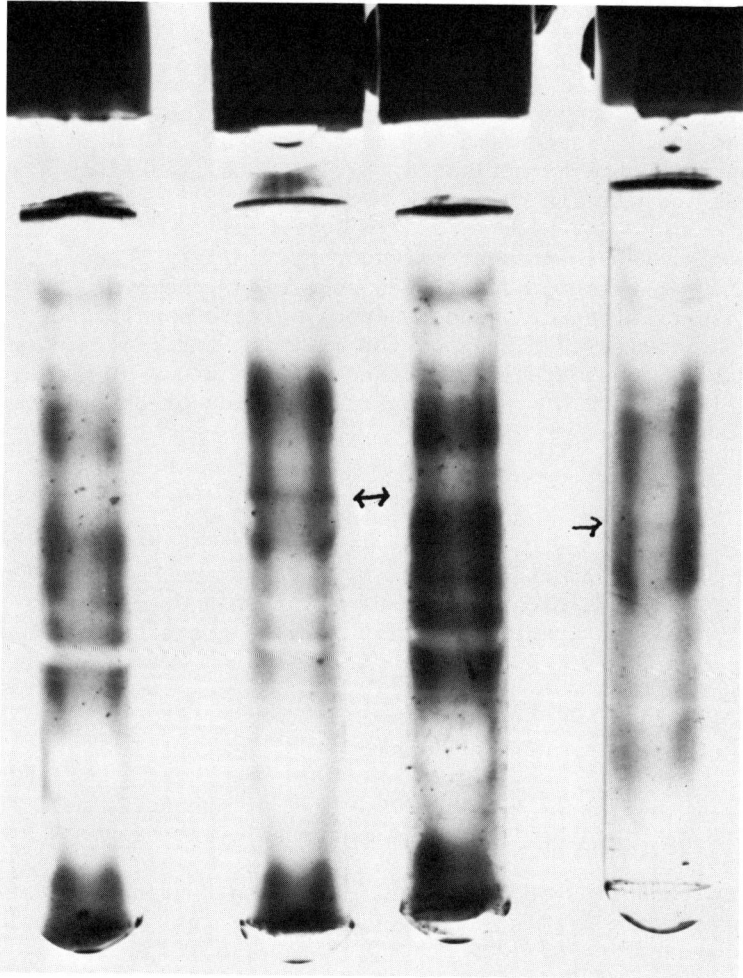

Figure 15. MAO band pattern in serum from children with Down's syndrome. Tube on left is control, while three tubes on right are from children with Down's syndrome.

would seem that different individuals variously classified as depressed have MAO patterns that are different from the normal patterns we have observed. Clearly, if these differences in MAO forms are indeed real (and further experiments will prove this), then the variations in the excretion of metabolites of both indolealkylamines and catecholamines seen in depression may in part be due to these differences in multiple forms.

We have also looked at the blood MAO patterns of children with Down's syndrome and compared them to normal patterns. Figure 15 shows the results. There seems to be at least one MAO band that does not appear in the normal child. We have now looked at six such children and all six have this extra band.

Admittedly, we can present only our preliminary observations with human MAO at this time. It does seem clear, however, that our consistent observations of age dependency, tissue specificity, and substrate sensitivity in tissue of the multiple forms of monoamine oxidase may have considerable importance in the study of mental disease in particular and of the biological function of this enzyme in general.

ACKNOWLEDGMENT

This work was supported in part by USPHS Grant MH 06415-13 and Department of Mental Hygiene, State of California Grant Number 68-2-34. Support from The Grant Foundation is also gratefully acknowledged.

REFERENCES

Brooke, M. H., and Engel, W. K. 1966. Use of phenazine methosulfate in enzyme histochemistry of human muscle biopsies. *Neurology* 16:986.

Eberle, E. D., and Eiduson, S. 1968. Effect of pyridoxine deficiency on aromatic L-amino acid decarboxylase in the developing rat liver and brain. *J. Neurochem.* 15:1071.

Eiduson, S. 1966. 5-Hydroxytryptamine in the developing chick brain: Its normal and altered development and possible control by end-product repression. *J. Neurochem.* 13:923.

Fellman, J. H., and Roth, E. S. 1965. The competitive inhibition of amine oxidase with special reference to the carcinoid syndrome. *Canad. J. Biochem.* 43:909.

Fine, I. H.; Kaplan, N. O.; and Kuftinec, D. 1963. Developmental changes of mammalian lactic dehydrogenases. *Biochemistry* 2:116.

Gomes, B.; Igaue, I.; Kloepfer, H. G.; and Yasunobu, K. T. 1969. Isolation and characterization of the multiple beef liver amine oxidase components. *Arch. Biochem. Biophys.* 132:16.

Gorkin, V. Z. 1963. Partial separation of rat liver mitochondrial amine oxidases. *Nature* 200:77.

Gorkin, V. Z.; Komisarova, N. V.; Lerman, M. I.; and Veryovkina, I. V. 1964. The inhibition of mitochondrial amine oxidases *in vitro* by proflavine. *Biochem. Biophys. Res. Commun.* 15:383.

Graham, R. C., and Karnovsky, M. J. 1965. The histochemical demonstration of monoamine oxidase activity by coupled peroxidatic oxidation. *J. Histochem. Cytochem.*

Hardegg, W., and Heilbronn, E. 1961. Oxidation of serotonin and tyramine by rat-liver mitochondria. *Biochem. Biophys. Acta* 51:553.

Kim, H. C., and D'Iorio, A. 1968. Possible isoenzymes of monoamine oxidase in rat tissues. *Canad. J. Biochem.* 46:295.

Latner, A. L., and Skillen, A. W. 1968. *Isoenzymes in Biology and Medicine*. London: Academic Press.

Markert, C. L., and Ursprung, H. 1962. The otogeny of isozyme patterns of lactate dehydrogenase in the mouse. *Develop. Biol.* 5:363.

Nagatsu, T.; Yamamoto, T.; and Harada, M. 1970. Purification and properties of human brain mitochondrial monoamine oxidase. *Enzymologia* 39:15.

Oswald, E. O., and Strittmatter, C. F. 1963. Comparative studies in the characterization of monoamine oxidases. *Proc. Soc. Exp. Biol. Med.* 114:668.

Otsuka, S., and Kobayashi, Y. 1964. A radioisotopic assay for monoamine oxidase determinations in human plasma. *Biochem. Pharmacol.* 13:995.

Ragland, J. B. 1968. Multiplicity of mitochondrial monoamine oxidases. *Biochem. Biophys. Res. Commun.* 31:203.

Schultz, G. A., and Ruth, R. F. 1968. The lactate dehydrogenases of the chicken: Estimation and repression during the development of lymphoid and other tissues. *Canad. J. Biochem.* 46:555.

Shih, J. C., and Eiduson, S. 1969. Multiple forms of monoamine oxidase in the developing brain. *Nature* 224:1305.

Smith, C. H., and Kissane, J. M. 1963. Distribution of forms of lactic dehydrogenase within the developing rat kidney. *Develop. Biol.* 8:151.

Spector, S.; Gordon, R.; Sjoerdsma, A.; and Udenfriend, S. 1967. End-product inhibition of tyrosine hydroxylase as a possible mechanism for regulation of norepinephrine synthesis. *Molec. Pharmacol.* 3:549.

Squires, R. F. 1968. Additional evidence for the existence of several forms of mitochondrial monoamine oxidase in the mouse. *Biochem. Pharmacol.* 17:1401.

Werle, E., and Röwer, F. 1952. Uber tierische und pflanzliche Monoaminoxydasen. *Biochem. Z.* 322:320.

Wuntch, T.; Chen, R. F.; and Vesell, E. S. 1970. Lactate dehydrogenase isozymes; kinetic properties at high enzyme concentrations. *Science* 167:63.

Youdim, M.B.H.; Collins, G.G.S.; and Sandler, M. 1969. Multiple forms of rat brain monoamine oxidase. *Nature* 223:626.

Youdim, M.B.H., and Sourkes, T. L. 1966. Properties of purified soluble monoamine oxidase. *Canad. J. Biochem.* 44:1397.

Youdim, M.B.H., and Sandler, M. 1967. Isoenzymes of soluble monoamine oxidase from human placental and rat liver mitochondria. *Biochem. J.* 105:43.

REGULATION OF CATECHOLAMINE BIOSYNTHESIS:

TYROSINE HYDROXYLASE AND DIHYDROPTERIDINE REDUCTASE

José M. Musacchio

New York University School of Medicine

New York, New York

It is generally accepted that catecholamines have an important role in the regulation of several brain functions, and there is increasing evidence that they may be involved in the development of certain affective disorders. Most of the agents used in the treatment for depression and mania are known to affect either the synthesis, storage, and release of catecholamines or the central adrenergic receptors. These brief considerations are sufficient to justify an examination of the enzymes that are considered important for the regulation of catecholamine biosynthesis.

The hydroxylation of tyrosine to DOPA is considered to be the rate-limiting step in catecholamine biosynthesis (Levitt et al. 1965). This step, however, is quite complex (Figure 1) and it is not known which of its components is actually the limiting factor. Tyrosine hydroxylase requires molecular oxygen and a reduced pteridine as cofactors (Nagatsu, Levitt, and Udenfriend 1964b; Brenneman and Kaufman 1964). Dihydropteridine reductase, the enzyme that reduces the pteridine cofactor, should also be considered part of the system, since the reduced pteridine cofactor is quite unstable. In order to understand the importance of the different components of this step, we will first discuss them separately and then examine the complete system.

Tyrosine hydroxylase. Tyrosine hydroxylase was isolated from the brain and adrenal medulla by Nagatsu, Levitt, and Udenfriend (1964 a and b). The enzyme was initially described as being particle-bound, and the fraction found soluble was considered to have been solubilized by prolonged homogenization. Contrary to these results, we found that rat and bovine adrenal tyrosine hydroxylase are not particle-bound (Musacchio 1967 and 1968). Independently,

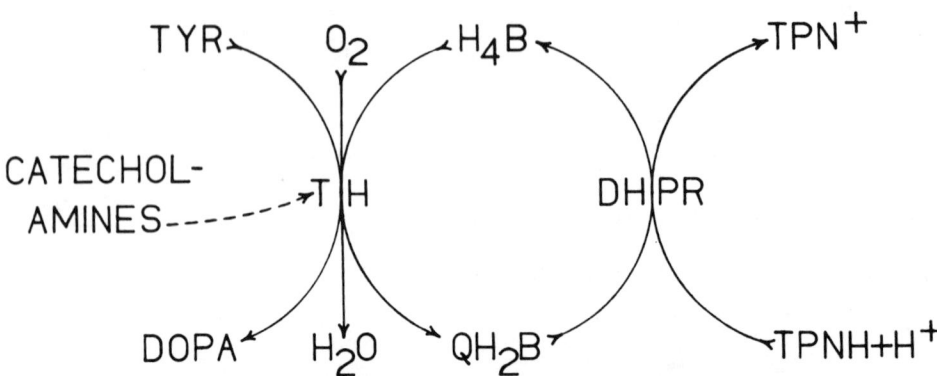

Figure 1. <u>Hydroxylation of tyrosine to DOPA</u>. TYR: tyrosine; TH: tyrosine hydroxylase; H_4B: tetrahydrobiopterin; QH_2B: quinonoid form of dihydrobiopterin; DHPR: dihydropteridine reductase. Catecholamine feedback inhibition is indicated by broken line.

Laduron and Belpaire (1968) have also concluded that bovine adrenal tyrosine hydroxylase is mainly localized in the high-speed supernatant fraction. The intracellular localization of this enzyme and its relation with the cytoplasmic or granular catecholamine pools may hold the answer to how catecholamine biosynthesis is controlled; it may also provide an explanation for the mechanism of action of certain pharmacological agents on catecholamine biosynthesis. We decided, therefore, to investigate the problem, using techniques specifically designed for subcellular distribution studies; in addition, since we found that tyrosine hydroxylase aggregates and sediments upon centrifugation, we also studied the phenomenon of aggregation and how it changes the apparent subcellular distribution of the enzyme.

The subcellular distribution of tyrosine hydroxylase was studied with sucrose density gradients. As Figure 2 shows, tyrosine hydroxylase is associated with the soluble fraction of the cell components; the chromaffin granules, indicated by the epinephrine peak at 1.6 to 1.8 M sucrose, contain only negligible amounts of tyrosine hydroxylase activity. Some tyrosine hydroxylase activity was found at the bottom of the gradient, in the pellet containing such coarse particles as unbroken cells, nuclei, and cell debris. The specific activity of tyrosine hydroxylase is highest in the soluble fraction and lowest in the chromaffin granule region (Table 1). This is another clear indication that the enzyme is not

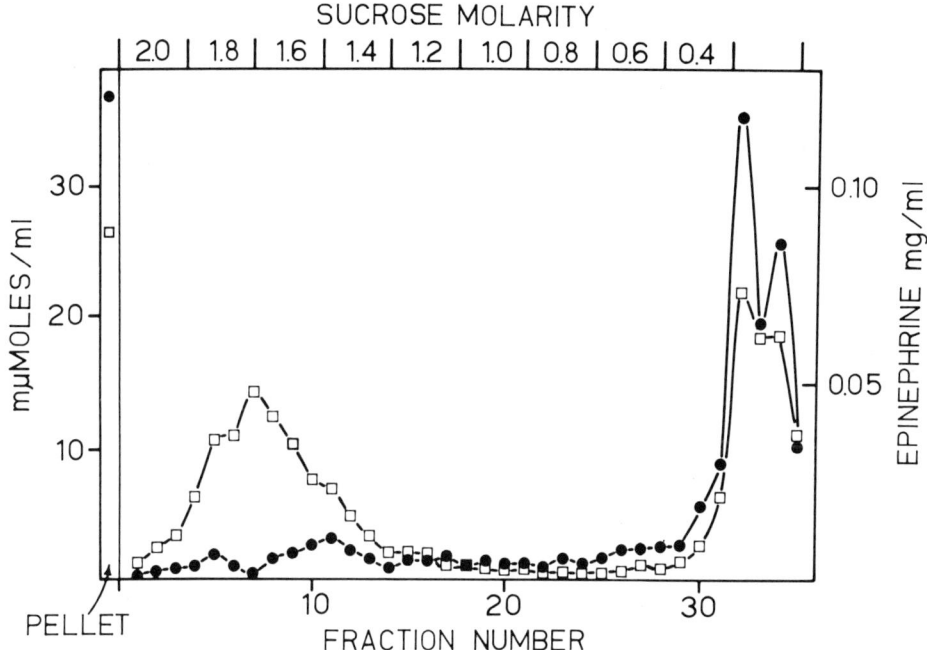

Figure 2. <u>Subcellular distribution of beef adrenal tyrosine hydroxylase and epinephrine.</u> Adrenal medullae were homogenized in five volumes of an isotonic KCl buffer. The sucrose molarity of the different gradient layers is indicated at top of figure; space at the right of 0.4 M sucrose indicates layer occupied by the homogenate and where the soluble components remain after centrifugation. Tyrosine hydroxylase activity (●) is expressed as mμmoles of tritiated water produced in 10 min/ml. Epinephrine concentration (□) is expressed as mg/ml (Wurzburger and Musacchio 1971).

associated with the chromaffin granules.

There are many types of artifacts that may obscure the subcellular distribution of an enzyme (de Duve 1964). We were especially concerned with ruling out two possibilities that could apparently alter the distribution of the enzyme if it were particle-bound: (1) leakage of tyrosine hydroxylase from the chromaffin granules, and (2) failure to detect particle-bound tyrosine hydroxylase.

The first possibility, that the enzyme could be located in the chromaffin granules *in vivo* and leak out during the tissue homogenization, is quite unlikely for the following reasons: (a) only a small percentage of the total enzyme activity is associated with the

TABLE 1

Distribution of Tyrosine Hydroxylase and
Epinephrine in a Sucrose Density
Gradient[a]

Fraction	Tyrosine Hydroxylase[b] %	Tyrosine Hydroxylase Specific Activity[c]	Epinephrine[d] %	TH/E[e]
Pellet	21.1	7.0	13.2	1.59
Chromaffin	10.8	2.5	33.0	0.32
Intermediate	4.2	3.3	5.7	0.73
Soluble	63.9	11.8	48.1	1.33
Homogenate		7.1		1.00

[a] Adrenal medullae were homogenized as described in Figure 2.
[b] Tyrosine hydroxylase activity of each fraction is expressed as percentage of total activity, which was 1,355 mµmoles of tritiated water produced in 10 min/gm of wet tissue.
[c] mµmoles of tritiated water produced in 10 min/mg protein.
[d] Epinephrine in each fraction is expressed as percentage of total content.
[e] Ratio between tyrosine hydroxylase and epinephrine percentages in each fraction (Wurzburger and Musacchio 1971).

chromaffin granules while they still retain a high percentage of the catecholamines. This lack of association between the chromaffin granules and tyrosine hydroxylase is well illustrated by the ratio between the percentage distribution of enzyme and catecholamines in each fraction, as it is shown by the results in Table 1. (b) If the enzyme were localized in the storage granules, different homogenization procedures should be expected to release different amounts of enzyme, which would produce different distribution patterns. The results of our experiments with different methods of homogenization indicate that the enzyme is extragranular (Wurzburger and Musacchio 1971). (c) The specific activity of tyrosine hydroxylase is lowest in the chromaffin region of gradients, even lower than in the total homogenate; in contrast, the specific activity is highest in the soluble fraction, the only fraction in which it increases after fractionation. Proteins known to be contained in the chromaffin granules, namely, chromogranin A and dopamine-β-hydroxylase, are recovered mainly from the granules, where their specific activities are the highest (Sage, Smith, and Kirshner 1967; Laduron and Belpaire 1968). This clearly is not the case with tyrosine hydroxylase.

The second possibility, that tyrosine hydroxylase could be particle-bound and undetectable, either because the enzyme was inaccessible to substrate, or because it was inhibited by the high catecholamine content of the particle, is quite unlikely. Several methods were used to disrupt subcellular particles, such as osmotic shock, dialysis against hypotonic buffers, treatment with Cutscum, and tryptic digestion. All these procedures failed repeatedly to activate hypothetical stores of tyrosine hydroxylase (Wurzburger and Musacchio 1971). These results are in agreement with our previous findings in which sonication and dialysis failed to activate any latent tyrosine hydroxylase in the adrenal chromaffin granules (Musacchio 1968).

The composition of the buffer used in the homogenization of the adrenal medullae also has a marked effect on the distribution of tyrosine hydroxylase between the coarse fraction of nuclei and cell debris and the low-speed supernatant fraction; a much larger proportion of the enzyme was found to precipitate with the coarse particles when sucrose instead of isotonic potassium chloride was used (Wurzburger and Musacchio 1971). This adsorption of tyrosine hydroxylase to coarse particles is exaggerated by using frozen instead of fresh adrenal glands. The effects of sucrose and freezing probably explain why the enzyme was originally described as particle-bound.

There are marked differences in some of the physicochemical characteristics of the enzyme, depending on the isolation procedure used. Tyrosine hydroxylase, sedimented after aggregation and adsorption to large particles, can be solubilized by tryptic digestion (Petrack, Sheppy, and Fetzer 1968), but this treatment produces an enzyme form that is much smaller than the native tyrosine hydroxylase. The sedimentation coefficients of native and trypsin-treated tyrosine hydroxylase were determined by sucrose density gradient centrifugation. Native tyrosine hydroxylase was found to have a sedimentation coefficient of 9.2 and that of the trypsin-treated enzyme was 3.4. The sedimentation coefficient and the Stokes radius of trypsin-treated tyrosine hydroxylase were used to calculate the molecular weight of this form of the enzyme, which was found to be 34,000. The molecular weight of the native form of the enzyme is about 140,000 to 150,000, indicating that the trypsin-treated enzyme is only a fragment of the native form (Musacchio *et al.* 1971).

TABLE 2

Effect of Dihydropteridine Reductase on DOPA Formation

	DOPA Formed (mµmoles)
Control	1.94
Dihydropteridine reductase added	24.90

Samples were incubated for one hour with 10 mµmoles of dimethyltetrahydropterin (Musacchio 1969).

The activity of tyrosine hydroxylase is inhibited *in vitro* by compounds with a catechol structure and this inhibition is competitive with the artificial pteridine cofactor (Udenfriend, Zaltzman-Nirenberg, and Nagatsu 1965; Ikeda, Fahien, and Udenfriend 1966). Norepinephrine, at concentrations of 1×10^{-3} M, produces a 50 percent inhibition of tyrosine hydroxylase activity when equal concentrations of the artificial pteridine cofactor are used. The *in vivo* cytoplasmic concentrations of catecholamine and natural cofactor are not known. However, since the cofactor content of the adrenal gland has been estimated as 0.5 to 2.0 µg/gm (Lloyd and Weiner 1970), the concentration of natural cofactor in the adrenal gland, assuming that it is uniformly distributed in the cells, can be roughly calculated between 2×10^{-6} M to 1×10^{-5} M. The *in vivo* feedback inhibition of tyrosine hydroxylase, therefore, will presumably require low concentrations of cytoplasmic catecholamines.

The structure of the natural cofactor is also important for the study of the regulation of catecholamine synthesis. In confirmation of the findings of Lloyd (1969), we have isolated a pteridine from beef adrenal medullae that has the fluorescent spectrum and the chromatographic characteristics of biopterin (Musacchio and Castellucci 1969). Ultimately, all the *in vitro* studies on the regulation of catecholamine biosynthesis will have to be confirmed by using the natural cofactor.

Dihydropteridine reductase. We have found a pteridine-reducing enzyme in beef adrenal glands that is capable of reducing the quinonoid form of dihydrobiopterin and several analogs (Musacchio 1969). The enzyme, like tyrosine hydroxylase, is located in the soluble fraction of the adrenal gland homogenate. It requires NADPH for activity and produces a several-fold increase in the production of DOPA when it is added to a tyrosine hydroxylase system in which the amount of pteridine cofactor is limiting (Table 2). This experiment, in which the total amount of DOPA produced is larger than the amount of pteridine added, clearly indicates that the enzyme is able to reduce the cofactor oxidized in the hydroxylation of tyrosine to DOPA. Dihydropteridine reductase can reduce the phenylalanine hydroxylase rat liver cofactor, the tyrosine hydroxylase beef adrenal cofactor, and the quinonoid form of dihydrobiopterin. It does not reduce biopterin and it is not inhibited by aminopterin and methotrexate; dihydropteridine reductase, therefore, is presumably different from tetrahydrofolate dehydrogenase (Musacchio 1969).

As will be discussed, dihydropteridine reductase, by changing the tissue levels of the reduced pteridine cofactor, could change the rate of catecholamine biosynthesis and the effectiveness of the catecholamine feedback inhibition.

Regulation of catecholamine biosynthesis. Experiments that are now classic have demonstrated that an increase in sympathetic nerve activity produces an acceleration of catecholamine biosynthesis in adrenal glands (Hökfelt and McLean 1950; Holland and Schümann 1956; Bygdeman and von Euler 1958) and in peripheral adrenergic nerves (von Euler and Hellner-Björkman 1955). The sympathetic nerve activity affects catecholamine biosynthesis at the level of the hydroxylation of tyrosine to DOPA, as demonstrated in the decentralized rat salivary glands (Musacchio and Weise 1965). These experiments demonstrated that the conversion of labeled tyrosine to norepinephrine was halved in the decentralized glands, while the conversion of DOPA and dopamine to norepinephrine was unchanged (Figure 3). Since then investigations have demonstrated repeatedly that increased sympathetic activity produces an increase in catecholamine synthesis from tyrosine (Oliverio and Stjärne 1965; Alousi and Weiner 1966; Gordon et al. 1966; Sedvall and Kopin 1967). The mechanism by which nerve activity may regulate catecholamine synthesis is not known, but there is increasing evidence that there is a feedback control mechanism.

The first indication that an elevated concentration of tissue catecholamines decreased its own synthesis was provided by Neff and Costa (1966). They demonstrated that the administration of a monoamine oxidase inhibitor produced a 50 percent decrease in norepinephrine synthesis rates in rat brain and heart. Alousi and Weiner (1966), by using a different approach, showed that norepinephrine is able to inhibit the synthesis of labeled catecholamines from labeled tyrosine in the guinea pig vas deferens; the amount of norepinephrine necessary for this inhibition was so small that it was chemically undetectable. From these experiments, Alousi and Weiner concluded that there is a small compartment of norepinephrine, presumably cytoplasmic, that is critical for the regulation of its

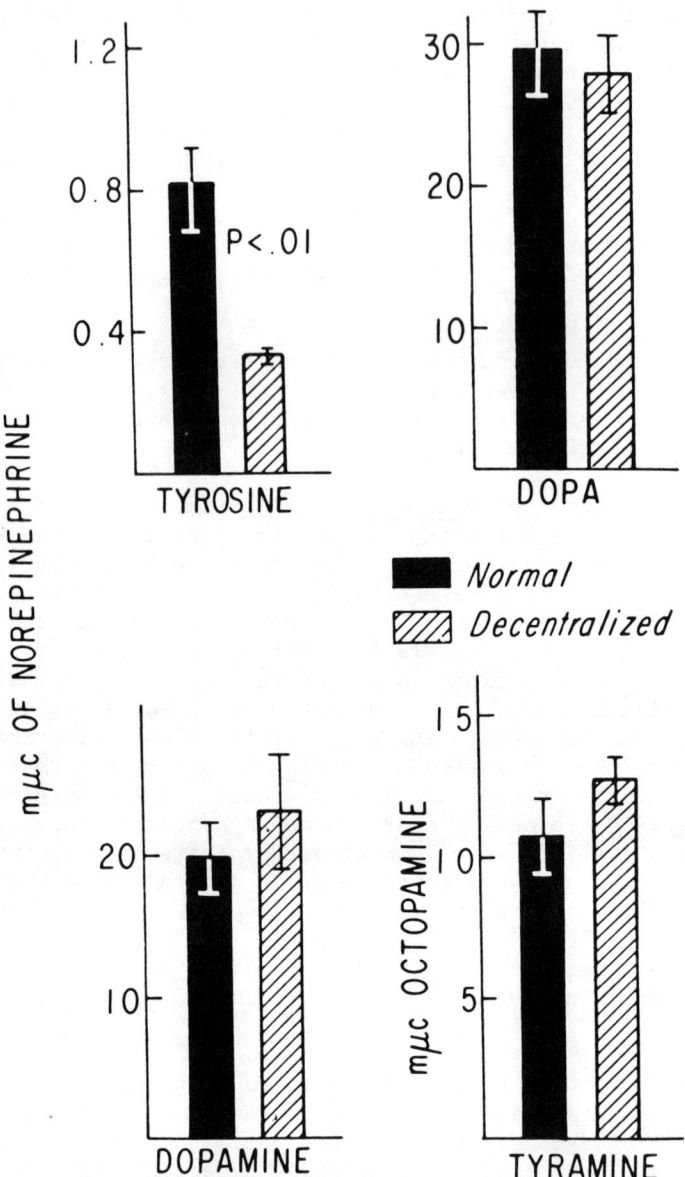

Figure 3. Nervous control of tyrosine hydroxylase activity.
^{3}H-norepinephrine or ^{3}H-octopamine levels in the intact and decentralized rat salivary gland one hour after administration of precursors are indicated at bottom of bars. Results are expressed as mμC of radioactive amine per salivary gland ± S.E.M. Six determinations are included in each group (Musacchio and Weise 1965).

own synthesis. This hypothesis is consistent with the findings that tyrosine hydroxylase is a cytoplasmic enzyme. Additional pharmacological evidence is now available strongly indicating that catecholamine biosynthesis is controlled, at least in part, by the concentration of cytoplasmic catecholamines (Weiner and Selvaratnam 1968; Kopin, Weise, and Sedvall 1969; Golstein, Ohi, and Backstrom 1970).

Tyrosine hydroxylase activity is inhibited 50 percent by 1×10^{-3} M norepinephrine, and this inhibition is competitive with the concentration of pteridine cofactor (Udenfriend, Zaltzman-Nirenberg, and Nagatsu 1965). The high concentration of catecholamines necessary to inhibit tyrosine hydroxylase *in vitro* produced some initial doubts regarding the physiological significance of the feedback regulatory mechanism. These doubts were unjustified, however, because the *in vitro* experiments were carried out with extremely high concentration of cofactor and, therefore, a very high concentration of catecholamines was necessary to produce inhibition. *In vivo* the pteridine cofactor levels are at least 100-fold lower than those used for the *in vitro* experiments. Furthermore, these levels refer to the concentration of total cofactor, reduced and oxidized; the concentration of reduced cofactor, which is the active form, is probably even lower. These considerations indicate that the feedback inhibition of tyrosine hydroxylase is most likely of physiological significance.

We have studied the interaction of the pteridine cofactor and catecholamines *in vitro*, in a complex system composed of tyrosine hydroxylase, dihydropteridine reductase, partially oxidized pteridine cofactor, etc. As can be seen in Figure 4, the rate of DOPA formation is a function of the concentration of dihydropteridine reductase. This system is quite sensitive to inhibition by catecholamines, since epinephrine at a concentration of 1×10^{-5} M produces a 50 percent inhibition of DOPA formation. These *in vitro* experiments provide further support to the hypothesis of feedback regulation of catecholamine synthesis. Futhermore, they suggest that the activity of dihydropteridine reductase not only can control the rate of catecholamine synthesis but can also antagonize the catecholamine inhibition of tyrosine hydroxylase.

As is indicated in Figure 5, thioproperazine and reserpine, administered *in vivo*, change the rate of catecholamine synthesis in rat caudate nucleus slices but they do not change the amount of tyrosine hydroxylase in the tissues (Besson *et al.* in preparation). The localization of tyrosine hydroxylase in the cytoplasm explains the changes in the rate of catecholamine synthesis produced by thioproperazine and reserpine. The inhibition of tyrosine hydroxylase activity produced by reserpine can be explained by an increase in cytoplasmic catecholamine concentration resulting from the inhibition of the granular uptake mechanism. When tyrosine hydroxylase

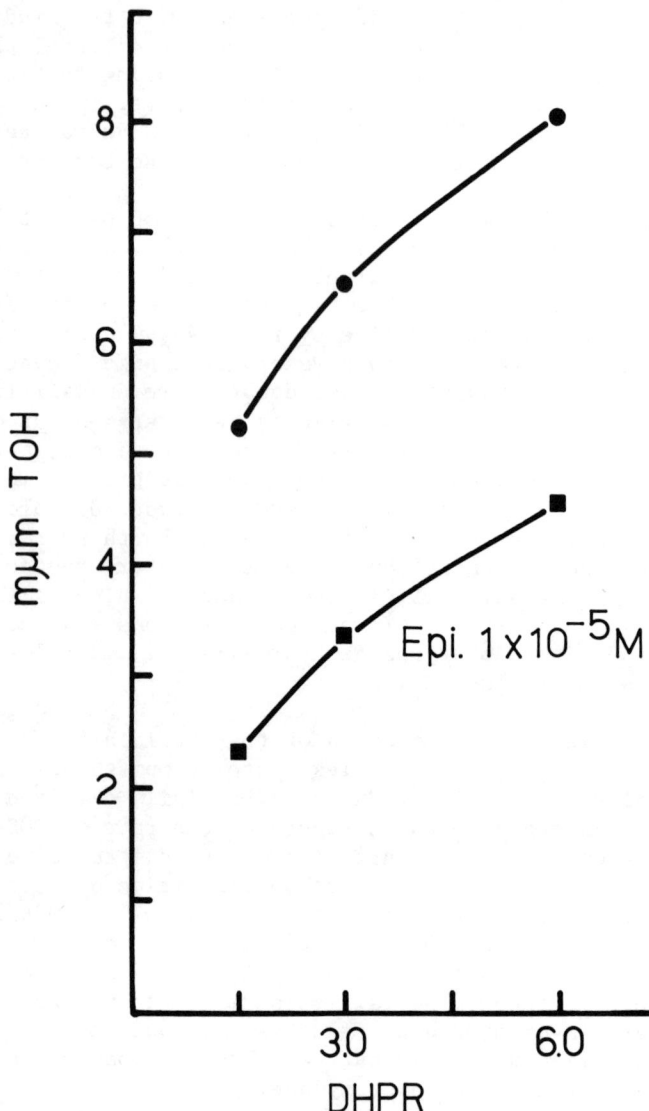

Figure 4. <u>Effect of dihydropteridine reductase and epinephrine on the formation of DOPA</u>. Tyrosine hydroxylase was incubated in the presence of different amounts of partially purified dihydropteridine reductase (DHPR), as is indicated on the abscissa. Incubation mixture contained 100 mµmoles of tyrosine-3,5-^{3}H, a TPNH-generating system, 100 mµmoles of freshly prepared dimethyldihydropterin and Tris-HCl buffer, pH 6.0. Epinephrine was added to the samples indicated up to a final concentration of 1×10^{-5} M. The formation of DOPA was measured by the formation of tritiated water (TOH).

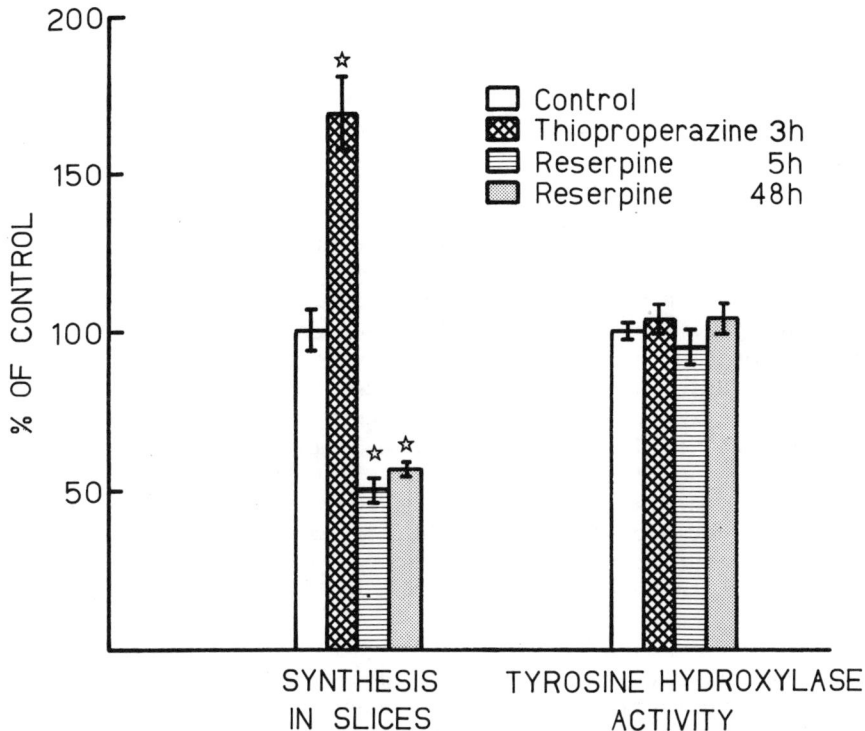

Figure 5. <u>Effect of thioproperazine and reserpine treatment on DOPA formation in caudate tissue slices and on purified tyrosine hydroxylase.</u> Rats were injected with 5 mg/kg of thioproperazine or reserpine at the times before sacrifice indicated in the figure; the rats receiving reserpine for 48 hours were also injected at 24 hours. Each result is the average of six determinations and they are expressed as the percentage ± S.E.M. of the control values (From Besson, Cheramy, Musacchio and Glowinski, in preparation).

is assayed after purification, no changes in activity are detected (Figure 5). The increase in catecholamine synthesis produced by thioproperazine can be explained by a decrease in cytoplasmic catecholamine concentration produced by a release of feedback inhibition brought about by an increase in dopamine output. The changes produced by thioproperazine in the tissue slices are not observed after isolation and purification of tyrosine hydroxylase, indicating once more that the spatial relationships and *in vivo* concentrations of substrate, cofactors, enzymes, and end-product in the cell are essential for the regulation of catecholamine synthesis.

In addition to the feedback control of catecholamine synthesis--which is involved in rapid changes in neurotransmitter demands--an additional mechanism exists for adaptation to long-lasting increases in neurotransmitter needs, namely, induction of tyrosine hydroxylase. Induction of tyrosine hydroxylase activity has been demonstrated in sympathetically innervated organs and in the brain (Mueller, Thoenen, and Axelrod 1969; Viveros *et al.* 1969; Thoenen, Mueller, and Axelrod 1969; Musacchio *et al.* 1969). Brain tyrosine hydroxylase activity cannot be induced as easily as adrenal or sympathetic nerve endings enzyme. Chronic electroshock treatment can produce a small but significant increase of tyrosine hydroxylase activity in the rat brain stem and cortex (Musacchio *et al.* 1969). Reserpine has been reported to produce an increase in rabbit brain stem tyrosine hydroxylase (Mueller, Thoenen, and Axelrod 1969). In the rat, treatment with reserpine for forty-eight hours does not produce any increase in tyrosine hydroxylase activity, but treatment for seven days with 2.5 mg/kg produces a 60 percent increase in brain stem but not in caudate tyrosine hydroxylase (Musacchio and Wurzburger, unpublished observation). The changes observed are probably due to neuronal hyperactivity associated with the stress produced by the chronic treatment with large doses of reserpine; if the changes were due to the direct action of reserpine on the neurons, the caudate tyrosine hydroxylase should have been increased, and this was not the case.

It is conceivable that dihydropteridine reductase could also be induced by long-lasting increases in neurotransmitter demands, but we will have to await more sensitive methods to detect the enzyme in order to explore this possibility.

SUMMARY

The regulation of catecholamine biosynthesis takes place at the hydroxylation of tyrosine to DOPA. This reaction is complex, and it is not known which of its components is rate-limiting. Tyrosine hydroxylase is located in the cell cytoplasm and its activity is inhibited by a cytoplasmic catecholamine pool. Since this inhibition is competitive with the levels of reduced pteridine cofactor, the levels of reduced cofactor--or the activity of dihydropteridine reductase -- may be an important determinant of the rate of catecholamine synthesis and of the catecholamine level at which the feedback inhibition will be effective.

ACKNOWLEDGMENTS

The author thanks Miss Gale L. D'Angelo and Mr. Robert J. Wurzburger for their excellent technical assistance.

This work was supported in part by Grant 5 RO 1 AM 13,128 from the National Institutes of Health. The author is Research Scientist Awardee of the PHS Grant 1-K2-MH-17,885.

REFERENCES

Alousi, A., and Weiner, N. 1966. The regulation of norepinephrine synthesis in sympathetic nerves: Effect of nerve stimulation, cocaine, and catecholamine-releasing agents. *Proc. Nat. Acad. Sci.* 56:1491.

Besson, M. J., Cheramy, A.; Musacchio, J. M.; and Glowinski, J. In preparation.

Brenneman, A. R., and Kaufman, S. 1964. The role of tetrahydropteridines in the enzymatic conversion of tyrosine to 3,4-dihydroxyphenylalanine. *Biochem. Biophys. Res. Commun.* 17:177.

Bygdeman, S., and von Euler, U. S. 1958. Resynthesis of catechol hormones in the cat's adrenal medulla. *Acta Physiol. Scand.* 44:375.

de Duve, C. 1964. Principles of tissue fractionation. *J. Theor. Biol.* 6:33.

von Euler, U. S., and Hellner-Björkman, S. 1955. Effect of increased adrenergic nerve activity on the content of noradrenaline and adrenaline in cat organs. *Acta Physiol. Scand.* 118:17.

Goldstein, M.; Ohi, Y.; and Backstrom, T. 1970. The effect of ouabain on catecholamine biosynthesis in rat brain cortex slices. *J. Pharmacol. Exp. Ther.* 174:77.

Gordon, R., Reid, J. V. O.; Sjoerdsma, A.; and Udenfriend, S. 1966. Increased synthesis of norepinephrine in the rat heart on electrical stimulation of the stellate ganglia. *Molec. Pharmacol.* 2:606.

Hökfelt, B., and McLean, J. 1950. The adrenaline and noradrenaline content of the suprarenal glands of the rabbit under normal conditions and after various forms of stimulation. *Acta Physiol. Scand.* 21:258.

Holland, W. C., and Schümann, H. J. 1956. Formation of catechol amines during splanchnic stimulation of the adrenal gland of the cat. *Brit. J. Pharmacol.* 11:449.

Ikeda, M.; Fahien, L. A.; and Udenfriend, S. 1966. A kinetic study of bovine adrenal tyrosine hydroxylase. *J. Biol. Chem.* 241:4452.

Kopin, I. J.; Weise, V. K.; and Sedvall, G. C. 1969. Effect of false transmitters on norepinephrine synthesis. *J. Pharmacol. Exp. Ther.* 170:246.

Laduron, P., and Belpaire, F. 1968. Tissue fractionation and catecholamines-II. *Biochem. Pharmacol.* 17:1127.

Levitt, M.; Spector, S.; Sjoerdsma, A.; and Udenfriend, S. 1965. Elucidation of the rate-limiting step in norepinephrine biosynthesis in the perfused guinea-pig heart. *J. Pharmacol. Exp. Ther.* 148:1.

Lloyd, T. A. 1969. Isolation of tyrosine hydroxylase cofactor from bovine adrenal medulla and sheep brain. *Fed. Proc.* 28:873.

Lloyd, T., and Weiner, N. 1970. Isolation and characterization of the tyrosine hydroxylase cofactor from bovine adrenal medulla. *Pharmacologist* 12:287.

Mueller, R. A.; Thoenen, H.; and Axelrod, J. 1969. Increase in tyrosine hydroxylase activity after reserpine administration. *J. Pharmacol. Exp. Ther.* 169:74

Musacchio, J. M. 1967. Subcellular distribution of adrenal tyrosine hydroxylase. *Pharmacologist* 9:210.

Musacchio, J. M. 1968. Subcellular distribution of adrenal tyrosine hydroxylase. *Biochem. Pharmacol.* 17:1470.

Musacchio, J. M. 1969. Beef adrenal medulla dihydropteridine reductase. *Biochem. Biophys. Acta* 191:485.

Musacchio, J. M., and Castellucci, L. B. 1969. Effect of adrenal medulla dihydropteridine reductase and tyrosine hydroxylase adrenal cofactor on DOPA formation. *Pharmacologist* 11:274.

Musacchio, J. M.; Julou, L.; Kety, S. S.; and Glowinski, J. 1969. Increase in rat brain tyrosine hydroxylase activity produced by electroconvulsive shock. *Proc. Nat. Acad. Sci.* 63:1117.

Musacchio, J. M., and Weise, V. K. 1965. Effects of decentralization on norepinephrine biosynthesis from tyrosine, DOPA and dopamine. *Pharmacologist* 7:156.

Musacchio, J. M.; Wurzburger, R. J.; and D'Angelo, G. L. 1971. Different molecular forms of bovine adrenal tyrosine hydroxylase. *Molec. Pharmacol.* 7:(#2), in press.

Nagatsu, T.; Levitt, M.; and Udenfriend, S. 1964a. Conversion of L-tyrosine to 3,4-dihydroxyphenylalanine by cell-free preparation of brain and sympathetically innervated tissues. *Biochem. Biophys. Res. Commun.* 14:543.

Nagatsu, T.; Levitt, M.; and Udenfriend, S. 1964b. Tyrosine hydroxylase: The initial step in norepinephrine biosynthesis. *J. Biol. Chem.* 239:2910.

Neff, V. H., and Costa, E. 1966. The influence of monoamine oxidase inhibition on catecholamine synthesis. *Life Sci.* 5:951.

Oliverio, A., and Stjärne, L. A. 1965. Acceleration of noradrenaline turnover in the mouse heart by cold exposure. *Life Sci.* 4:2339.

Petrack, B.; Sheppy, F.; and Fetzer, V. 1968. Studies on tyrosine hydroxylase from bovine adrenal medulla. *J. Biol. Chem.* 243:743.

Sage, H. J.; Smith, W. J.; and Kirshner, N. 1967. Mechanism of secretion from the adrenal medulla. *Molec. Pharmacol.* 3:81.

Sedvall, G. C., and Kopin, I. J. 1967. Influence of sympathetic denervation and nerve impulse activity of tyrosine hydroxylase in the rat submaxillary gland. *Biochem. Pharmacol.* 16:39.

Thoenen, H.; Mueller, R. A.; and Axelrod, J. 1969. Trans-synaptic induction of adrenal tyrosine hydroxylase. *J. Pharmacol. Exp. Ther.* 169:249.

Udenfriend, S.; Zaltzman-Nirenberg, P.; and Nagatsu, T. 1965. Inhibitors of purified beef adrenal tyrosine hydroxylase. *Biochem. Pharmacol.* 14:837.

Viveros, O. H.; Arqueros, L.; Connett, R. J.; and Kirshner, N. 1969. Mechanism of secretion from the adrenal medulla. *Molec. Pharmacol.* 5:60.

Weiner, N., and Selvaratnam, I. 1968. The effect of tyramine on the synthesis of norepinephrine. *J. Pharmacol. Exp. Ther.* 161:21.

Wurzburger, R. J., and Musacchio, J. M. 1971. Subcellular distribution and aggregation of bovine adrenal tyrosine hydroxylase. *J. Pharmacol. Exp. Ther.* in press.

BEHAVIORAL, METABOLIC, AND ENZYMATIC STUDIES OF A BRAIN INDOLEETHYLAMINE N-METHYLATING SYSTEM

Arnold J. Mandell, Bruce Buckingham, and David Segal

School of Medicine, University of California, San Diego

La Jolla, California

Although there have been many good reasons to look for a brain indoleamine N-methylating enzyme since the introduction of the Harley-Mason amine methylation hypothesis of schizophrenia (Osmond and Smythies 1952) and Axelrod's exciting and systematic elucidation of various amine-methylating enzymes in the central nervous system (Axelrod 1965), our own particular interests in this field started in 1964 when we were studying the effect of the intravenous infusion of various amine precursors on sleep patterns in man. We reported a 5-hydroxytryptophan (5-HTP)-induced increase in rapid eye movement sleep (Mandell, Mandell, and Jacobson 1965). At the same time we noted that occasionally there was a disruption of sleep during 5-HTP infusions, with episodes of bizarre mentation. Whereas 5-hydroxytryptophan alone in small doses (150 mg i.v. over 6 to 8 hours) would usually produce some degree of sedation in our subjects, higher doses (200 mg or more), or smaller doses given in combination with a monoamine oxidase inhibitor as a pretreatment before intravenous amino acid load produced behavioral and psychic activation. We then became aware of the wide variety of studies by a number of investigators (Kety 1961; Pollin, Cardon, and Kety 1961; Kline, Simpson, and Sacks 1967; Himwich et al. 1970) that demonstrated similar reversals of the indoleamino acid-produced sedation with monoamine oxidase inhibitor pretreatment.

The Harley-Mason hypothesis quite generally states that some mental illness might result from a normal biogenic amine being methylated in an unusual way or to an unusual extent to produce hallucinogenic amines and resulting behavioral aberrations. Derived from the studies of the relative peripheral and central pharmacological potency of various O-and N-methylated amines, it has been a seductive hypothesis indeed. Although attention generated by this hypothesis generally focused on such phenylethylamines as mescaline or dimethoxyphenylethylamine, the theory can be examined just as well within the context of the indoleethylamines. Following Axelrod's elucidation of many similar amine-methylating systems in the brain, and a number of studies of induced behavioral aberrations with indoleamino acid loads accompanied by pretreatment with monoamine oxidase inhibitors, it was natural to speculate about the possibility that an indoleethylamine might be N-methylated if its normal pathway of oxidative deamination were blocked.

Having noted these observations while doing sleep research, we began to search for a dependable animal model manifesting this behavioral effect in order to begin to study some of its neurochemical correlates. We chose the newborn White Leghorn chick because of its reduced blood-brain barrier to peripherally administered amines during its first thirty days of life, as well as the stereotypy of its behavioral responses to drugs. Following behavioral work on the chick, we did correlative isotopic 5-hydroxytryptophan turnover studies with and without a monoamine oxidase inhibitor. Then we addressed the problem more directly by searching for the presence of an indoleethylamine N-methyltransferase enzyme in the chick brain. We then extended our studies to search for this enzyme in various mammalian experimental animals including man, and we have recently begun to study the behavioral affects of methylated indoleethylamines in rats. These studies were done in an attempt to get a coherent description of the availability, characteristics, and importance of an indoleethylamine N-methylating system in the brain. The following is a brief summary of our work to date.

METHODS

Behavioral studies on five-day-old White Leghorn chicks were carried out following loads of 5-hydroxytryptophan administered intravenously into the jugular vein with and without pargyline hydrochloride (5 mg/kg) pretreatment, using an activity platform connected through a cumulative counter to a multichannel kymograph (Mandell, Mandell, and Jacobson 1965). Behavioral evaluation of the relative central potencies of bufotenine and O-methylbufotenine administered intraventricularly in freely moving adult male albino rats (weight, 300 grams) was carried out using the technique of Segal and Mandell (1970).

Metabolic turnover studies were done in the whole brain and the blood content of labeled 5-HTP, 5-hydroxytryptamine (5-HT), bufotenine (BUFO), and 5-hydroxyindoleacetic acid (5-HIAA) in thirty White Leghorn cockerels that received 5-hydroxytryptamine-2-^{14}C (10.5 mCi/mmole). Animals receiving 5-HT were killed three minutes

after injection, and those receiving 5-HTP were decapitated thirty
minutes after injection. The radioactivity of the metabolites was
determined by solvent extraction, ultracentrifugation, thin layer
chromatography (TLC), and scintillation counting. The brains were
removed rapidly, weighed, and homogenized in acidified ethanol
(0.01 percent HCl) maintained at 4° C. Blood was treated in a similar manner. In addition, the lung tissue of four animals was collected. Ten milligrams of ascorbic acid and 10 to 30 µg of appropriate carriers (5-HTP + 5-HT ± BUFO ± 5-HIAA) were added during the
extraction procedure. An equal amount of water was added and the
sample frozen briefly. The extracts were thawed and centrifuged at
75,000 x G (4° C) for ninety minutes. The supernatant was lyophilized and resolubilized in 0.5 ml of the cold acidified ethanol.
A 10 percent aliquot of the concentrated extract was chromatographed
bidimensionally on cellulose TLC using the solvent system of meth-
anol-butanol-benzene-water-formic acid (40:30:20:10:1) in the first
dimension, and all of these except formic acid in the second dimension. The compounds were visualized under ultraviolet light after
ferricyanide oxidation and ethylenediamine condensation, or after
spraying with a modified Ehrlich's reagent (10 percent p-dimethyl-
aminobenzaldehyde). The areas of cellulose in which 5-HTP, 5-HT,
BUFO, and 5-HIAA were located, collected, and placed in vials containing PPO (2,5-diphenyloxazole, 0.5 gm/100 ml toluene) as liquid
scintillation medium and thixotropic gel powder (Cab-O-Sil, Packard),
thoroughly mixed in a shaker, and counted in a Beckman LS II liquid
scintillation spectrometer with external standard quench corrections.
Counts per minute (count/min) recorded on data tape were converted
to disintegrations per minute (dpm) and the data further computed
using the Beckman Omega Data Reduction System. In addition to the
known indole metabolites, two additional areas on the chromatograms
of blood and liver were occasionally found to contain low amounts
of ^{14}C-containing material. These spots are at present unidentified
and not included in the chemical analyses.

Enzyme assays were carried out on tissue from brains of chick,
rat, sheep, and man. The three human brain specimens were collected
as follows: One piece of brain tissue was taken from the prefrontal
cortical area of a 54-year-old woman during a neurosurgical decom-
pression procedure following a cerebral hemorrhage. A second piece
of tissue was taken from the parietal cortical area of a 5-day-old
infant during a shunting procedure for congenital hydrocephalus.
Regional human brain studies were done on tissue from a third brain
from a 17-year-old boy who died suddenly of a testicular carcinoma.
The brain was removed and the various pieces homogenized and frozen
within two hours following death. The enzyme assay for indoleethylamine N-methyltransferase in some experiments was done using a method
characterized by a high blank due to the poor specificity of the
procedure involving isoamyl alcohol extraction of radioactive product (Morgan and Mandell 1969). A less polar and therefore more

specific solvent for extraction was substituted for isoamyl alcohol by using tryptamine as the substrate. This permitted the use of toluene or n-heptane as the extraction solvent of radioactive methylated product and resulted in a more sensitive assay with a much reduced background.

Our most recently used assay was done as follows: Brain tissue was homogenized at high speed in a blender for sixty seconds in 0.1 M K_2PO_4 buffer (made up of a mixture of sodium mono and dibasic phosphates, pH 7.9) 1/1.5, w/v. This was centrifuged at 50,000 x G for twenty minutes. The supernatant was used as "homogenate" in some of our assays. Further purification by ammonium sulfate precipitation was carried out with the 40-60 percent ammonium sulfate precipitate as the enzyme source. This was purified further by using Sephadex G-100 and G-200 columns equilibrated with the 0.1 M K_2PO_4 buffer. A typical assay incubation mixture contained 100 µl of 0.1 M K_2PO_4 buffer, 50 µl containing 2 µM of tryptamine (as the hydrochloride), 100 µl of enzyme preparation (containing 0.1 to 0.5 mg protein), and 50 µl of a solution of S-adenosylmethionine (SAM)-^{14}C-methyl that contained 130,000 cpm and 20 mµM of SAM. The final volume of the incubation mixture was 300 µl. Incubation at 37° produced toluene-extractable radioactivity in a linear fashion with time, protein concentration, and substrate level. The reaction was stopped by adding 0.5 ml of sodium borate buffer (0.5 M, pH 10). The product was extracted by the addition of 5 ml of toluene, shaken in Vortex shaker for forty-five seconds and centrifuged at 900 x G for three minutes. The tube was then pertubated slightly to break up the existing emulsion and centrifuged again at 900 x G for three minutes. The samples were then placed in a freezer (-20° C) for at least three hours. Then the toluene phase was poured into counting vials containing toluene-based fluor with 10 percent Biosolv BBS-3, and counted in a Beckman LS-250 scintillation counter with external standard quench corrections. Specific product radioactivity was determined by chromatography and scintillation counting following pooling of toluene extracts and lyophilization with known carriers (indole known standards were obtained from J. Biel of Aldrich Chemical). Chromatography of products was done by cellulose thin layer chromatography and various solvent systems.

RESULTS

Our laboratory, among others, has reported that in the young chick in which 5-hydroxytryptamine enters the central nervous system, systemically administered 5-HT produces behavioral and physiological signs of sedation that are similar to natural sleep, differing only in the degree of muscular relaxation (Mandell and Spooner 1969). In our hands, this is a monotonic, dose-dependent phenomenon. Figure 1 shows the rather typical sleeping posture induced in a baby chick by

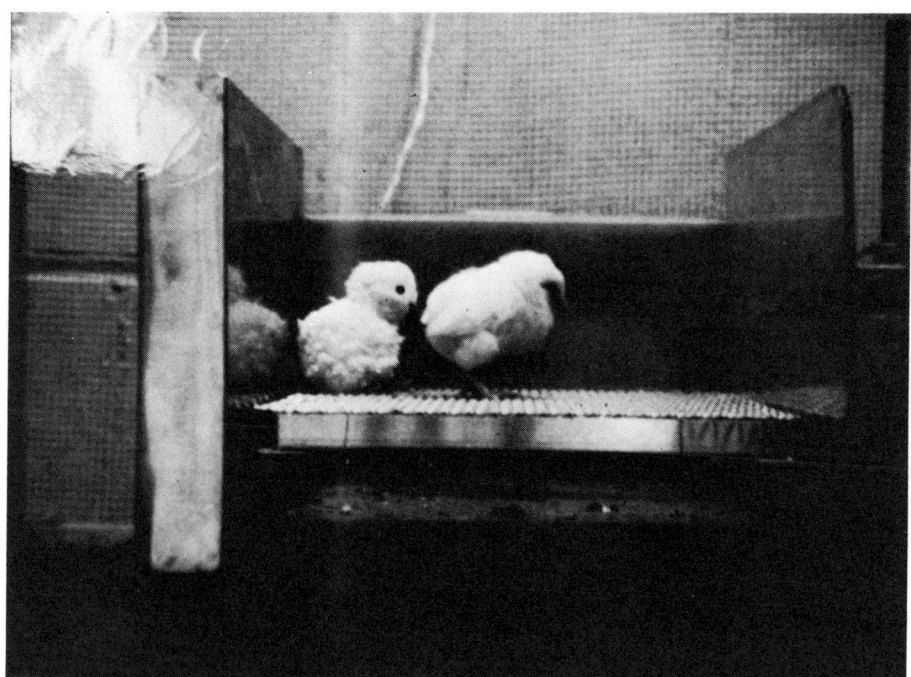

Figure 1. Typical response of chick to intravenous administration of 5-HT. Note relatively normal sleep posture and wing attitude. This is a monotonic, dose-dependent phenomenon.

intravenous 5-HT administration. The effect of this dose of 5-HT (0.1 mmole/kg) could become a peculiar kind of hyperactive state and bizarre posture (Figure 2) by pretreatment with a monoamine oxidase inhibitor, pargyline hydrochloride (5 mg/kg). In addition to hyperactivity, propulsive gait, and aggressive pecking, there was an interesting wing posture which has been seen as a rather unique response by chicks to the administration of either hallucinogens or high doses of amphetamines. Dimethyltryptamine and bufotenine, particularly, produced this sort of wing-spread posture. Since the 5-HT alone could not produce this phenomenon at any dose level, it is tempting to speculate that the bizarre posture and behavior might involve a mechanism other than 5-HT conservation alone induced by the monoamine oxidase inhibitor. In his well-known 1961 report in *Science*, Axelrod suggested the presence of an enzyme in rabbit lung (a nonspecific N-methyltransferase) that could function in the speculated shunt diagrammed in Figure 3. The question was, of course,

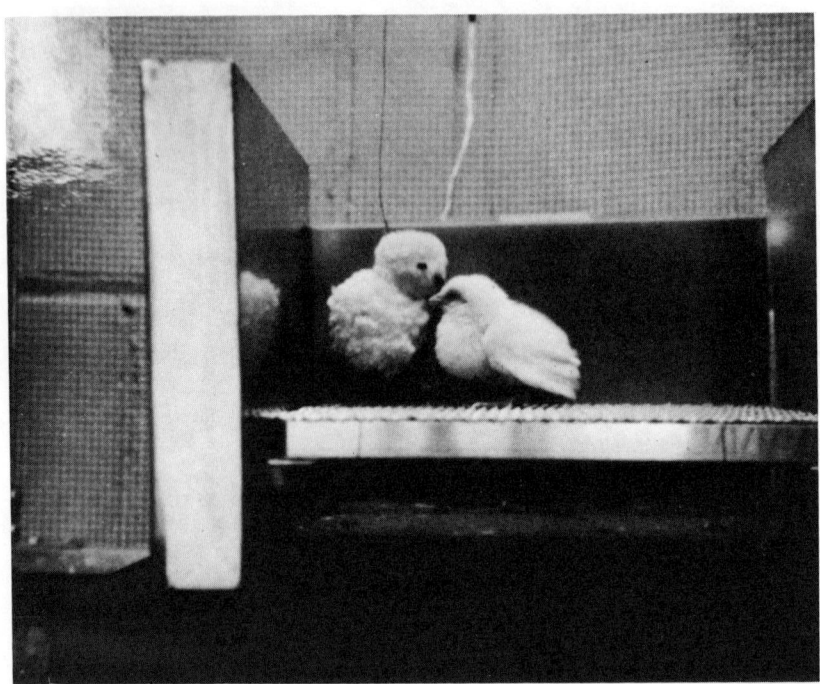

Figure 2. Typical response of chick when the intravenous administration of 5-HT was preceded by dose of a monoamine oxidase inhibitor (pargyline hydrochloride, 5 mg/kg). Note particularly the splayed attitude of wings. This response was quite characteristic of the actions of methylated indolealkylamines such as dimethyltryptamine and bufotenine.

whether a demonstrable increase or presence of an N-methylated indoleethylamine could be noted when behavioral activation was induced by the administration of an indoleamino acid following a monoamine oxidase inhibitor. As described before, ^{14}C-5-hydroxytryptophan was administered intravenously to chicks with and without pargyline hydrochloride (5 mg/kg). Figure 4 demonstrates metabolic reflections of monoamine oxidase inhibition (an increase in radioactive serotonin and a decrease of 5-hydroxyindoleacetic acid) associated with a doubling of radioactive bufotenine. The actual amount of radioactivity was relatively small, with a relatively high degree of variance. These results seemed far from striking. Figure 5 represents the results of the same kind of chemical determination done in the lung of the chick. Here the increase in bufotenine radioactivity seemed to

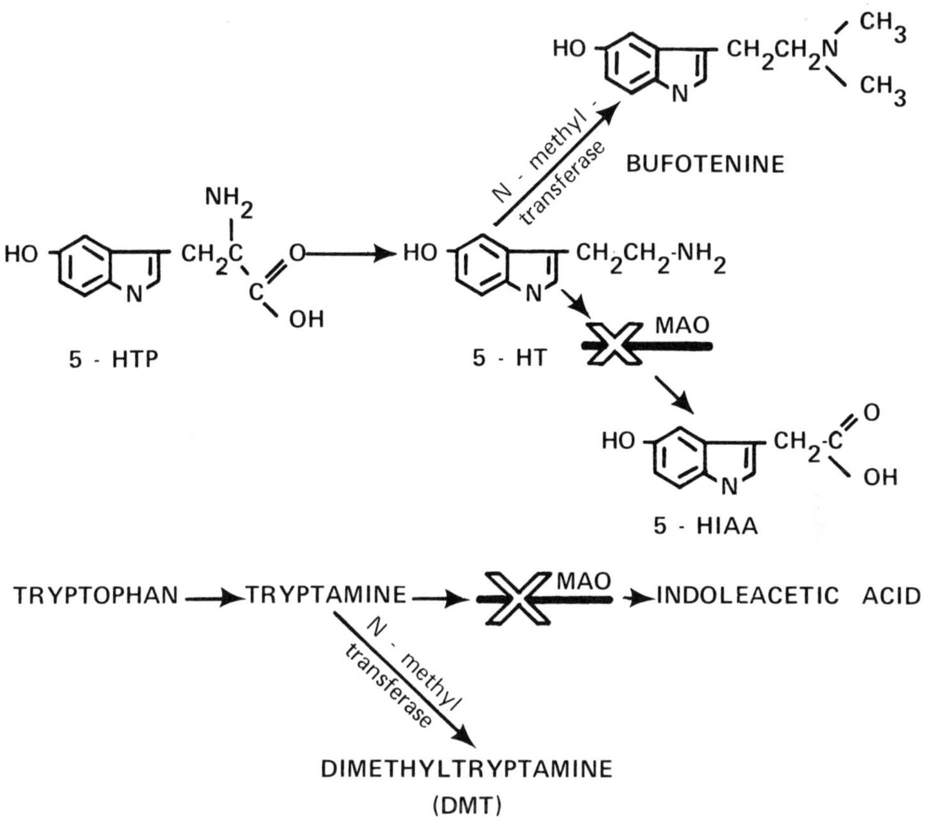

Figure 3. Diagrammatic representation of mechanisms speculated to underlie the reversal of 5-HT-induced sedation with monoamine oxidase inhibitor pretreatment. It is hypothesized that inhibition of the normal oxidative degradation of the indolealkylamines leads to more substrate being shunted through previously insignificant transmethylation pathways.

be considerably larger. It was not possible, at this stage of the chick's maturity, to determine whether the brain's radioactive bufotenine came from the lungs or the brain.

We took another approach to this problem. We attempted to find an enzyme capable of N-methylating indoleethylamines in the brain itself. Although Axelrod had not reported such a brain enzyme, he nonetheless had worked out enough parameters in similar transmethyl-

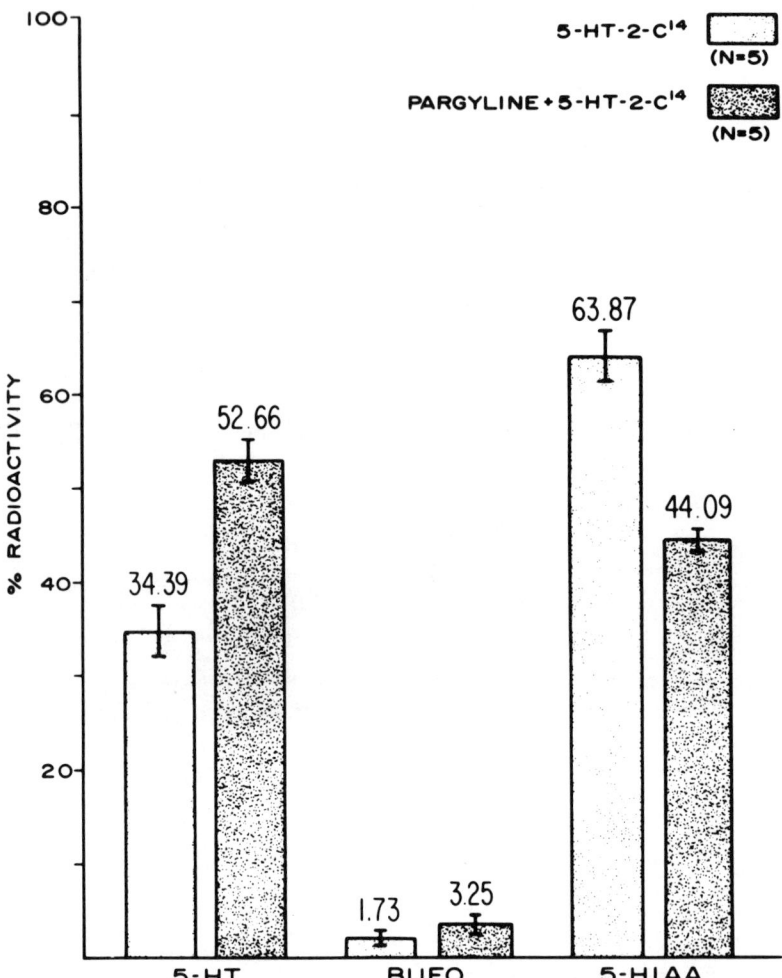

Figure 4. Metabolic distribution of radioactivity in brain following infusion of 10 μM/kg of 5-HT-2-^{14}C with and without monoamine oxidase inhibitor pretreatment. Note expected increase in radioactive 5-HT, decrease in radioactive 5-HIAA, and accompanying increase in labeled bufotenine. This latter change failed to reach significance.

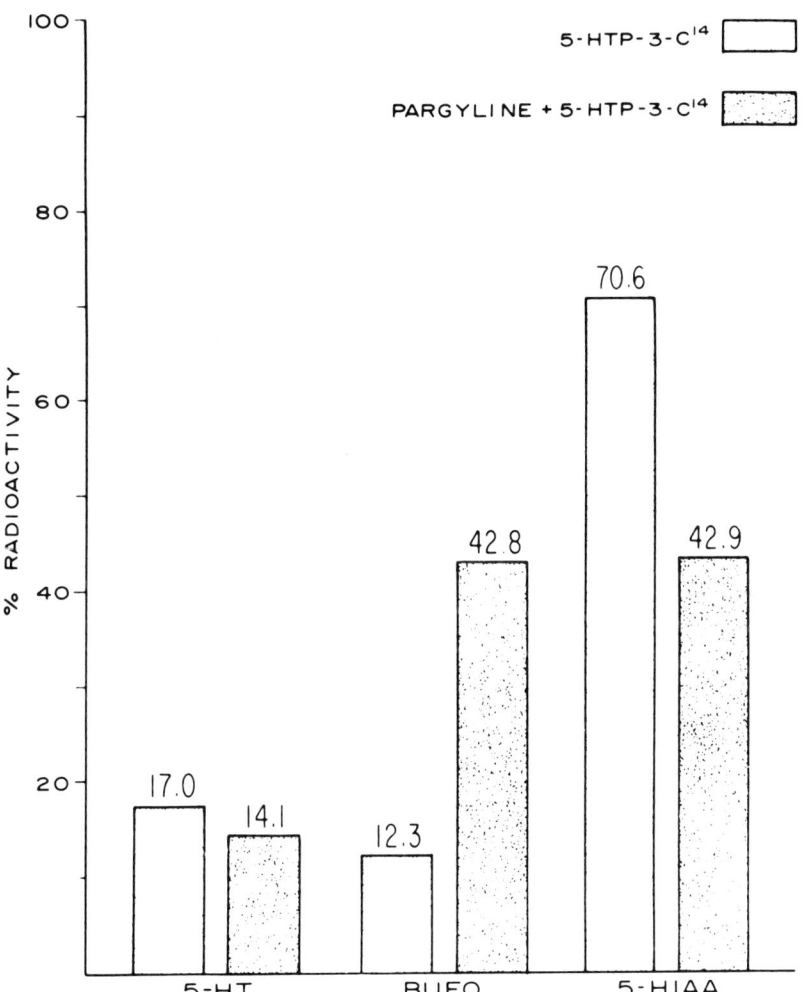

Figure 5. Experimental results, similar to Figure 4, in chick lung. Note larger increase in radioactive bufotenine.

ase assays (histamine, catecholamines, and nucleic acids) that we felt that we could begin to look for such an enzyme in chick brain. A wide variety of assay techniques were tried, and our newest version is described in some detail in the "Methods" section. Our initial studies showed that chick brain "homogenate" could catalyze the production of isoamyl alcohol-extractable radioactivity from S-adenosylmethionine-^{14}C-methyl, which was a function of the indoleamine substrate level, was linear with time and protein concentration, and that this activity was capable of being enriched about ten-fold using ammonium sulfate precipitation and a Sephadex G-200 column. Table 1 demonstrates this progressive enrichment using isoamyl alcohol-extractable radioactivity as the dependent variable.

Using a discontinuous sucrose gradient of 0.32 M, 0.8 M, and 1.2 M sucrose, centrifugation of wide-clearance brain homogenate at 100,000 x G for ninety minutes evidenced two peaks of indoleethylamine N-methyltransferase activity in the supernatant and the supramitochondrial particulate fraction (Figure 6). Table 2 is a summary of our studies of the substrate specificity for N-transmethylation of chick brain homogenate. Note that four indoleethylamines seem capable of being methyl acceptors in this system. Table 3 summarizes the regional specific activity in the rat brain, using isoamyl alcohol-extractable radioactivity. Recent studies of sheep brain in our laboratory have indicated that the caudate, which has relatively low activity in this study on rats, seems to show remarkably high enzyme activity in the sheep.

Table 4 represents perhaps one of the more interesting aspects of our studies of brain indoleethylamine N-methyltransferase activity. It seems that this kind of enzyme activity is demonstrable in human brain. It is interesting that the amygdala, medulla, and uncus have the highest specific activity of the parts measured. I apologize for the irregularity of this brain dissection; it occurred because of the limits of time and arrangements in the university morgue. Since only a small amount of human brain material was available, an attempt was made to get some idea whether this human brain enzyme activity was specific for indoleethylamines, or whether it resembled the nonspecific aromatic amine N-methylating system described by Axelrod in 1961. Table 5 shows that 100,000 x G supernatant fraction of the homogenate had relatively high activity for indoleethylamines and low activity for the phenylethylamines and histamine. Fractionation by ammonium sulfate precipitation (35 to 45 percent) led to a decrease in histamine N-methyltransferase activity, relatively no change in phenylethylamine N-methyltransferase activity, and relatively higher values for the indoleethylamine substrates. These findings suggest substrate specificity for indoleethylamines. Holding the ionic strength constant, the pH optimum for the N-methylation of serotonin was determined using the 100,000 x G supernatant fraction of human brain homogenate (Figure 7). This

TABLE 1

Activity of Indoleethylamine N-Methyltransferase
from Whole Chick Brain

ENZYME SOURCE	SPECIFIC ACTIVITY*
Supernatant fraction of whole brain homogenate	0.26
45% – 55% saturated $(NH_4)_2SO_4$ precipitate	0.87
Sephadex gel filtration fraction	2.54

*Activity is expressed as mµM N-methylserotonin formed per milligram of protein per 90 minutes.

TABLE 2

Substrate Specificity of Chick Brain
Indoleethylamine N-Methyltransferase

SUBSTRATE	RELATIVE ACTIVITY %
5-Hydroxytryptamine	100
5-Methoxytryptamine	88
Tryptamine	60
N-Methyltryptamine	47
Normetanephrine	6
5-Hydroxy-N,N-dimethyltryptamine	--

Enzyme source was Sephadex G-200 column eluate, the fraction containing 0.1 mg of protein.

TABLE 3

Regional Specific Activity of Rat Brain
Indoleethylamine N-Methyltransferase*

REGION	SPECIFIC ACTIVITY**
Medulla	364 ± 48.7
Cerebellum	354 ± 33.1
Pons	299 ± 49.6
Mesencephalon	258 ± 26.0
Olfactory Bulb	158 ± 43.3
Hypothalamus	154 ± 12.3
Amygdala	152 ± 12.8
Occipital Pole	143 ± 19.5
Caudate	121 ± 21.3
Frontal Pole	105 ± 22.0

*N = 6. 5-HT as substrate and isoamyl alcohol as product extraction solvent.

**Mean ± S.E.M. as mμM of 5-HT methylated/gm/hr.

TABLE 4

Regional Specific Activity of Human Brain
Indoleethylamine N-Methyltransferase*

BRAIN	REGION	SPECIFIC ACTIVITY**	SOURCE
Infant male	parietal cortex	95	biopsy
Adult female	frontal cortex	103	biopsy
Adolescent male	frontal cortex	<30	two hours postmortem
	orbital surface of frontal lobe	69	
	ventral midbrain (long tracts included)	74	
	amygdala	136	
	medulla	189	
	uncus	218	

*5-HT was substrate and isoamyl alcohol the product extraction solvent. Each value is mean of three determinations.

**mµM of 5-HT methylated/gm/hr.

TABLE 5

Substrate Affinities of Methylating
Enzymes in Human Brain Homogenate*

SUBSTRATE	FRACTION	
	100,000 x G SUPER.	$NH_4 SO_4$; 35-45%
5-HT	100	100
Tryptamine	95	111
N-methyl-5-HT	94	79
N-methyltryptamine	62	55
Norepinephrine	0	7
Normetanephrine	41	40
Histamine	1110	134

*Brain homogenate relative to 35 to 45 percent ammonium sulfate cut for various biogenic amine methyl acceptors (see text). 5-HT as reference substrate (i.e., equal to 100 percent).

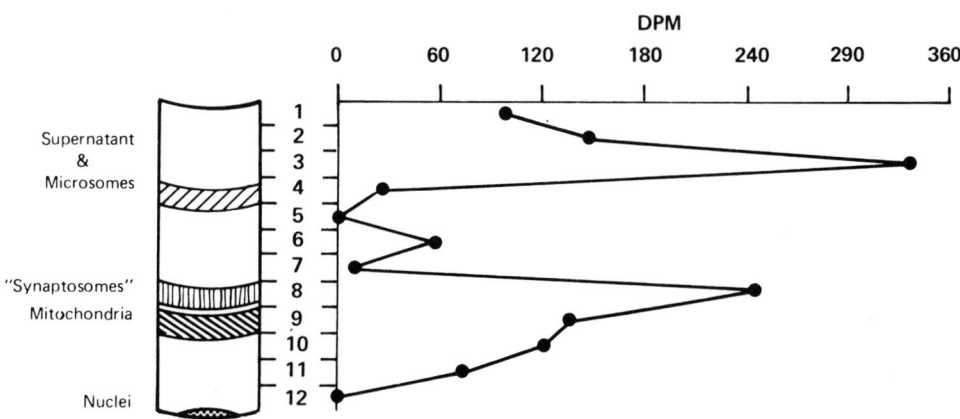

Figure 6. Subcellular localization in chick brain of indoleethylamine N-methyltransferase. Incubation mixture contained 50 μl of serial 3-ml fractions from the sucrose gradient. 5-HT was the substrate. The three layers of sucrose were 0.32 M, 0.8 M, and 1.2 M sequentially. The gradient was centrifuged at 100,000 x G for 90 minutes.

was the same as was demonstrated by Axelrod for lung enzyme.

Because of the shortage of human brain material, we have recently switched to using sheep brain. Table 6 summarizes studies of the relative substrate specificity of the brain enzyme from sheep brain during enrichment procedures. We are currently using tryptamine as the indoleamine substrate and toluene extraction of product. This increases the sensitivity and decreases the blanks. During these purification procedures, it seems that the indoleethylamine N-methyltransferase activity increases while the histamine decreases, and the phenylethylamine fails to make a significant appearance in these experiments. It seems that indoleethylamine N-methyltransferase is discriminable from other already known brain N-methyltransferases. This activity was linear over time, for protein and substrate concentration within the constraints of the reaction conditions described in the previous section. Boiled enzyme demonstrated no activity. The Km for SAM was 2×10^{-5}. The Km for 5-HT was 9×10^{-4}. The Ki for chlorpromazine was 10^{-3}, and for lithium 2×10^{-4}.

Chromatograms of the toluene-extractable radioactivity, lyophilized and spotted on cellulose thin layer chromatographic plates, were run in three solvent systems: isopropanol-H_2O-NH_4OH (50:50:3);

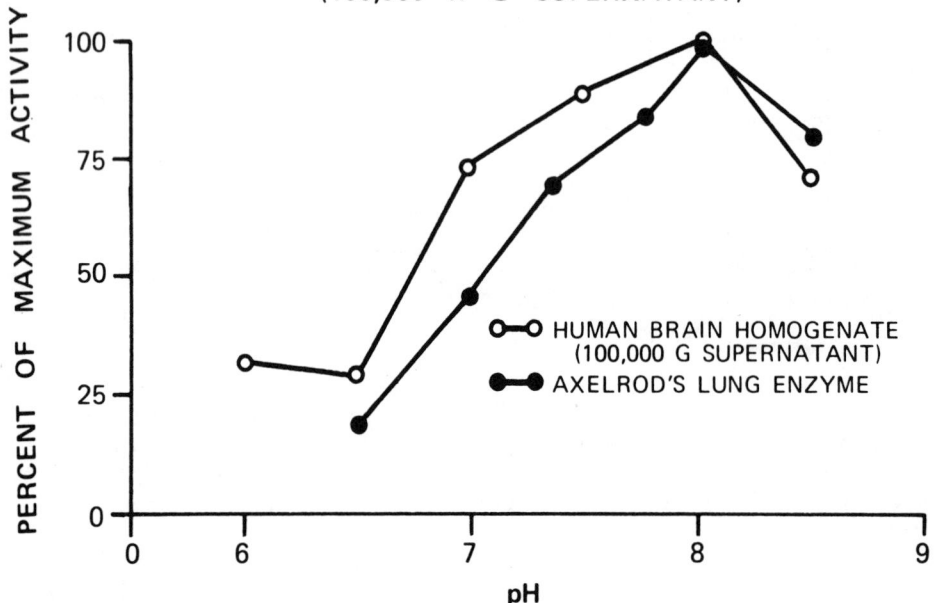

Figure 7. The pH optimum for human brain indoleethylamine-N-methyltransferase activity. Note similarity to Axelrod's lung enzyme (Axelrod 1961).

TABLE 6

Substrate Specificity and Purification of Mammalian Brain Indoleethylamine N-Methyltransferase (Sheep)*

SUBSTRATES	SPECIFIC ACTIVITIES OF FRACTIONS**		
	100,000 x G Super.	35-45% NH_4SO_4	G-200
Tryptamine	0.22	0.86	2.13
Histamine	7.13	1.23	0.17
Normetanephrine	0.04	–	–
Norepinephrine	–	–	–

*Enzyme was purified with ammonium sulfate precipitation and Sephadex G-200 column fractionation. Values below 0.02 mμM/mg/hour were regarded as zero.

**as mμM of substrate methylated/mg protein/hour.

isopropanol-H_2O-NH_4OH (100:10:2.5) and 8 percent NaCl in H_2O. Tryptamine, monomethyltryptamine, and dimethyltryptamine were seen as contiguous in one dimension, with a radioactive peak occurring in the area of monomethyltryptamine (Figures 8, 9, and 10). The first chromatogram is elegantly clean (Figure 8). The second and third systems (Figures 9 and 10) are not as clear. What seem to be multiple products have confused us somewhat, especially in light of the linearity of product-radioactivity with incubation time of the assay. I believe it is safe to say that, in terms of the chromatography of products, we have more work to do.

Since it seems that less than one-tenth of one percent of an isotopic dose of bufotenine enters the brain of an animal possessing a fully matured blood-brain barrier (Himwich 1969), it is not surprising that reports of the central actions of this agent have been negative (Turner and Merlis 1959). The structure of bufotenine is so similar to O-methylbufotenine (a known potent hallucinogen at 600 µg/dose; Gessner *et al.* 1960), that we guessed that the blood-brain barrier-crossing ability of the two compounds accounted for the difference in their potency. We believed that if we could eliminate the blood-brain barrier as a factor, we might find bufotenine to be very close in potency to its more lipid-soluble methylated congener. Using intraventricular infusions of both compounds in freely moving rats (Segal and Mandell 1970), and monitoring the drug-induced motor activity, we were able to demonstrate that bufotenine is somewhat more centrally active than O-methylbufotenine in producing hyperactivity (Figure 11). In addition, bufotenine produced bizarre boxing motions in the rat rather consistently at these low doses. Thus it seems that bufotenine, if produced in the brain, may be a potent biological agent.

CONCLUSION

We have presented some highly suggestive evidence that there may be an indoleethylamine N-methyltransferase enzyme in mammalian brain that can turn serotonin into N-methylated derivatives that may be biologically active. The enzyme is relatively low in specific activity and has a relatively high Km. One can argue that, with a Km in the 10^{-3} range, serotonin would never be in concentration high enough for the enzyme to function, or that serotonin in the brain might never reach a level at which the function of this enzyme might be physiologically significant. This may be true under normal circumstances. During a state such as chronic amphetamine intoxication, however, or during treatment with a monoamine oxidase inhibitor, it is possible that such an indoleethylamine-methylating shunt could become kinetically feasible. It is tempting to speculate that the amphetamine psychoses might result from such a mechanism following the amphetamine-induced inhibition of monoamine oxidase. Another

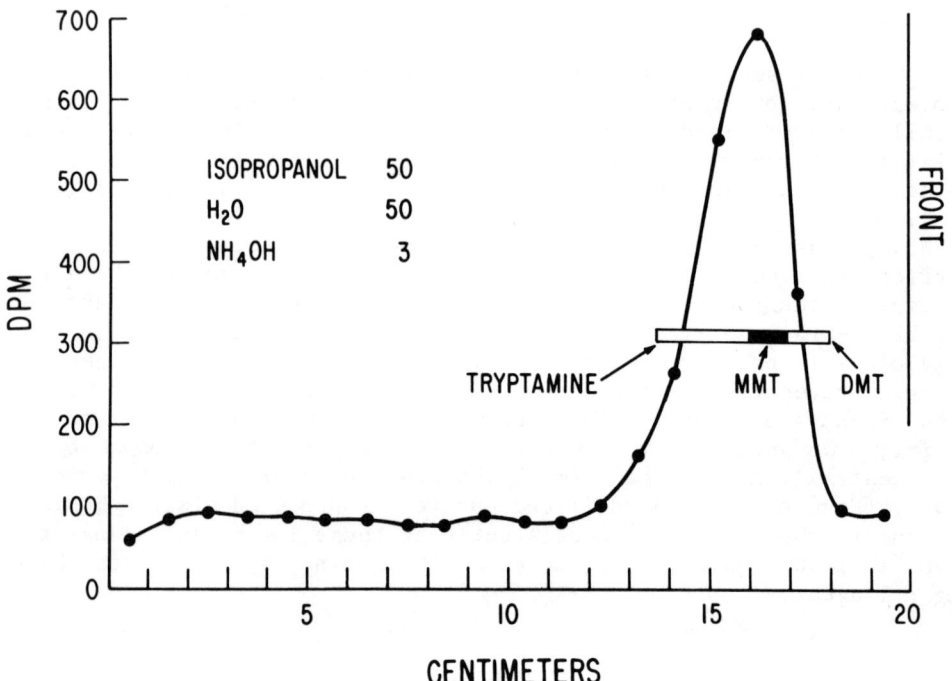

Figure 8. Cellulose thin layer chromatography in one dimension of toluene-extractable radioactivity following assay of sheep brain indoleethylamine N-methyltransferase, using tryptamine as substrate. Enzyme source was Sephadex G-200 column eluate which was 20X enriched from whole brain homogenate.

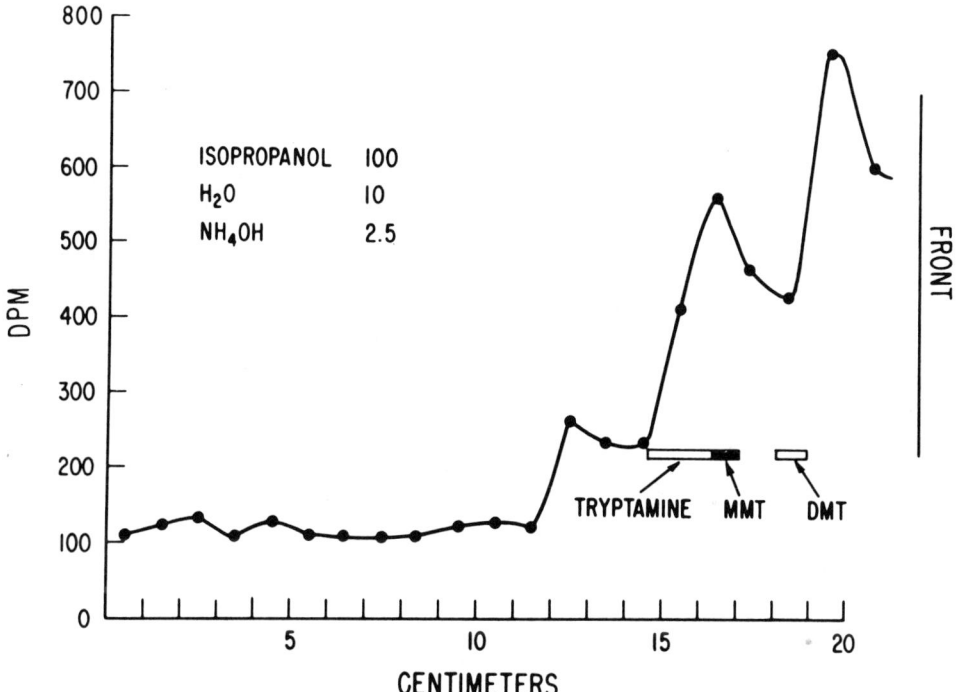

Figure 9. Cellulose thin layer chromatography of toluene-extractable radioactive product(s) as in Figure 8, with another set of solvent ratios.

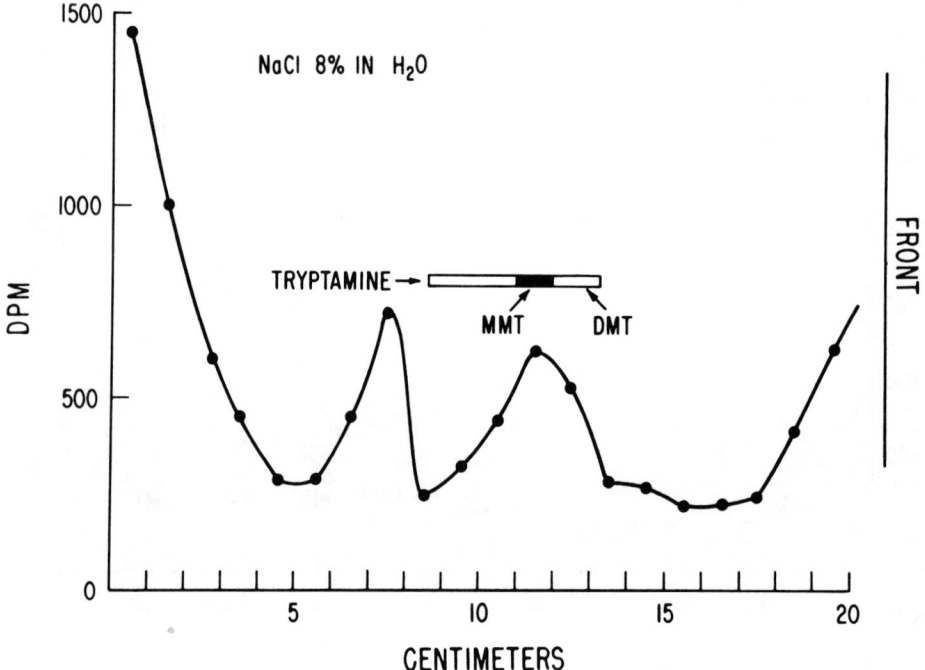

Figure 10. Cellulose thin layer chromatography of toluene-extractable radioactive product(s) as in Figure 8, with another solvent system.

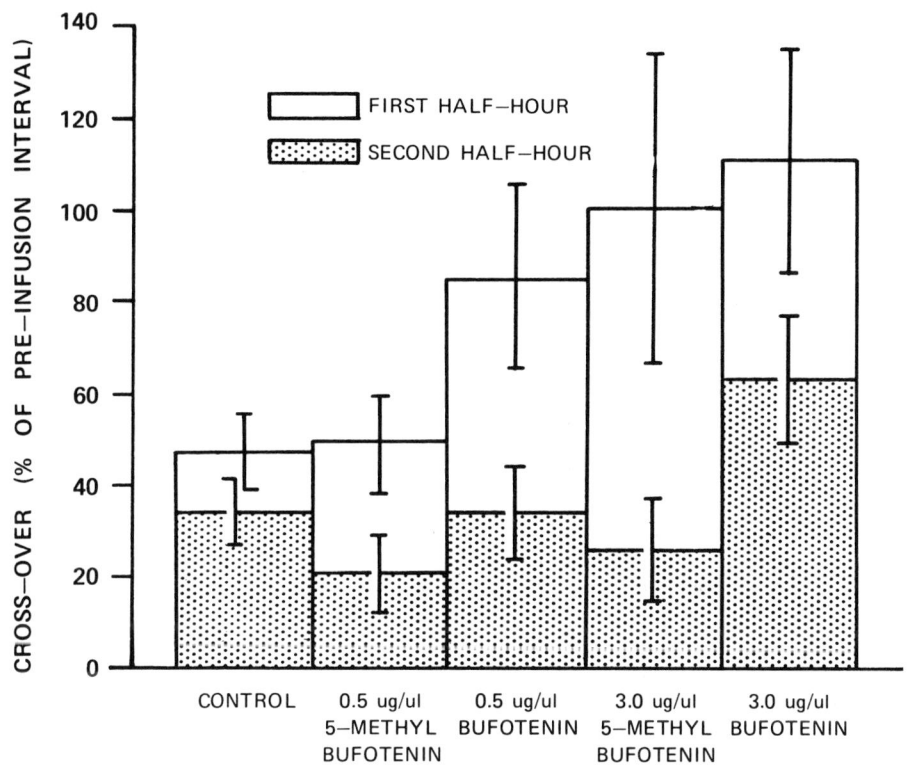

Figure 11. Effects on gross motor activity of intraventricular infusion of bufotenine and 5-methylbufotenine in freely moving rats. N = 6. Infusion rate was 1 μl/3 minutes. Note comparability of the potency of these two compounds when the blood-brain barrier is removed as a factor.

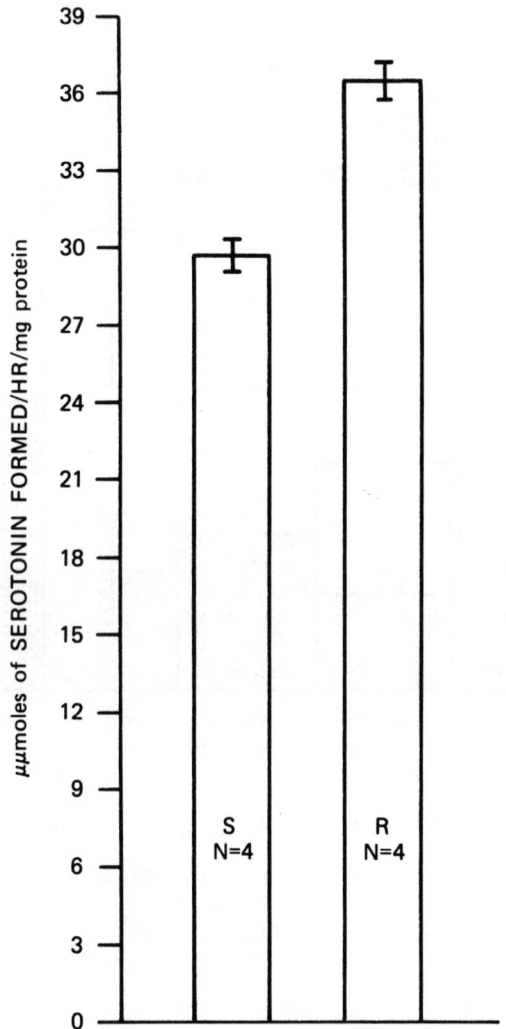

Figure 12. Effect of 1.5 mg/kg of reserpine given subcutaneously in two injections, twelve hours apart, on pons-midbrain tryptophan hydroxylase activity. See text.

possibility for the development of circumstances that could lead to unusual increases in serotonin substrate levels is currently being explored in our laboratories--that of a drug- or behavior-induced increase in tryptophan hydroxylase activity. Figure 12 shows preliminary data from this work. In this adaptation of the tryptophan hydroxylase assay of Ichiyama et al. (1970), note that reserpine administration can increase the specific activity of this rate-limiting enzyme in the biosynthesis of serotonin. Perhaps other drugs and conditions can do this as well. A third possibility for an indoleethylamine substrate reaching meaningful concentrations for transmethylation would be its shift in subcellular location to a pool that would be protected from monoamine oxidase and be available for transmethylation. This possibility is difficult to explore experimentally. Since the mono- and dimethylated tryptamines are poor substrates for brain monoamine oxidase (Blaschko and Levine 1966), it seems that once the indoleethylamines are N-methylated they can resist degradation long enough to be physiologically significant. We have recently demonstrated that methylated indoleamines competitively inhibit the oxidative deamination of serotonin by monoamine oxidase *in vitro*. Perhaps once this methylation process is allowed to begin, it could propagate itself.

ACKNOWLEDGMENT

Supported by National Institute of Mental Health Grant MH-14360-04.

REFERENCES

Axelrod, J. 1961. Enzymatic formation of psychotomimetic metabolites from normally occurring compounds. *Science* 134:343.

Axelrod, J. 1965. The formation and metabolism of physiologically active compounds by N and O methyltransferases. In *Transmethylation and Methionine Biosynthesis*. S. K. Shapiro and F. Schlenk (eds.). Chicago: University of Chicago Press, p. 71.

Blaschko, H., and Levine, W. G. 1966. Metabolism of indolealkylamines. In *5-Hydroxytryptamine and Related Indolealkylamines*. V. Erspamer (ed.). New York: Springer-Verlag.

Gessner, P. K.; Khairallah, P. A.; McIsaac, W. M.; and Page, I. H. 1960. The relationship between the metabolic fate and pharmacological actions of serotonin, bufotenine and psilocybin. *J. Pharmacol. Exp. Ther.* 130:126.

Himwich, H. 1969. Personal communication.

Himwich, H. E.; Narasimachari, N.; Heller, B.; Spaide, J.; Haskovec, L.; Fujimori, M.; and Tabushi, K. 1970. Comparative behavioral and urinary studies on schizophrenics and normal controls. In *Biochemistry of Brain and Behavior*. R. E. Bowman and S. P. Datta (eds.). New York: Plenum Press, p. 207.

Ichiyama, A.; Nakamura, S.; Nishizuka, Y.; and Hayaishi, O. 1970. Enzymic studies on the biosynthesis of serotonin in mammalian brain. *J. Biol. Chem.* 245:1699.

Kety, S. S. 1961. Possible relation of central amines to behavior in schizophrenic patients. *Fed. Proc.* 20:4.

Kline, N. S.; Simpson, G.; and Sacks, W. 1967. Amines and amine precursors combined with a monoamine oxidase inhibitor in the treatment of depression. In *Neuropsychopharmacology*. New York: Excerpta Medica Foundation, p. 343.

Mandell, A. J. 1970. Drug induced alterations in brain biosynthetic enzyme activity--a model for adaptation to the environment by the central nervous system. In *Biochemistry of Brain and Behavior*. R. E. Bowman and S. P. Datta (eds.). New York: Plenum Press, p. 97.

Mandell, M.; Mandell, A. J.; and Jacobson, A. 1965. Biochemical and neurophysiological studies of paradoxical sleep. In *Recent Advances in Biological Psychiatry*, vol. VII. J. Wortis (ed.). New York: Plenum Press, p. 115.

Mandell, A. J., and Spooner, C. E. 1969. An N,N-indole transmethylation theory of the mechanism of MAOI-indole amino acid load behavioral activation. In *Schizophrenia--Current Concepts and Research*. D. V. Sankar (ed.). New York: PJD Pub., p. 496.

Morgan, M., and Mandell, M. 1969. Indole(ethyl)amine N-methyltransferase in the brain. *Science* 165:492.

Osmond, H., and Smythies, J. R. 1952. Schizophrenia: A new approach. *J. Mental Sci.* 98:309.

Pollin, W.; Cardon, P. V.; and Kety, S. S. 1961. Effects of amino acid feedings in schizophrenic patients treated with iproniazid. *Science* 133:104.

Segal, D. S., and Mandell, A. J. 1970. Behavioral activation of rats during intraventricular infusion of norepinephrine. *Proc. Nat. Acad. Sci. U.S.A.* 66:289.

Turner, W. J., and Merlis, S. 1959. Effect of some indolealkylamines in man. *Arch. Neurol. Psychiat.* 81:121.

TRANSMETHYLATION PROCESSES IN SCHIZOPHRENIA

F. Antun, D. Eccleston, and J. R. Smythies

Department of Psychiatry, University of Edinburgh, and
Medical Research Council, Brain Metabolism Unit

Edinburgh, Scotland

It is generally agreed today that the etiology of schizophrenia is compounded of a genetically determined predisposition, in the form of some vulnerable enzyme system or systems in the brain possibly concerned with reactions to stress, together with various environmental factors that determine whether the genotype is actually expressed as the phenotype. There is very little information, however, on what the biochemical lesion is, and only a handful of hypotheses about what the lesion could be. The so-called transmethylation hypothesis is based on the observation made in 1950 by Harley-Mason, Osmond, and Smythies that mescaline is an O-methyl derivative of dopamine. Many other psychotomimetic drugs have been discovered since then, and most of these are either O-methyl, or N-methyl (or both) derivatives of the central neurotransmitters, noradrenaline, dopamine and serotonin.

The transmethylation theory simply states that schizophrenia may be associated with a defective enzyme system concerned in transmethylation reactions, so that toxic levels of some psychotomimetic agent builds up in the brain. The enzyme, N-methyltransferase, has been discovered in brain (Mandell 1971), and several groups have reported the detection of dimethyltryptamine in the body fluids of schizophrenic patients (e.g., Tanimukai *et al.* 1970).

I will discuss (1) the experimental data, (2) the transmethylation hypothesis in more detail, and (3) some recent work on transmethylation in the brain brought about by methionine.

The Data

When we consider what the alleged biochemical fault in schizophrenia may be, we find, alas, very few facts on which to build. Fifty years of research have yielded the following meager harvest relevant to the transmethylation hypothesis.

(a) Many workers have reported that schizophrenics are less reactive to histamine than normal people. This may be seen most clearly by measuring the size of the wheal produced by an intradermal injection of histamine. It is consistently smaller in schizophrenics than in normal people and returns to normal size upon clinical remission.

(b) Seymour Kety and his group then at the National Institute of Mental Health found that some chronic schizophrenics react with an acute psychosis to methionine plus an inhibitor of the enzyme, monoamine oxidase. Other schizophrenic patients, clinically indistinguishable from the former, do not react at all. This observation was confirmed by several groups, and the monoamine oxidase inhibitor was shown to be unnecessary (Smythies and Antun 1970; Antun *et al.* 1971); the active agent is the methionine. This period of acute psychosis is often followed by a period of clinical remission.

(c) Schizophrenic patients also react more commonly than normal with an acute psychosis to antabuse, a drug given to chronic alcoholics to prevent their drinking.

(d) The drugs that alleviate schizophrenic symptoms--that is, the phenothiazines and butyrophenones--have a wide range of biological activity, but one of their most potent effects is in inhibiting the adrenergic synapses in the central nervous system and, in particular, the dopamine receptors.

(e) The drugs that can produce an acute psychosis (a "bad trip") in normal people--that is, the hallucinogens like d-LSD and mescaline--have been shown to inhibit brain serotonin mechanisms and to potentiate certain adrenergic mechanisms.

Interpretation of the Data

These are the clues currently available, and we can ask, meager as they are, whether they suggest the nature of the metabolic lesion-- or, at least, what system in the brain might be involved. The evidence presented in sections (c) and (d) suggests that schizophrenia may be associated with an overactive central adrenergic system and, in particular, with the mechanisms involving dopamine. Antabuse nonspecifically inhibits the enzyme that converts dopamine to noradrenaline, and thus it tends to raise levels of brain dopamine. Recent experiments have linked brain dopamine to the control of psychomotor aspects of behavior. Raising the level of brain dopamine in animals leads to restless, agitated behavior. The evidence in section (e) implicates a possible blockade of central serotonin transmission. Thus it may be that schizophrenia is associated with an overactive adrenergic system and an underactive serotonin system in the brain.

It is now thought that these central amine neurons play key roles in the brain's control of behavior and of emotional reactions. It is well known that the classical syndrome of depression is associated with low levels of brain serotonin and norepinephrine, and that it may indeed be induced by such agents as reserpine that deplete the brain's store of these amines. In Parkinsonism, which is characterized as much by poverty of movement and emotional expression as by the familiar tremor and rigidity, brain levels of dopamine are greatly lowered. In cats treated with p-chlorophenylalanine (PCPA), which specifically blocks the formation of brain serotonin, there are gross disturbances of behavior, including certain electroencephalographic (EEG) changes in the form of peculiar spikes from loci deep in the brain that are not dissimilar from spikes claimed to have been recorded from such regions in schizophrenics.

We can now ask a second question. If this is the case, what factor or factors are responsible for depressing the central serotonin mechanisms and stimulating the central adrenergic mechanisms? Clearly there could be a number of different reasons. But the simplest is to suppose that the schizophrenic is producing an endotoxin that acts like LSD. If we study the list of compounds that can induce this sort of psychotic reaction (as distinct from the delirium induced by such agents as atropine), we can observe that many of them are methylated derivatives of the central neurotransmitters, serotonin and noradrenaline (Figure 1). Tryptamine is converted into the powerful hallucinogenic drug, dimethyltryptamine (DMT), by adding two methyl groups on the nitrogen atom, and serotonin is converted into an even more powerful hallucinogen by putting two methyl groups on the nitrogen and one on the oxygen atom. Mescaline, dimethoxymethylamphetamine (DOM) (which is some one-hundred times as potent as mescaline), and related compounds are all O-methyl derivatives of dopamine. It is therefore interesting to note that one of the normal metabolic routes for the inactivation of catecholamines is by methylation of one of its hydroxyls (Figure 1). The methyl group for all these conversions is taken from methionine, and this immediately suggests an explanation for the data in sections (a) and (b).

In our pilot studies we have recently shown *in vivo* that methionine donates methyl groups to catechol metabolites. For, if

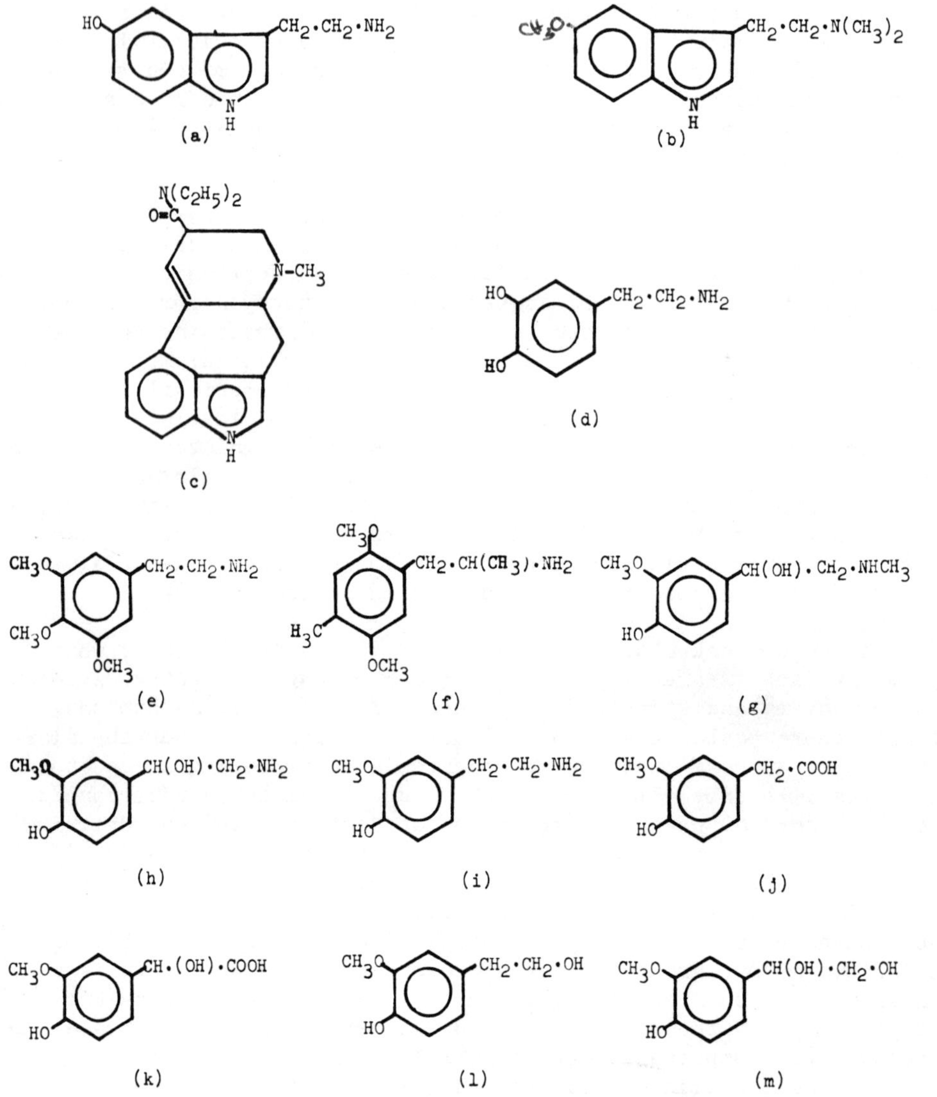

Figure 1. (a) serotonin; (b) dimethyltryptamine (DMT); (c) d-LSD; (d) dopamine; (e) mescaline; (f) DOM; (g) metanephrine; (h) normetanephrine; (i) 3-methoxytyramine; (j) homovanillic acid (HVA); (k) 3-methoxy-4-hydroxymandelic acid (VMA); (l) 3-methoxy-4-hydroxyphenylethanol (MHPT); (m) 3-methoxy-4-hydroxyphenylglycol (MHPG).

schizophrenics have an overactive methylating enzyme or, more plausibly, an underactive demethylating enzyme--since most metabolic disorders are associated with weak or absent enzymes--then, adding more active methyl groups in the form of methionine would put more pressure on the already faltering mechanism. In addition, the normal method of inactivating histamine is by N-methylation. There are known enzymes in the body that will remove methyl groups. The proper action of one, or a series of them, may normally protect the brain from accumulating dangerous psychotoxic compounds related to DMT. In support of this idea, unconfirmed reports (Israelstam et al. 1970) have been published stating that, following ingestion of methionine with its active methyl group radioactively labeled, the release of radioactive CO_2 is slower in schizophrenics than in normal controls-- suggesting an overactive methylating pool. Another report, also unconfirmed so far (Heath, Nesselhof, and Timmons 1966), claims that schizophrenics are highly resistant to the methionine antimetabolite, methionine sulphoximine (MSO).

In normal people MSO at a dosage of over 200 mg per day produces an acute delirium with slow waves in the EEG. This can be prevented by giving methionine in a ratio of 19 parts to 1. In our series of ten schizophrenics no such reaction occurred, some even showed an apparent alleviation of symptoms, and none developed any EEG abnormality. This suggests that inhibition of the excess methylation balance in the schizophrenic by MSO may actually be beneficial. Thus, either too much or too little methylation seems to result in psychotic responses. This correlates with two other reports (but is denied by still others) that it is possible to detect DMT and related psychotoxins in the urine of schizophrenic patients. There is no increase in vanillylmandelic acid (VMA)--the methylated metabolites of adrenaline--in the urine of schizophrenics, however, nor can this be shown to increase following methionine administration. The main difference between VMA and 3-methoxy-4-hydroxyphenylglycol (MHPG) is that the former comes from bodily tissues and the latter from brain metabolism. Any psychotoxin in schizophrenia, however, is more likely to be a derivative of DMT than of mescaline, because the former are much more potent than the latter. Lastly, chlorpromazine, a phenothiazine, has been shown to inhibit the enzyme that adds the methyl group to the nitrogen of tryptamine to make DMT, and this enzyme has been reported to be present in brain.

It is quite possible, of course, that this explanation is not correct. Methionine could produce this result by other mechanisms-- for example, by upsetting the general amino acid balance of the body (excess methionine will do this better than any other amino acid), or by its role in other metabolic systems of which it has several. It is also possible that the defect in schizophrenia lies in some yet undiscovered biochemical mechanism, but an approach along these lines can hardly lead to an active research program.

We will now report on some recent work carried out at Edinburgh.

After the isolation and purification of catechol-O-methyltransferase (COMT) and catechol-N-methyltransferase (CNMT) from animal biological tissues, Axelrod and his group demonstrated that both enzymes were capable of methylating catecholamines *in vitro* when they were incubated with S-adenosyl-L-methionine, the active form of L-methionine.

Although these findings indicate that L-methionine is the methyl donor in *in vitro* experiments, no one has demonstrated that such transfer of a methyl group takes place *in vivo*. For our experimental model we concentrated on the O-methylated metabolites of dopamine and noradrenaline [i.e., homovanillic acid (HVA); 3-methoxytyramine (MTYR); 3-methoxy-4-hydroxyphenylethanol (MHPT); 3-methoxy-4-hydroxymandelic acid (VMA); 3-methoxy-4-hydroxyphenylglycol (MHPG); normetanephrine (NMN), and metanephrine (MN)] (Figure 1). Our aim was to demonstrate the transfer of the methyl group from L-methionine to each of the above O-methylated metabolites, both centrally and peripherally.

Methylation in the CNS

Male albino rats were injected through the tail vein with L-methionine-^{14}C-methyl (60 mCi/mM, 12.5 μCi/rat). After two hours they were killed by cervical fracture, decapitated, and the brains removed. The brains were homogenized with 4% perchloric acid (PCA) and centrifuged. The supernatants were decanted and saved for the estimations.

Acids. The acids were extracted from the supernatants with ethyl acetate, back-extracted into 1M pH 10 borate buffer, and re-extracted from the buffer at pH 1 into ethyl acetate. The ethyl acetate extracts were blown down to small volumes and applied, together with markers of authentic HVA and VMA, to chromatography paper. The chromatograms were developed by descending chromatography in two solvent systems--(a) isobutyl methyl ketone:4% formic acid (10:1 v/v); (b) chloroform:methanol:ammonia sp. gr. 0.88 (12:7:1 v/v). The results are shown in Figure 2.

Alcohols. The remaining supernatants were incubated for twenty-four hours with sulphatase enzyme to hydrolyse the MHPG sulphate conjugate. The hydrolysates were then passed over columns filled with an anion exchange resin (AG1-X4-Cl form). The effluents were saved for the determination of the O-methylated catechols, and the eluates containing the alcohols were blown to a small volume under vacuum and applied to chromatography paper, together with markers of authentic MHPG and MHPT. The chromatograms were developed in the

TRANSMETHYLATION PROCESSES IN SCHIZOPHRENIA

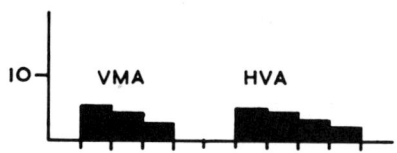

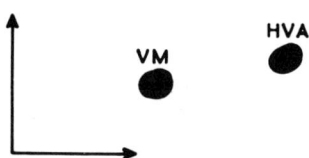

Figure 2. Form of chromatogram and counts expressed as dpm on 1-cm strips for 3-methoxy-4-hydroxymandelic acid (VMA), and homovanillic acid (HVA)--from CNS.

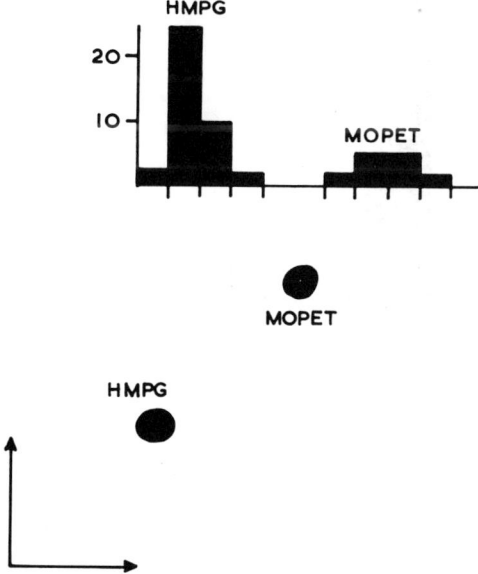

Figure 3. As in Figure 2 for 3-methoxy-4-hydroxyphenylglycol (MHPG) and 3-methoxy-4-hydroxyphenylethanol (MHPT)--from CNS.

same solvent systems used for the acids. The results are shown in Figure 3.

O-methylated catechols. The effluents from the anion exchange resin were passed over columns of CG-50 (NH_4^+ form) cation exchange resin. The columns were washed with water, then eluted with 3N ammonia. The eluates were blown down to small volumes under vacuum and were applied, together with markers of authentic NMN, MN, and MTYR, to silica-gel thin layer plates, 20 x 20 cm. Two-dimensional chromatography with two solvent systems (isopropyl alcohol-ammonia, 5% [4:1]; benzene-acetic acid-water [62.5:35:15]) were used to develop the chromatograms. The results are shown in Figure 4.

The O-methylated metabolites were localized by spraying the developed chromatograms with diazotized *p*-nitroaniline (saturated solution in 0.5 N HCl), then with 5% sodium hydroxide in ethanol. The spots were cut out in 1 x 4 cm strips in the case of the acids and alcohols, and scraped into 1 x 4 cm portions in the case of the O-methylated catechols. The strips and scrapings were then counted by liquid scintillation against blanks.

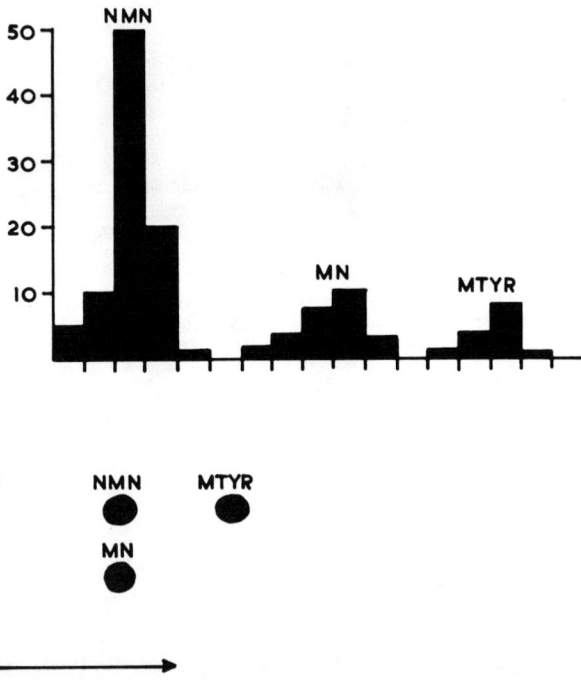

Figure 4. As in Figure 2 for normetanephrine (NMN), metanephrine (MN), and 3-methoxytyramine (MTYR)--from CNS.

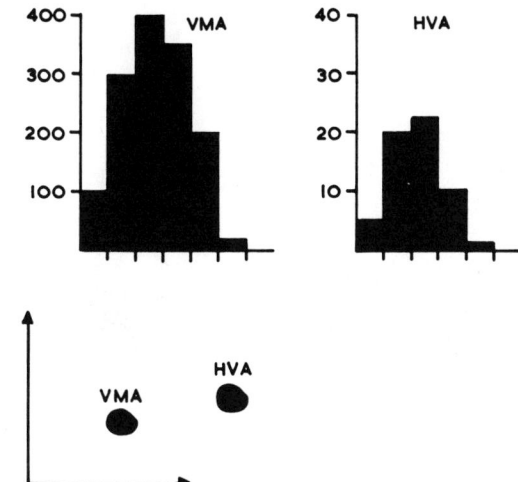

Figure 5. As in Figure 2--from whole body.

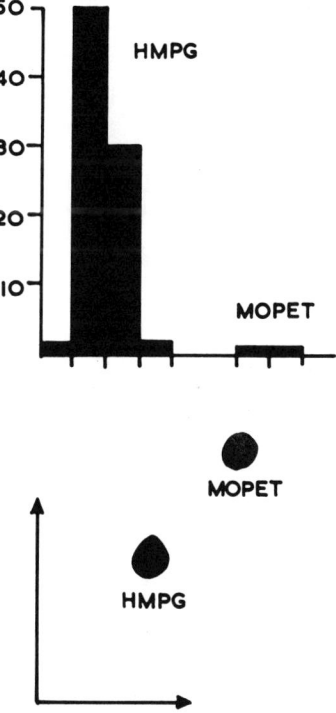

Figure 6. As in Figure 3--from whole body.

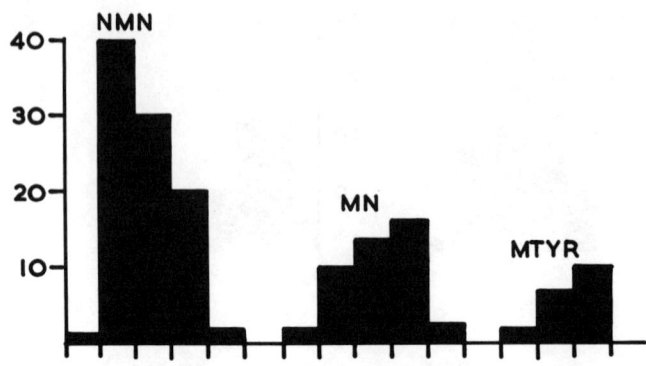
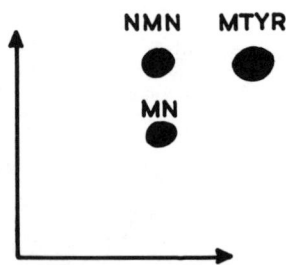

Figure 7. As in Figure 4--from whole body.

Total Body Methylation

Albino male rats were injected through the tail vein with 12.5 µCi of L-methionine-^{14}C-methyl (60 mCi/mM). They were then placed in metabolic cages for 24-hour urine collection.

The urines were then adjusted to pH 1 and processed in the same way as the brain homogenates, except for the hydrolysates of which samples were incubated with a mixture of sulphatase enzyme and glucoronidase enzyme to hydrolyse the MHPG and metanephrine conjugates, respectively. The results are shown in Figure 5 (acids), Figure 6 (alcohols), and Figure 7 (O-methylated catecholamines).

DISCUSSION

As can be seen from the results, the major central O-methylated metabolites found were normetanephrine and MHPG; amounts of the other O-methylated metabolites were insignificant. These values only represent the levels of O-methylated metabolites at one specific time, and they do not necessarily reflect the actual levels and turnover of these metabolites.

In observing the results representing total body methylation, one finds, as expected, that VMA is the major O-methylated metabolite. NMN and MHPG, on the other hand, were found in smaller amounts. Although the NMN represents release from peripheral stores (since NMN does not cross the blood-brain barrier), the MHPG, depending on the size of the peripheral noradrenaline pool, comes mainly from brain. Thus, our pilot studies have been able to demonstrate the probable transfer of the ^{14}C-methyl group from L-methionine to the above-mentioned metabolites. Since methionine contributes methyl groups to a host of metabolites in the body, we are now in the process of testing the probability of this transfer with various separation procedures in order to be absolutely certain of the authenticity of these O-methylated metabolites.

REFERENCES

Antun, F.; Burnett, G.; Cooper, A. J.; Daly, R. J.; and Smythies, J. R. 1971. *J. Psychiat. Res.* in press.

Heath, R. G.; Nesselhof, W. Jr.; and Timmons, E. 1966. D,L-methionine-d,l-sulphoximine effects in schizophrenic patients. *Arch. Gen. Psychiat.* 14:213.

Israelstam, D. M.; Sargent, T.; Finley, N. N.; Winchell, H. S.; Fish, M. B.; Motto, J.; Pollycove, M.; and Johnson, A. 1970. Abnormal methionine metabolism in schizophrenic and depressive states: a preliminary report. *J. Psychiat. Res.* 7:185.

Mandell, A. J.; Buckingham, B.; and Segal, D. 1971. Behavioral, metabolic, and enzymatic studies of a brain indoleethylamine N-methylating system. This volume.

Rosenthal, D., and Kety, S. (eds.) 1968. *The Transmission of Schizophrenia.* Oxford: Pergamon Press.

Smythies, J. R. 1970. *Brain Mechanisms and Behaviour.* Oxford: Blackwell.

Smythies, J. R. 1971. The chemical anatomy of synaptic mechanisms. *Int. Rev. Neurobiol.* vol. 14, in press.

Smythies, J. R., and Antun, F. 1970. The biochemistry of psychosis. *Scottish Med. J.* 15:34.

Tanimukai, H.; Ginther, R.; Spaide, J.; Bueno, J. R.; and Himwich, H. E. 1970. Detection of psychotomimetic N,N-dimethylated indolamines in the urine of four schizophrenic patients. *Brit. J. Psychiat.* 117:421.

EFFECTS OF DRUGS ON CATECHOLAMINE SYNTHESIS

Irwin J. Kopin

Laboratory of Clinical Science
National Institute of Mental Health

Bethesda, Maryland

Although the exact role of catecholamines in brain function is not clearly established, it is becoming increasingly evident that dopamine and norepinephrine do play important roles in control of movement, in determining affective state and alertness, and in neuroendocrine relationships. Utilization of catecholamines by neurons is associated with increased rates of synthesis, so that levels of the amines are altered only slightly compared to changes in their rates of utilization and replacement. Estimates of synthesis rates may, therefore, be more useful than determination of catecholamine levels in assessing changes in neuronal function.

Several methods for estimating the rate of amine synthesis in brain and other tissues have been used to study the effects of drugs or procedures on catecholamine utilization. These procedures provide useful information for assessing changes in rate of amine synthesis, but certain assumptions must be simplified to interpret such data in terms of absolute synthesis rates. In calculating absolute synthesis rate, such assumptions as a single, uniformly mixed pool of norepinephrine in the tissues, the lack of effect of drugs that inhibit synthesis on utilization rates, the maintenance of a steady state, the source (and specific activity) of the tyrosine precursor, etc. may be subject to question. In spite of such reservations about assumptions implicit in the various methods, it is likely that reasonable approximations are obtained and that changes in ap-

---

This article was written by Dr. Kopin in his private capacity. No official support nor endorsement by the U. S. Public Health Service is intended nor should be inferred.

parent rates of synthesis obtained reflect actual changes in these rates; that is, they do not seem to be artifacts of effects that alter the degree of validity of the assumptions. Thus, if a drug or procedure changes the rate of appearance of radioactive norepinephrine formed from labeled tyrosine, then it will alter, in the same direction, the apparent rate of turnover calculated from the disappearance of labeled amine or of endogenous amine, when synthesis is inhibited.

The effects of drugs on catecholamine turnover may be understood most easily by first reviewing current concepts of the function of the adrenergic neuron and the processes involved in the synthesis, storage, release, inactivation, and metabolism of the neurotransmitter. The biosynthesis of norepinephrine involves the sequential action of three enzymes (Figure 1). The first of these, tyrosine hydroxylase, converts tyrosine to 3,4-dihydroxyphenylalanine (DOPA), and it is believed to be rate-limiting (Levitt et al. 1965). Its activity seems to be modulated by feedback control, presumably by cytoplasmic catecholamines competing with a tetrahydropteridine cofactor of the enzyme (Ikeda, Fahien, and Udenfriend 1965). Drugs may diminish norepinephrine synthesis directly by acting on tyrosine hydroxylase, or indirectly by affecting the levels of cytoplasmic catecholamines.

Decarboxylation of DOPA to 3,4-dihydroxyphenylethylamine (dopamine) by aromatic L-amino acid decarboxylase (Lovenberg, Weissbach, and Udenfriend 1962) is rapid, and usually DOPA is not present in significant quantity. This step is not rate-limiting, and only under circumstances of almost complete inhibition of this enzyme is the overall rate of catecholamine synthesis diminished. Dopamine is formed in the cytoplasm; since dopamine-β-hydroxylase is located inside the storage vesicles (Viveros et al. 1969), the amine must enter, or be transported into, the vesicle before conversion to norepinephrine. Dopamine-β-hydroxylase is not usually rate-limiting, but under conditions of accelerated DOPA formation it may become a limiting factor in norepinephrine synthesis.

Norepinephrine in the storage vesicles seems to be bound as a complex with a specific protein (chromogranin), magnesium ion + and adenosine triphosphate. Drugs may interfere with binding by interfering with the mechanism of binding or by replacing the physiologic catecholamine. The process for release of the neurotransmitter by a nerve impulse is not clearly defined, but it seems to require calcium ions and to involve emptying of the contents of the vesicles into the synaptic cleft. Drugs may prevent release of the transmitter by interfering with the sequence of events that transduces a nerve impulse into neurotransmitter release. This diminution of norepinephrine utilization may indirectly reduce the rate of transmitter synthesis.

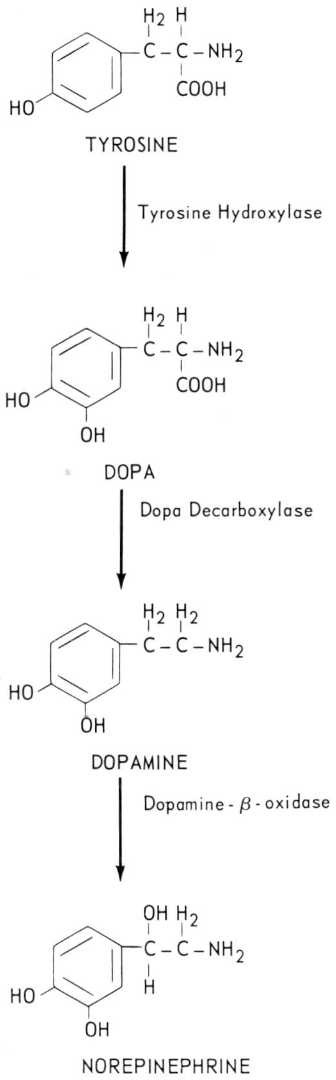

Figure 1. Biosynthesis of norepinephrine.

After release into the synaptic cleft, the transmitter acts on receptor sites of the postsynaptic membrane. Interference with this action may lead to reflex acceleration of presynaptic neuronal activity and thereby enhance amine synthesis. Termination of the action of the transmitter substance is necessary for the next nerve impulse to be effective. Amine uptake by a specific transport process into the presynaptic neuron seems to be the major source of inactivation at the adrenergic synapse (Axelrod and Kopin 1969). The amine can then be stored in the synaptic vesicles for reuse. Interference with such reuptake might lead to accelerated replacement of the neurotransmitter and enhanced amine synthesis. Inhibition of reuptake might cause prolonged action of the released transmitter, however, and lead to reflex reduction in presynaptic neuronal activity that would tend to reduce utilization. These opposite effects of inhibition of uptake on synthesis rates tend to cancel each other, and there may be no net effect on synthesis.

Catecholamines are substrates for monoamine oxidase and catechol-O-methyltransferase (Figure 2). The route of metabolism de-

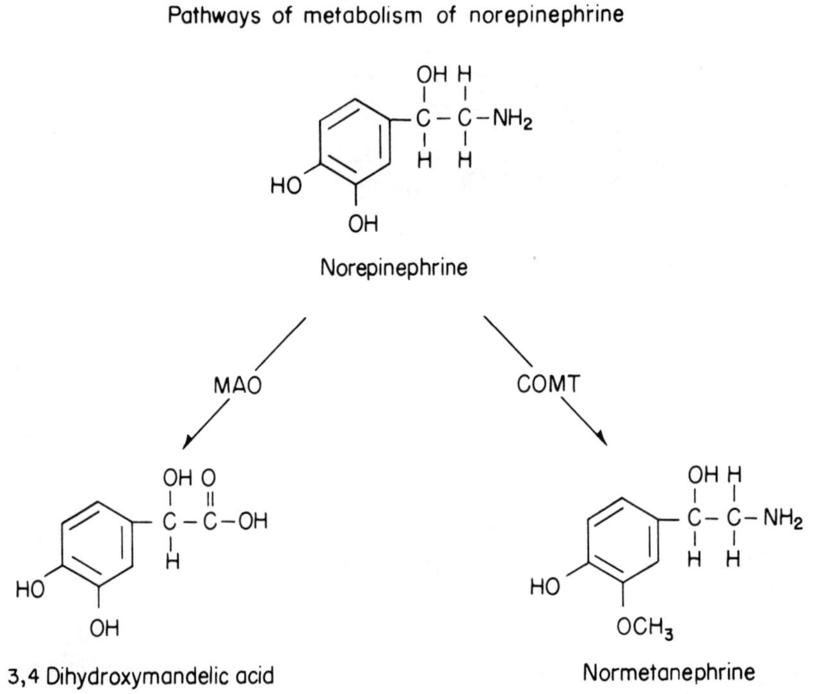
Pathways of metabolism of norepinephrine
Norepinephrine
MAO
COMT
3,4 Dihydroxymandelic acid
Normetanephrine

Figure 2

pends upon the site of release from the storage vesicles. Norepinephrine that leaks out of the vesicles or is released into the cytoplasm of the neuron is destroyed mainly by deamination; extraneuronally released norepinephrine is metabolized by catechol-O-methyltransferase, in either the postsynaptic cell or the liver and kidney after reaching the circulation (Axelrod and Kopin 1969).

Based on these concepts of the adrenergic neuron, the effects of drugs on norepinephrine synthesis rates may be related to their mechanism of action at a molecular level. First to be considered are the drugs that directly inhibit the processes involved in catecholamine biosynthesis (Table 1). Since tyrosine hydroxylase is the enzyme that usually limits the rate of catecholamine synthesis, this is the most effective site at which to inhibit synthesis. A number of analogs of tyrosine (α-methyltyrosine, 3-iodotyrosine, etc.) are effective competitive inhibitors of the enzyme (Udenfriend, Zaltzman-Nirenberg, and Nagatsu 1965). Catechol derivatives decrease activity of the enzyme by competition with its tetrahydropteridine cofactor and, as indicated earlier, $_{may}$ control the rate of DOPA formation by this mechanism.

DOPA decarboxylase is present in great abundance, and only relatively complete inhibition of this enzyme interferes with catecholamine biosynthesis. Decaborane seems to inhibit synthesis of catecholamines at this site by reducing the enzyme-pyridoxal complex (Merritt, Schultz, and Wykes 1964). Several α-methyl aromatic amino acids are both substrates and competitive inhibitors of decarboxylase (Sourkes 1954), but they do not inhibit the enzyme sufficiently to interfere with catecholamine biosynthesis.

Drugs that interfere with transport of dopamine into the vesicle prevent access of the substrate to dopamine-β-hydroxylase and thereby interfere with norepinephrine biosynthesis. Reserpine is bound by the vesicles, presumably in the membrane, and it blocks uptake of dopamine (Kirshner, Rorie, and Kamin 1963) as well as enhancing release of norepinephrine. This drug diminishes conversion of dopamine to norepinephrine by this mechanism. Similarly, chlorpromazine and metaraminol have actions at the vesicular membrane, and they interfere with conversion of dopamine to norepinephrine.

Dopamine-β-hydroxylase is a copper-containing enzyme, and it is inhibited by chelating agents such as diethyldithiocarbamate (Kaufman and Friedman 1965). Isosteres of dopamine act as competitive inhibitors. These drugs may interfere with norepinephrine synthesis, particularly when the rate of formation of the catecholamine is accelerated.

In addition to their direct effects on the enzymes and vesicular transport process involved in catecholamine biosynthesis, drugs

Table 1

DIRECT INHIBITION OF PROCESSES INVOLVED

IN CATECHOLAMINE BIOSYNTHESIS

Inhibited	Inhibitor	Mechanism
Tyrosine hydroxylase	α-Methyltyrosine Iodotyrosine Catechol	Competition with tyrosine Competition with tetrahydropteridine
Decarboxylase	α-Methyldopa Benzylhydrazines Benzyloxyamines Decaborane	Competition with substrate or pyridoxin Noncompetitive act on apoenzyme or coenzyme Reduction of enzyme
Dopamine transport	Phenylethylamines Reserpine	Competitive ?
Dopamine-β-hydroxylase	Phenylethylamine and isosteres Dithiocarbamate	Competition with substrate Chelate copper ion

may influence norepinephrine formation indirectly (Table 2). Since cytoplasmic levels of catecholamines influence tyrosine hydroxylase activity by feedback inhibition, drugs that increase free, intraneuronal cytoplasmic catecholamines would be expected to inhibit catecholamine biosynthesis. Monoamine oxidase inhibitors diminish the rate of catecholamine biosynthesis (Costa and Neff 1966), presumably as a result of blocking the destruction of cytoplasmic catecholamines. Amines related to phenylethylamine that contain either a β-hydroxyl group or a catechol moiety can displace norepinephrine from its vesicular storage sites (Musacchio, Weise, and Kopin 1967).

Table 2

INDIRECT EFFECTS OF DRUGS ON CATECHOLAMINE BIOSYNTHESIS

Mechanism	Agents

Decrease release from nerve ending (inhibit)
  Decrease nerve impulses
    Reflex
    Block excitation
  Block release mechanism
	
	Adrenergic stimulants
	Ganglionic blocking agents
	Bretylium, lithium

Increase intraneuronal cytoplasmic catecholamines (inhibit)
  Inhibit destruction
  Release norepinephrine into cytoplasm and/or inhibit uptake into vesicles
	
	Monoamine oxidase inhibitors
	Reserpine
	Phenylethylamines

Increase release from nerve ending (accelerate)
  Increase impulses reflexly
  Decrease reuptake
	
	Receptor blockers (phenoxybenzamine)
	Tricyclic antidepressants

The resultant increase in cytoplasmic norepinephrine inhibits tyrosine hydroxylation. Phenylethanolamine derivatives may also compete with dopamine for uptake into the dopamine-β-hydroxylase-containing vesicles and thereby interfere with norepinephrine formation. The phenylethylamine precursors of these compounds compete with dopamine for the enzyme, as well as for the vesicular transport system (Weiner and Selvaratnam 1968). They may interfere with β-hydroxylation of dopamine, either by competing directly for the enzyme or by preventing access of dopamine to the hydroxylating enzyme which is confined to the vesicle. When binding sites become available, catecholamine levels in the cytoplasm are reduced and synthesis is accelerated. Thus, false transmitters at first interfere with catecholamine synthesis and, later, when catecholamine stores are being repleted, norepinephrine synthesis is accelerated (Kopin, Weise, and Sedvall 1969).

Similarly, reserpine indirectly diminishes catecholamine biosynthesis by interfering with norepinephrine binding. Norepinephrine is released into cytoplasm, and tyrosine hydroxylation is inhibited (Weiner 1970). Furthermore, as indicated above, reserpine diminishes uptake of dopamine into the vesicles and prevents formation of norepinephrine at the β-hydroxylation step. When the effects of reserpine on vesicular uptake are reversed, cytoplasmic levels of catecholamines diminish and norepinephrine formation is accelerated (Weiner 1970).

Lithium ions seem to enhance uptake of norepinephrine by synaptosomes (Colburn et al. 1967), to diminish release of norepinephrine from electrically stimulated brain slices (Katz, Chase, and Kopin 1968), and to accelerate turnover of the catecholamine in brain (Corridi et al. 1967). Treatment with lithium alters the metabolism of norepinephrine so that deamination seems to be enhanced and O-methylation diminished. These variant effects, however, are not inconsistent if lithium interferes with intravesicular binding of the catecholamine. This would result in destruction by deamination and diminution of release by depolarization but still accelerate turnover.

Drugs blocking the receptor by diminishing synaptic efficacy would be expected to produce a reflexive compensatory increase in presynaptic neuronal activity that would be reflected in increased utilization of the neurotransmitter. Such a mechanism has been postulated to explain the elevated levels of homovanillic acid and the accelerated synthesis and turnover of dopamine in the brains of animals treated with chlorpromazine (Carlsson and Lindqvist 1963; Laverty and Sharman 1965). When receptor blockade is accompanied by inhibition of presynaptic uptake, the effects on net release and utilization would be expected to be magnified. Thus, phenoxybenzamine, which inhibits norepinephrine reuptake as well as its action on α-receptors, produces marked acceleration of norepinephrine synthesis and results in elevation of levels of tyrosine hydroxylase (Thoenen, Mueller, and Axelrod 1969).

Blockade of uptake might be associated with enhanced utilization and synthesis of the neurotransmitter but if the receptor were not blocked, potentiation of the released amine would be expected. This could result in a compensatory decrease in the rate of neuronal activity and diminished transmitter release. The net effect of diminished uptake in the absence of receptor blockade might therefore result in little, if any, alteration of transmitter synthesis. This might explain why drugs such as imipramine may produce only small and transient effects on synthesis of norepinephrine and still result in an increased level of synaptic transmitter or altered rate of nerve firing.

The relationship of psychoactive drugs to alterations in the synthesis and utilization of catecholamines has provided an attractive array of evidence supporting the hypothesis that these amines play an important role in brain function and have been the basis for hopes that such agents may be useful in treating a wide variety of psychiatric and neurological disorders. It is hoped that further elucidation of the role of amines in psychiatric disorders may lead to appropriate therapeutic agents to correct the metabolic bases of mental illness, addictive or tolerant states (e.g., amphetamine) or other disorders in which abnormalities of amine metabolism are found.

REFERENCES

Axelrod, J., and Kopin, I. J. 1969. Uptake, storage, release and metabolism of noradrenaline in sympathetic nerves. In *Progress in Brain Research*, vol. 31. K. Akert and P. G. Waser (eds.). Amsterdam: Elsevier Publishing Company, p. 21.

Carlsson, A., and Lindqvist, M. 1963. In vivo decarboxylation of α-methyl-dopa and α-methyl-metatyrosine. *Acta Pharmacol. Toxicol.* 20:140.

Colburn, R. W.; Goodwin, F. K.; Bunney, W. E.; and Davis, J. M. 1967. Effect of lithium on the uptake of noradrenaline by synaptosomes. *Nature* 215:1395.

Corridi, H.; Fuxe, K.; Hökfelt, T.; and Schou, M. 1967. Effect of lithium on cerebral monoamine neurones. *Psychopharmacologia* 11:345.

Costa, E., and Neff, N. H. 1966. Isotopic and non-isotopic measurements of the rate of catecholamine biosynthesis. In *Biochemistry and Pharmacology of the Basal Ganglia*. E. Costa, L. J. Cote, and M. D. Yahr (eds.). New York: Rover Press, p. 141.

Ikeda, M.; Fahien, L. A.; and Udenfriend, S. 1966. A kinetic study of bovine adrenal tyrosine hydroxylase. *J. Biol. Chem.* 241:4452.

Katz, R. I.; Chase, T. N.; and Kopin, I. J. 1968. Evoked release of norepinephrine and serotonin from brain slices. Inhibition by lithium. *Science* 162:466.

Kaufman, S., and Friedman, S. 1965. Dopamine-β-hydroxylase. *Pharmacol. Rev.* 17:71.

Kirshner, N.; Rorie, N.; and Kamin, D. L. 1963. Inhibition of dopamine uptake *in vitro* by reserpine administration *in vivo*. *J. Pharmacol. Exp. Ther.* 141:285.

Kopin, I. J.; Weise, V. K.; and Sedvall, G. C. 1969. Effect of false transmitters on norepinephrine synthesis. *J. Pharmacol. Exp. Ther.* 170:246.

Laverty, R., and Sharman, D. F. 1965. Modification by drugs on the metabolism of 3,4-dihydroxyphenylethylamine, noradrenaline and 5-hydroxytryptamine in the brain. *Brit. J. Pharmacol.* 24:759.

Levitt, M.; Spector, S.; Sjoerdsma, A.; and Udenfriend, S. 1965. Elucidation of the rate-limiting step in norepinephrine biosynthesis in the perfused guinea pig heart. *J. Pharmacol. Exp. Ther.* 148:1.

Lovenberg, W.; Weissbach, H.; and Udenfriend, S. 1962. Aromatic L-amino acid decarboxylase. *J. Biol. Chem.* 237:89.

Merritt, J. H.; Schultz, E. J.; and Wykes, A. A. 1964. Effect of decaborane on the norepinephrine content of rat brain. *Biochem. Pharmacol.* 13:1364.

Musacchio, J. M.; Weise, V. K.; and Kopin, I. J. 1967. Mechanism of norepinephrine binding. *Nature* 205:606.

Sourkes, T. L. 1954. Inhibition of dihydroxyphenylalanine decarboxylase by derivatives of phenylalanine. *Arch. Biochem. Biophys.* 51:444.

Thoenen, H.; Mueller, R. A.; and Axelrod, J. 1969. Trans-synaptic induction of adrenal tyrosine hydroxylase. *J. Pharmacol. Exp. Ther.* 169:249.

Udenfriend, S.; Zaltzman-Nirenberg, P.; and Nagatsu, T. 1965. Inhibitors of purified beef adrenal tyrosine hydroxylase. *Biochem. Pharmacol.* 14:837.

Viveros, O. H.; Arqueros, L.; Connett, R. J.; and Kirshner, N. 1969. Mechanism of secretion from the adrenal medulla. Studies of dopamine-β-hydroxylase as a marker for catecholamine storage vesicle membranes in rabbit adrenal glands. *Molec. Pharmacol.* 5:60.

Weiner, N. 1970. Regulation of norepinephrine biosynthesis. *Ann. Rev. Pharmacol.* 10:273.

Weiner, N., and Selvaratnam, I. 1968. The effect of tyramine on the synthesis of norepinephrine. *J. Pharmacol. Exp. Ther.* 161:21.

PHARMACOLOGICAL IMPLICATIONS OF THE EFFECTS OF AMPHETAMINE AND ITS ANALOGS ON THE TURNOVER RATE OF TISSUE CATECHOLAMINES

E. Costa, M. K. Naimzada, and A. Revuelta

Laboratory of Preclinical Pharmacology
National Institute of Mental Health
St. Elizabeths Hospital
Washington, D. C.

It is now well established that an acute paranoid psychosis may follow d-amphetamine administration (Young and Scoville 1938). Hence, Connell (1958), Bell (1965), and Kety (1967) have proposed this psychosis as a model for the study of affective disorders and schizophrenia. A better understanding of the biochemical factors involved in the actions elicited by d-amphetamine may increase the practical utility of this model. The picture that has emerged from our studies in rats on the biochemical correlates of the pharmacological effects of d-amphetamine can be summarized as follows:

1. d-Amphetamine depletes central and peripheral norepinephrine (NE) stores when injected in doses ten-fold greater than those required to increase exploratory motor activity (0.3 mg/kg i.v.); the doses of d-amphetamine decreasing brain NE content, however, fail to deplete striatal dopamine (DA) (Costa and Groppetti 1970a; Groppetti, Naimzada, and Costa 1971).

2. The d-amphetamine doses depleting brain NE also cause accumulation of p-hydroxynorephedrine in peripheral and central noradrenergic neurons. Since the biological half-life of p-hydroxynorephedrine concentrations in rat brain is twenty times longer than that of d-amphetamine, this metabolite persists in brain tissue longer than its parent compound (Groppetti and Costa 1969). Similar findings were independently reported by Brodie et al. (1969).

3. The persistent localization of p-hydroxynorephedrine in central and peripheral noradrenergic neurons parallels the long-lasting depletion of NE (Costa and Groppetti 1970a).

4. After a single peritoneal injection of 3 to 10 mg/kg of d-amphetamine, the pharmacological responses, including stereotype behavior and increase of locomotor activity, have disappeared 24 to 36 hours earlier than the depletion of NE. This finding suggests that the time course of the depletion of brain NE is unrelated to that of the pharmacological effects (hyperthermia, increase of motor activity, stereotype behavior, and anorexia) (Costa and Groppetti 1970b).

The discrepancy between the time course of the effects of d-amphetamine on behavior and brain biochemistry has kept us from concurring with the view that the central actions of d-amphetamine can be explained satisfactorily by its indirect sympathomimetic action, which biochemically is defined as the ability of d-amphetamine to release NE from nerve terminals. Before dismissing the working hypothesis that the action of d-amphetamine on noradrenergic nerves explains the pharmacological actions of d-amphetamine, we have tested whether this correlation could be substantiated by investigating the action of d-amphetamine on the turnover rate of brain norepinephrine and dopamine. We have found that the motor activity increase elicited by threshold doses of d-amphetamine is accompanied by an acceleration of turnover rate of striatum DA (Costa and Groppetti 1970a; Groppetti, Naimzada, and Costa 1971).

Although it is generally agreed that the rate of catecholamine turnover might be a measure of the efflux rate of the monoamine from nerve terminals onto postsynaptic receptors (see references in Costa and Neff 1970), the opinions of several investigators diverge when they are asked to define kinetically the compartmentation of NE stores in nerve terminals. Hence, some authors believe that in nerve terminals NE is stored in several compartments; others, although they recognize the complexities of the morphology of nerve terminals, insist on a simplified model comprising a single kinetic compartment (see references in Costa 1970). Operationally, the latter concept seems consistent with the present methodology and results. In fact, there is no direct kinetic evidence to reject the assumption that a single kinetic compartment open at both ends is a suitable model to describe the function of adrenergic nerve terminals. Recent papers conclude, however, that a two-compartment system is consistent with an apparent preferential release of newly synthesized NE from the brainstem neurons of rats receiving a foot shock (Thierry, Blanc, and Glowinski 1970).

TURNOVER RATE OF NE AND DA STORES IN TISSUES OF RATS

INJECTED WITH d-AMPHETAMINE

We estimated the effects of various doses of d-amphetamine on the turnover rate of NE by calculating the conversion index of L-tyrosine-3,5-^{3}H (Sp. Act. 31 Ci/mmole) in various tissue samples from animals killed 25 minutes after receiving 1 mCi/kg of the amino acid intravenously. The conversion index was calculated from

$$\frac{\text{dpm CA}}{\text{S.A.}_T} = \text{m}\mu\text{mol CA (conversion index)}$$

where CA is the catecholamine under study and S.A.$_T$ is the specific activity of tissue tyrosine (Groppetti, Naimzada, and Costa 1971). These experiments unequivocally show that 0.2 mg/kg i.v. of d-amphetamine injected 15 minutes before killing the rats and 10 minutes after injecting the label fails to change the turnover rate of NE in tel-diencephalon; this dose of d-amphetamine, however, increases the conversion index of heart NE (Table 1). The intraven-

TABLE 1

Conversion Index of L-Tyrosine-3,5-^{3}H into Catecholamines in Various Tissues of Rats Receiving Various Intravenous Doses of d-Amphetamine

mg/kg	Conversion Index (mµmol/gm/25 min)		
	Striatum DA	Tel-diencephalon NE	Heart NE
Saline (5 ml/kg) (10)	13.5 ± 1.8	0.58 ± 0.054	0.66 ± 0.02
0.2 (5)	9.0 ± 1.3	0.70 ± 0.083	0.97 ± 0.023*
0.3 (5)	25.0 ± 2*	0.47 ± 0.04	---

Rats received 1 mCi/kg i.v. of L-tyrosine-3,5-^{3}H and either saline or d-amphetamine 10 minutes later. The animals were killed 25 minutes after the injection. The specific radioactivity of tyrosine and catecholamines was assayed according to the method of Costa *et al.* (1968). Neither the steady-state concentration of DA nor that of NE is changed by either dose of d-amphetamine listed above.

*$p < 0.05$ when compared to saline-treated animals.

Number of animals in parentheses.

ous injection of 0.3 mg/kg, but not that of 0.2 mg/kg, of d-amphetamine increases the conversion index of striatum DA (Table 1). In these experiments we measured the steady-state level and the specific activity of tissue tyrosine; both parameters were not changed by either dose of d-amphetamine. The specific activity of tissue tyrosine in all the animals included in Table 1 was several times greater than the specific activity of either NE or DA found in the same tissue. Extrapolating from the conversion index reported in Table 1, we might infer that 0.2 mg/kg of the drug causes an indirect sympathomimetic effect only in cardiac tissues, whereas 0.3 mg/kg causes an activation of the dopaminergic nerve endings in striatum, but not of noradrenergic nerve terminals in tel-diencephalon.

CENTRAL EFFECTS OF d-AMPHETAMINE

Table 2 reports the effects of various doses of d-amphetamine on food intake and body temperature. The various responses were measured in groups of four rats each at 15, 30, and 60 minutes after drug injection. Motor and rearing activities were monitored continuously while rats were housed one in each of eight compartments of an I.R. Electronic Motility Meter (Metron Co., Sweden). Food intake was measured by weighing the food consumed by rats habituated (during the preceding 15 days) to eat their daily food intake within two hours.

TABLE 2

Pharmacological Responses at 15 Minutes after Various Intravenous Doses of d-Amphetamine

mg/kg	Motor Activity	Rearing Activity	Food Intake	Body Temperature
0.1	Normal	Normal	--	Normal
0.2	Normal	Normal	Decreased	Normal
0.3	Increased	Increased	Decreased	Normal
0.5	Increased	Increased	Decreased	Increased

The various responses are recorded in Table 2 as an increase or decrease when they were statistically significant from control ($p < 0.05$). These data show that 0.3 mg/kg i.v. of d-amphetamine is a threshold dose to increase locomotor and rearing activity, but that 0.2 mg/kg is already anorexigenic. These two doses of d-amphetamine neither cause hyperthermia nor decrease the concentrations of dopamine, norepinephrine, and serotonin (5-HT) in the various tissues studied. In comparing the data listed in Tables 1 and 2, we can conjecture that the increase of exploratory behavior elicited by d-amphetamine may be associated with a step-up of the turnover rate of striatum DA.

To investigate the biological significance of such a relationship further, we studied the following:

1. The biochemical correlates of the central actions of l-amphetamine.

2. The biochemical correlates to the pharmacological effects of three drugs chemically and pharmacologically related to amphetamine: aminorex, phenmetrazine, and p-Cl-amphetamine.

3. The effects of fenfluramine on brain monoamines.

BIOCHEMICAL CORRELATES OF SOME CENTRAL ACTIONS OF l-AMPHETAMINE

The data shown in Table 3 indicate that an l-amphetamine dose three times greater than that of d-amphetamine (Table 1) fails to alter the conversion of L-tyrosine-3,5-^{3}H into striatum DA. Both compounds fail to change the turnover rate of tel-diencephalic NE.

The methodology adopted for the experiments reported in Tables 3 and 4 compares with that employed for the experiments listed in Tables 1 and 2. The data reported in Tables 3 and 4 suggest that a dose of l-amphetamine three times greater than that of d-amphetamine fails to increase locomotor activity and to change the turnover rate of striatum DA. Since l-amphetamine decreases food intake and elicits hyperthermia, we might infer that these responses do not depend on an action of l-amphetamine on tel-diencephalic axons that store either DA or NE. Indirectly, these findings with l-amphetamine substantiate our tentative conclusion that the increase of motor activity elicited by d-amphetamine coincides with an increase of the turnover rate of striatum DA.

TABLE 3

Conversion of L-Tyrosine-3,5-^{3}H into Striatum DA
and Tel-diencephalic NE after Intravenous Injection of
1 mg/kg of ℓ-Amphetamine

Tissue	Amine	Conversion Index (mµmol/gm/25 minutes)	
		Saline	ℓ-Amphetamine
Striatum	DA	(8) 14.9 ± 0.53	(5) 14.8 ± 1.3
Tel-Diencephalon	NE	(8) 0.38 ± 0.05	(11) 0.39 ± 0.04

Rats received 1 mCi/kg i.v. of L-tyrosine-3,5-^{3}H and either saline or ℓ-amphetamine 10 minutes later. The animals were killed 25 minutes after injection. The specific radioactivity of tyrosine and catecholamines was assayed according to the method of Costa et al. (1968). Neither the steady-state concentrations of DA nor those of NE were changed by this dose of ℓ-amphetamine.

Number of animals in parentheses.

TABLE 4

Pharmacological Responses at 15 Minutes after
Intravenous Injection of ℓ-Amphetamine

Motor Activity	Rearing Activity	Food Intake	Body Temperature
Normal	Normal	Decreased	Increased

TABLE 5

Pharmacological Responses at 15 Minutes after Various Doses
of Aminorex, p-Cl-Amphetamine, and Phenmetrazine

Drug	mg/kg i.v.	Pharmacological Responses		
		Motor Activity	Food Intake	Body Temperature
Aminorex	0.25	Increased	Decreased	Normal
	0.50	Increased	Decreased	Increased
	1.0	Increased	Decreased	
p-Cl-Amphet-amine	0.3	Normal	Normal	
	0.6	Increased	Normal	Decreased
	1.2	Increased	Decreased	Normal
Phenmetrazine	1	Increased	Decreased	Normal
	2	Increased	Decreased	Increased

BIOCHEMICAL CORRELATES OF SOME CENTRAL ACTIONS
OF AMINOREX, PHENMETRAZINE, AND p-Cl-AMPHETAMINE

Phenmetrazine, p-Cl-amphetamine, and aminorex are chemically related to d-amphetamine and they mimic the central actions of this drug (compare data in Tables 2 and 5). The pharmacological profile of aminorex and phenmetrazine mimics closely that of d-amphetamine. In contrast, p-Cl-amphetamine differs from the latter pharmacologically because it elicits hypothermia. As will be shown later in this report, the biochemical effects of aminorex and phenmetrazine differ from those of d-amphetamine; in turn, the biochemical changes elicited by p-Cl-amphetamine differ from those elicited by aminorex, phenmetrazine, and d-amphetamine.

We injected rats intraperitoneally with various doses of phenmetrazine and aminorex and found that the concentrations of brainstem 5-HT and NE, heart NE, tel-diencephalic 5-HT and NE, and striatum DA did not change six hours after drug injection. As reported by Sanders-Bush and Sulser (1970), p-Cl-amphetamine depleted brain 5-HT. We then examined the concentrations in brain parts of NE, DA, and 5-HT at various times after injecting almost toxic doses of these compounds. We found that, after 8 mg/kg i.p. of p-Cl-amphetamine, the tel-diencephalic content of 5-HT is decreased by 50 percent or more in 2 to 24 hours. In contrast, the 5-HT content of brainstem is increased by about 30 percent between 1 and 2 hours after the drug injection, and returns to control values at about 4 hours. Other reports have suggested that the depletion of brain 5-HT elicited by p-Cl-amphetamine is due to a blockade of 5-HT synthesis (Sanders-Bush and Sulser 1970). Indirectly our findings cast some doubt on such an interpretation, as it would be difficult to explain the increase of the concentrations of brainstem 5-HT elicited by p-Cl-amphetamine as being due to tryptophan hydroxylase inhibition. The effects of this drug on brain 5-HT are reminiscent of that of fenfluramine (Costa, Groppetti, and Revuelta 1970); perhaps further experimentation may reveal a unified mechanism for the action of these two drugs on brain 5-HT concentrations. Moreover, we found that NE and DA concentrations of tel-diencephalon, brainstem, striatum, and heart are not affected by this dose of p-Cl-amphetamine. Considering that this dose of p-Cl-amphetamine is about twelve times greater than the dose required to elicit central stimulation (Table 5), and keeping in mind that corresponding doses of d- and ℓ-amphetamine would deplete tissue catecholamine concentrations, it is surprising that NE concentrations of heart and of the brain parts analyzed are unaffected by p-Cl-amphetamine, a chemical analog of amphetamine. When a similar experiment is carried out with corresponding doses of d-amphetamine, the concentration of brain and heart NE is decreased longer than 24 hours while the concentration of 5-HT in brainstem and tel-diencephalon remains unchanged (Costa and Groppetti 1970a and b). Hence, we can conclude that the effects of p-Cl-amphetamine on tissue monoamine stores are quite different from those of d-amphetamine.

Rats received 10 mg/kg of aminorex intraperitoneally, a dose 40 times greater than that capable of causing anorexia and increasing the locomotor activity (Table 5). This dose of aminorex failed to change the concentrations of NE and DA in tel-diencephalon and that of NE in brainstem, lung, and heart. The 5-HT concentrations of tel-diencephalon were unchanged but those of brainstem appeared elevated; this change was statistically significant at a single time point, two hours after the aminorex injection.

We finally studied the effects of phenmetrazine (20 mg/kg i.p.)

on the 5-HT, DA, and NE content of tel-diencephalon, brainstem, striatum, lung, and heart of rats. This drug resembles aminorex and fails to decrease tissue levels of these monoamines. Like aminorex, phenmetrazine tends to elevate the tissue levels of brainstem 5-HT, but in our study this elevation was statistically significant only one hour after the phenmetrazine injection.

Table 6 reports the results of our study of the effects of aminorex, phenmetrazine, and p-Cl-amphetamine on the conversion index of L-tyrosine-3,5-^{3}H into catecholamines in striatum, brainstem, tel-diencephalon, and heart. The data reported in Table 6 show that aminorex (0.25 mg/kg i.v.) increases the conversion index of striatum DA and tel-diencephalic NE, whereas the injection of p-Cl-amphetamine (0.6 mg/kg i.v.) not only accelerates the conversion of tyrosine into striatum DA and tel-diencephalic NE, but also increases the conversion of tyrosine into brainstem NE. In contrast, phenmetrazine (1 mg/kg i.v.) selectively increases the conversion of tel-diencephalic tyrosine into NE. None of these three drugs at the doses used affected the conversion of tyrosine into heart NE. We have not yet studied the conversion of L-tryptophan-^{3}H into tissue 5-HT, but we have measured the concentrations of tel-diencephalic and brainstem 5-HT in the same animals included in Table 6. We found that these drugs, including p-Cl-amphetamine at the doses listed in Table 6, fail to change the 5-HT concentrations of these tissues.

EFFECT OF FENFLURAMINE ON BRAIN MONOAMINES

Fenfluramine (N-ethyl-α-methyl-3 trifluoromethylphenylethylamine) is chemically related to d-amphetamine but is devoid of central stimulatory effects in man (Oswald 1970) and in animals (Boissier et al. 1965). This pharmacological peculiarity has suggested that fenfluramine may be devoid of many of the unwanted side effects elicited by d-amphetamine when used in man as an anorexigenic drug. In rats, fenfluramine depresses exploratory activity and its toxicity does not increase with animal aggregation (LeDouarec and Neveu 1970). We found that fenfluramine causes a depletion of 5-HT from tel-diencephalon which lasts longer than one might have expected from the biological half-life of fenfluramine (Costa, Groppetti, and Revuelta 1970). The depleting effects of fenfluramine do not extend to brainstem, stomach, and heart stores of 5-HT. Fenfluramine increases the turnover rate of tel-diencephalic 5-HT, but such an acceleration could not be detected in the 5-HT stores of brainstem, heart, and stomach (Costa et al. 1970).

We have measured the concentrations of fenfluramine metabolites radiochemically and by gas chromatography-mass spectrometry in various tissues after trimethylsilylheptafluorobutyryl derivatization of ethyl acetate and ethyl ether extracts of tissue homogenates (Mor-

TABLE 6

Conversion Index of L-Tyrosine-3,5-^{3}H into Catecholamines in Various Tissues of Rats Receiving Intravenously Aminorex, p-Cl-Amphetamine, and Phenmetrazine

Drug	mg/kg	CONVERSION INDEX (mµmol/gm/25 minutes)			
		Striatum DA	Brainstem NE	Tel-diencephalon NE	Heart NE
Saline	5 ml/kg (5)	11.4 ± 0.45	1.55 ± 0.26	0.52 ± 0.054	0.76 ± 0.12
Aminorex	0.25 (5)	19.6 ± 2.5*	2.20 ± 0.10	0.73 ± 0.044†	0.87 ± 0.077
Phenmetrazine	1 (5)	12.9 ± 0.7	1.96 ± 0.14	0.80 ± 0.054†	0.89 ± 0.044
p-Cl-Amphetamine	0.6 (5)	18.1 ± 1.5†	2.48 ± 0.24*	0.79 ± 0.054†	1.01 ± 0.16

Rats received 1 mCi/kg i.v. of L-tyrosine-3,5-^{3}H and either saline or d-amphetamine 10 minutes later. The animals were killed 25 minutes after injection. The specific radioactivity of tyrosine and catecholamines was assayed according to the method of Costa et al. (1968). Neither the steady-state concentration of DA nor that of NE is changed by aminorex, phenmetrazine, or p-Cl-amphetamine.

*$p < 0.05$
†$p < 0.01$

gan, Cattabeni, and Costa 1970). Fenfluramine and norfenfluramine have been detected in brain 24 hours after the administration of l-fenfluramine but only norfenfluramine was present 24 hours after l-fenfluramine administration, when the brain 5-HT concentrations still seemed to be lower than those of control rats. It seems possible, therefore, that norfenfluramine can deplete 5-HT stores, but it is unlikely that the drug displaces 5-HT in a manner similar to that invoked for NE by the amphetamine metabolite, p-OH-norephedrine. Furthermore, since the turnover rate of 5-HT is not reduced after fenfluramine, it is possible that a direct action on the membranes of serotonergic neurons is involved in this depletion. Only high doses of fenfluramine cause a depletion of catecholamine stores in brain and heart but the time course of this depletion coincides with that of tissue levels of fenfluramine (Costa, Gropetti, and Revuelta 1970).

CONCLUSIONS

The data discussed in this paper tend to negate the hypothesis that an effect on brain noradrenergic neurons in the tel-diencephalon is solely responsible for the increase of motor activity elicited by d-amphetamine and its analogs (aminorex, p-Cl-amphetamine, and phenmetrazine) in the rat. Such an indirect activity might be invoked for some compounds but not for all of them (Tables 1 and 6). In particular, 0.3 mg/kg i.v. of d-amphetamine increases motor activity but does not change the turnover rate of tel-diencephalic NE.

If we were to consider only d-amphetamine, we could actually show that a stereoisomeric specificity links the effects of this drug on motor activity and striatum DA turnover rate. The l-isomer in doses three times as great as of the d-isomer does not increase motor activity and fails to accelerate the turnover rate of striatum DA. The threshold doses of d-amphetamine for the increase of striatum DA turnover rate and the increase of motor activity seem quite similar (Tables 1 and 2). Such a relationship, however, does not apply to the other amphetamine-like drugs studied.

Phenmetrazine increases motor activity without changing the turnover rate of striatum DA. Using as background information the data of this report, it is impossible to propose a unified theory correlating biochemical and pharmacological effects of the amphetamine analogs studied. They all seem to affect the turnover of brain catecholamines, but their selectivity of action seems to vary within different catecholaminergic neuronal systems. Perhaps some clarification is in order. An important difference should be emphasized between the behavioral effects elicited by d-amphetamine and the other amphetamine-like drugs included in this report. Aminorex, phenmetrazine, and p-Cl-amphetamine fail to elicit the stereotype behavior which is part of the pharmacological profile of d-amphetamine (Randrup and Munkvad 1966). It may be important, therefore, to clarify whether either the action of d-amphetamine on dopaminergic neurons or the persistent accumulation of p-OH-norephedrine might be the two biochemical actions that can be associated with stereotype behavior. Pretreatment of rats with desmethylimipramine, however, abolishes the formation of p-OH-norephedrine but actually prolongs the duration of the stereotype behavior elicited by d-amphetamine (Costa and Groppetti 1970b). Moreover, the increase of motor activity elicited by d-amphetamine cannot be associated with an increase of turnover of tel-diencephalic NE because this effect cannot be brought in evidence in the tel-diencephalon of rats receiving a dose of d-amphetamine sufficient to increase motor activity. The formation and accumulation in brain of p-hydroxynorephedrine, a long-lasting amphetamine metabolite, may mask the acceleration of NE turnover in tel-diencephalon by selectively localizing in NE axons where it functions as a false transmitter (see references in Costa and Groppetti 1970a and b). If this were the case, then we could explain why d-amphetamine, unlike aminorex, p-Cl-amphetamine, and phenmetrazine, fails to accelerate the turnover rate of tel-diencephalic NE stores.

Our study also shows that anorexia and hyperthermia are unrelated to an increase of the turnover rate of catecholamines. Actually, the anorexic effects of fenfluramine may suggest that they result from a direct effect of these drugs on a brain postsynaptic receptor which we have not yet defined. Finally, we would like to recall that many investigators have suggested on several occasions that the stereotype behavior is the counterpart in rats of the acute psychoses observed in man after continuous self-administration of high doses of d-amphetamine. Our experience would tend to limit the validity of such an extrapolation. This derives from an inference; phenmetrazine does not elicit stereotype behavior in rats, yet it can cause psychosis in man.

SUMMARY

1. The minimal d-amphetamine dose to elicit an increase of motor activity in rats also accelerates the turnover rate of striatum dopamine but not that of tel-diencephalic norepinephrine.

2. These biochemical and pharmacological effects exhibit a powerful stereoisomeric specificity.

3. Rats injected with minimal doses of phenmetrazine, aminorex, and p-Cl-amphetamine to elicit an increase of motor activity exhibit an increase of turnover rate of tel-diencephalic norepinephrine. The turnover of striatum dopamine fails to increase after phenmetrazine but not after the other two amphetamine-like compounds.

4. p-Cl-amphetamine depletes brain serotonin in tel-diencephalon but fails to deplete the concentration of serotonin in brainstem.

5. Fenfluramine, which resembles p-Cl-amphétamine in regard to the effects on brain serotonin stores, fails to increase motor activity and actually decreases it.

6. The anorexigenic action of all the drugs studied cannot be related to their indirect action on catecholaminergic nerve terminals.

7. Stereotype behavior of rats cannot be observed after large doses of p-Cl-amphetamine, aminorex, and phenmetrazine but is present after d- and ℓ-amphetamine administration.

REFERENCES

Bell, D. S. 1965. Comparison of amphetamine psychosis and schizophrenia. *Brit. J. Psychiat.* 111:701.

Boissier, J. R.; Simon, P.; Fichelle, J.; and Hervouet, E. 1965. Action psychoanalytique de quelques anorexigenes dérivés de la phénéthylamine. *Thérapie* 20:297.

Brodie, B. B.; Cho, A. K.; Stefano, P.J.E.; and Gessa, G. L. 1969. On mechanisms of NE release by amphetamine and tyramine and tolerance to their effects. In *Advances in Biochemical Psychopharmacology*, vol. 1. E. Costa and P. Greengard (eds.). New York: Raven Press, p. 219.

Connell, P. H. 1958. Amphetamine psychosis. *Maudsley Monographs*, No. 5. London: Chapman and Hall, p. 62.

Costa, E. 1970. Simple neuronal models to estimate turnover rate of noradrenergic transmitters *in vivo*. In *Advances in Biochemical Psychopharmacology*, vol. 2. E. Costa and E. Giacobini (eds.). New York: Raven Press, p. 169.

Costa, E., and Groppetti, A. 1970a. Biosynthesis and storage of catecholamines in tissues of rats injected with various doses of d-amphetamine. In *Amphetamines and Related Compounds; Proceedings of the Mario Negri Institute for Pharmacological Research*. E. Costa and S. Garattini (eds.). New York: Raven Press, p. 231.

Costa, E., and Groppetti, A. 1970b. Relationships between biochemical and pharmacological responses elicited by d-amphetamine. Presented at the symposium, Current Concepts on Amphetamine Abuse, Duke University, North Carolina, in press.

Costa, E., and Neff, N. H. 1970. Estimation of turnover rates to study the metabolic regulation of the steady-state level of neuronal monoamines. In *Handbook of Neurochemistry*, vol. 4. A. Lajtha (ed.). New York: Plenum Publ. Co., p. 45.

Costa, E.; Spano, P. F.; Groppetti, A.; Algeri, S.; and Neff, N. H. 1968. Simultaneous determination of tryptophan, tyrosine, catecholamines and serotonin specific activity in rat brain. *Atti. Accad. Med. Lombard.* 23:1100.

Costa, E.; Groppetti, A.; and Revuelta, A. 1970. Action of fenfluramine on monoamine stores of rat tissues. *Brit. J. Pharmacol.*, in press.

Groppetti, A., and Costa, E. 1969. Tissue concentrations of p-hydroxynorephedrine in rats injected with d-amphetamine: Effect of pretreatment with desipramine. *Life Sci.* 8:653.

Groppetti, A.; Naimzada, M. K.; and Costa, E. 1971. Evidence for a stereoisomeric effect of (+)amphetamine on the striatum dopamine turnover rate and motor activity. *J. Pharmacol. Exp. Ther.*, submitted for publication.

Kety, S. S. 1967. The hypothetical relationships between amines and mental illness: A critical synthesis. In *Amines and Schizophrenia.* H. E. Himwich, S. S. Kety, and J. P. Smythies (eds.). New York: Pergamon Press, p. 271.

LeDouarec, J. C., and Neveu, C. 1970. Pharmacology and biochemistry of fenfluramine. In *Amphetamine and Related Compounds; Proceedings of the Mario Negri Institute for Pharmacological Research.* E. Costa and S. Garattini (eds.). New York: Raven Press, p. 75.

Morgan, C. D.; Cattabeni, F.; and Costa, E. 1970. Methamphetamine and their metabolites and monoamine concentrations in rat tissue. *J. Pharmacol. Exp. Ther.*, submitted for publication.

Oswald, I. 1970. Effects on sleep of amphetamine and its derivatives. In *Amphetamines and Related Compounds; Proceedings of the Mario Negri Institute for Pharmacological Research.* E. Costa and S. Garattini (eds.). New York: Raven Press, p. 865.

Randrup, A., and Munkvad, J. 1966. Role of catecholamines in the amphetamine excitatory response. *Nature* 211:540.

Sanders-Bush, E., and Sulser, F. 1970. Biochemical considerations on the mode of action of p-chloroamphetamine. In *Amphetamines and Related Compounds; Proceedings of the Mario Negri Institute for Pharmacological Research.* E. Costa and S. Garattini (eds.). New York: Raven Press, p. 865.

Thierry, A.-M.; Blanc, G.; and Glowinski, J. 1970. Preferential utilization of newly synthesized norepinephrine in the brain stem of stressed rats. *Europ. J. Pharmacol.* 10:139.

Young, D., and Scoville, W. B. 1938. Paranoid psychosis in narcolepsy and the possible danger of benzedrine treatment. *Med. Clin. N. Amer.* 22:637.

STUDIES ON THE MECHANISM OF ACTION OF

6-METHOXYTETRAHYDRO-β-CARBOLINE IN ELEVATING BRAIN SEROTONIN

Beng T. Ho, Dorothy Taylor, and William M. McIsaac

Texas Research Institute of Mental Sciences
Houston, Texas

Over many years, the involvement of biogenic amines in the mediation of depression has been substantiated. Still remaining to be answered is the question whether low brain serotonin (5-HT) or norepinephrine (NE) is specifically responsible for this abnormal state. The evidence that elevating the level of brain 5-HT alleviates depression was first presented by Coppen, Shaw, and Farrell (1963). They reported that administration of tryptophan to depressed patients potentiated the antidepressant action of a monoamine oxidase (MAO) inhibitor. Additional elaboration on this subject was presented by Glassman (1969). If resolution of the problem as to the function of these amines lies in the differential elevation of a specific amine, then it would seem desirable to have an agent that would specifically elevate only one brain amine.

During the screening of a number of our synthetic β-carbolines for their effect on brain amine levels, we discovered one compound that consistently produced a preferential rise of brain 5-HT levels over those of NE. This compound, 6-methoxy-1,2,3,4-tetrahydro-β-carboline (6-MeO-THBC) (Figure 1), when injected into mice or rats

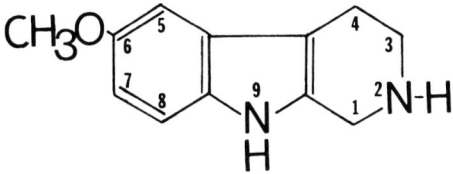

Figure 1. Structure of 6-methoxy-1,2,3,4-tetrahydro-β-carboline (6-MeO-THBC).

intraperitoneally at 50 mg/kg, gave an approximately four-fold increase in brain 5-HT, while the brain NE levels of animals were not vastly altered. This paper reports our studies on the mechanism of action of 6-MeO-THBC.

METHODS

Female Yale-Swiss mice weighing between 18 to 20 gm or male Sprague-Dawley rats weighing 180 to 220 gm were used. Unless otherwise specified, animals were injected intraperitoneally with 6-MeO-THBC in 50 percent propylene glycol or its hydrochloride salt in saline, and they were sacrificed after 2 hours. Control animals were given the vehicle only. One brain from each rat or a pool of three mouse brains was homogenized in 0.01 N HCl.

Determination of NE, 5-HT, and 5-HIAA. 5-HT and NE were extracted according to the method of Wiegland and Perry (1961). Fluorescence of 5-HT in 3 N HCl was measured at 540 nm (activation 295 nm), and that of NE was measured by the formation of trihydroxyindole as reported by Shore and Olin (1958) and read at 500 nm (activation 400 nm). In animals receiving 5-HTP (Table 1), brain 5-HT was measured by the method of Bogdanski et al. (1956). For 5-HIAA measurement, a combined fluorometric method of Gialcalone and Valzelli (1966) and Udenfriend, Weissbach, and Brodie (1958) was used.

Determination of enzyme activities. Monoamine oxidase: Brains from the animals receiving 6-MeO-THBC hydrochloride were homogenized with 10 parts of 0.25 M sucrose, and MAO activities were assayed *in vitro* using tryptamine-2-^{14}C as substrate (Ho et al. 1968).

Tryptophan pyrrolase: Livers from the starved animals were homogenized in 0.14 M KCl containing NaOH and L-tryptophan, then centrifuged to obtain a supernatant of "cell sap." Allopurinol was dissolved in 2 drops of 5N NaOH, then immediately neutralized with 6N HCl and diluted with water; 6-MeO-THBC hydrochloride was dissolved in water. The compound was added to the enzyme preparation and the enzyme activity measured by a modified method of Knox (1955).

Tryptophan hydroxylase: Brain homogenates from the animals receiving 6-MeO-THBC hydrochloride were prepared in 0.05 M phosphate buffer, pH 7.4, and were assayed *in vitro* by converting the substrate, tryptophan-^{14}C, first to 5-HTP-^{14}C, then by decarboxylation to 5-HT-^{14}C [a modified procedure of Lovenberg, Jequier, and Sjoerdsma (1967)].

5-HTP decarboxylase: Tissues from the animals receiving 6-MeO-THBC hydrochloride were homogenized in 0.05 M phosphate buffer, pH 7.4. The enzyme activity was measured using the modified procedure of Snyder and Axelrod (1964) with 5-HTP-^{14}C as substrate.

TABLE 1

Effects of 6-MeO-THBC, 5-HTP, and Pargyline on Distribution of 5-HT and NE in Discrete Areas of Rat Brain

Percentage Increase from Control

Region	6-MeO-THBC-treated		5-HTP-treated		Pargyline-treated	
	5-HT	NE	5-HT	NE	5-HT	NE
Cerebellum	1,363	13.8	736	51.7	45.5	65.5
Cortex	524	22.8	229	14.3	61.8	65.7
Pons and Medulla	286	13.8	204	- 1.7	133	84.5
Hypothalamus and Thalamus	255	- 5.4	141	-52.7	87.9	67.6
Midbrain	108	14.7	197	41.2	150	79.4
Whole Brain	429	26.5	232	0	102	109

Rats receiving pargyline (150 mg/kg) intraperitoneally in isotonic saline or D,L-5-HTP (100 mg/kg) intraperitoneally in the same vehicle were sacrificed after 2 hours and 30 minutes respectively.

Isolation of particulate and supernatant fractions from brains.
The two fractions were prepared according to a modified procedure of Giarman, Freedman, and Schanberg (1964).

Isolation of platelets. Platelet-rich plasma was obtained by centrifuging the blood at 80 x g for 20 minutes at 0° C. Separation of the platelets was then done according to the procedure of Crawford and Rudd (1962).

RESULTS AND DISCUSSION

The result of a time study showed that a maximum increase of the 5-HT level occurred two hours following intraperitoneal administration of 6-MeO-THBC to mice (Figure 2). The levels declined sharply thereafter, but a 40 percent increase above control levels was still observed eight hours after injection and the normal level was returned to normal when it was measured at twenty-four hours. In contrast to 5-HT, the levels of NE in brain were not substantially affected by 6-MeO-THBC. This was judged by the findings that, at the two-hour period when the increase of 5-HT was about 290 percent above the controls, there was no increase of NE.

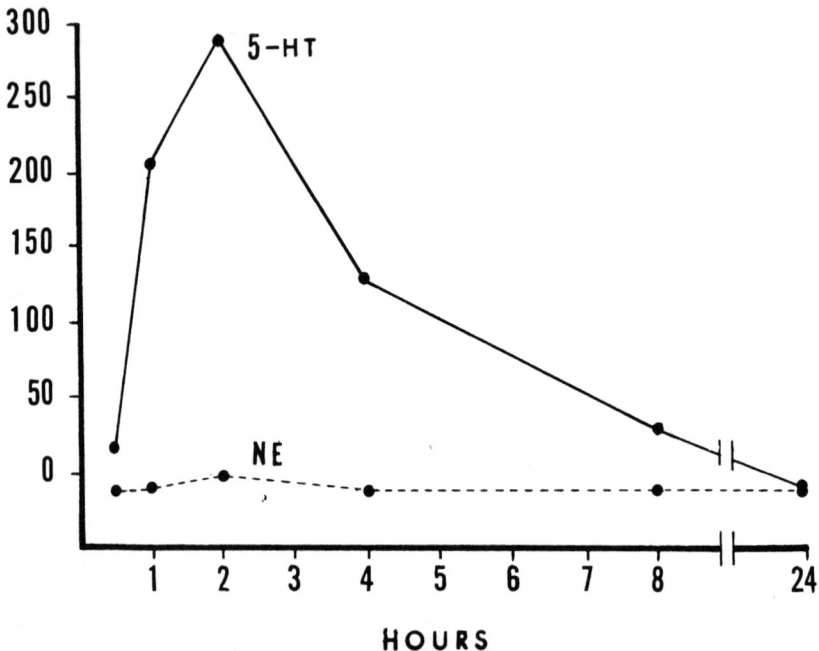

Figure 2. Effect of intraperitoneal administration of 6-MeO-THBC on the levels of 5-HT and NE in mouse brain. Nine animals were used at each time interval.

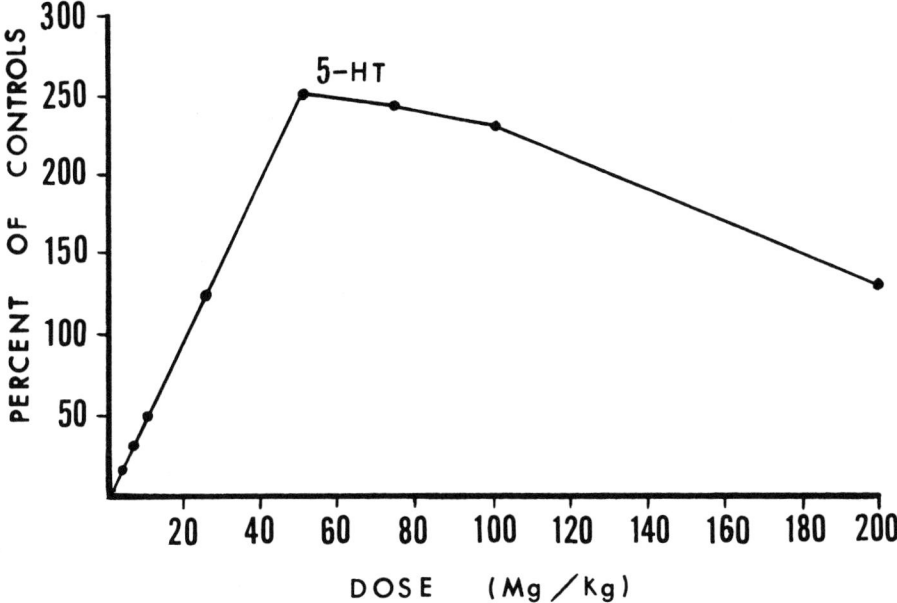

Figure 3. Effect of increasing intraperitoneal doses of 6-MeO-THBC on the levels of 5-HT in mouse brain.

The dose-response curve for 6-MeO-THBC showed a linear relationship in the increase of 5-HT up to 50 mg/kg (Figure 3). The effect became less pronounced as the dose was increased beyond 50 mg/kg and at 200 mg/kg, which was very close to the LD_{50} (230 mg/kg), the compound exerted only one-half of the effect observed with 50 mg/kg.

The effects of 6-MeO-THBC on the regional distribution of 5-HT and NE in rat brains were determined after an intraperitoneal injection of 50 mg/kg of the compound (Table 1). While the levels of norepinephrine in various regions of the brain were relatively unaffected, 6-MeO-THBC caused substantial increases of serotonin in all the discrete areas measured, the largest percentage increases being found in the cerebellum and cortex. The pattern of serotonin elevation in different regions closely resembled that observed when 100 mg/kg of 5-hydroxytryptophan (5-HTP) was administered intraperitoneally, but was dissimilar to that observed with 150 mg/kg of pargyline, a monoamine oxidase inhibitor. Pargyline caused moderate increases in both serotonin and norepinephrine levels in all the regions studied, and the largest percentage increases in serotonin were not in the cerebellum and cortex.

In studying the effects of 5-HT on subcellular distribution in mouse brain, 6-MeO-THBC was compared with pargyline (Table 2). The latter increased the amount of 5-HT in the particulate fraction or the "bound" 5-HT, but had little effect on the supernatant 5-HT. The action of 6-MeO-THBC in elevating brain 5-HT was predominantly on the particulate fraction, and a 682 percent increase from the controls was actually observed. The compound, however, was found to cause a 58 percent decrease of "free" 5-HT in the supernatant. The results obtained with 6-MeO-THBC were quite similar to those reported by Giarman et al. (1964) when 5-HT was injected intraperitoneally into rats and the amine level in brains was measured after 10 minutes.

Either preventing the metabolism of serotonin or enhancing its biosynthesis could cause the increase of the amine in brain (Figure 4). Our studies on the mechanism of action of 6-MeO-THBC were then directed toward these possibilities.

No significant change in the activity of monoamine oxidase was observed in mice treated with 6-MeO-THBC (Table 3). This was in agreement with our previous *in vitro* finding that the β-carboline was only a very weak inhibitor of the enzyme (Ho et al. 1958). Further supporting data were obtained by measuring brain 5-hydroxy-

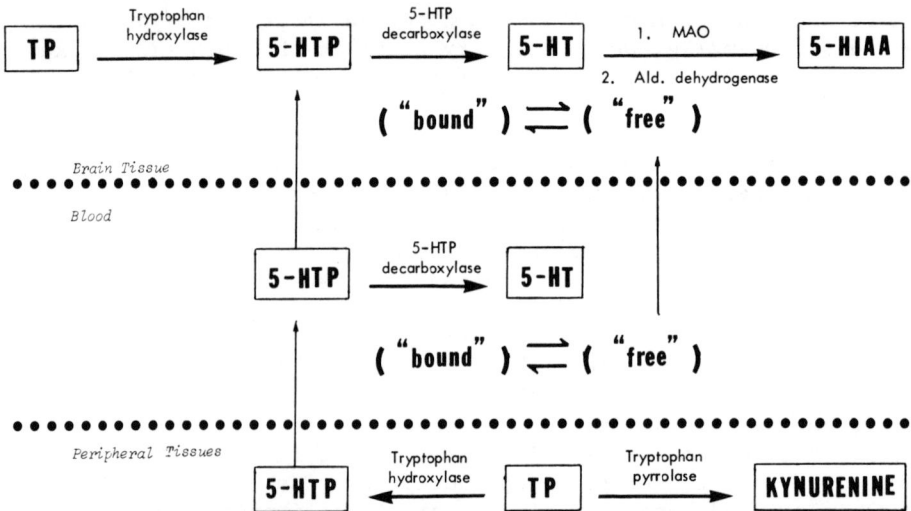

Figure 4. Synthesis and disposition of 5-HT and precursors. Proposed mechanism of the elevation of brain 5-HT by 6-MeO-THBC.

TABLE 2

Effect of 6-MeO-THBC and Pargyline on Subcellular
Distribution of 5-HT in Mouse Brain

Treatment	5-HT (µg/gm brain)*			Percentage Change from Controls	
	Total	Particulate	Supernatant	Particulate	Supernatant
Controls (50% propylene glycol)	0.89 ± 0.01	0.61 ± 0.00	0.28 ± 0.01		
6-MeO-THBC (50 mg/kg)	4.86 ± 0.07	4.74 ± 0.07	0.12 ± 0.00	682	-58
Controls (saline)	0.86 ± 0.03	0.58 ± 0.04	0.28 ± 0.02		
Pargyline (150 mg/kg)	1.19 ± 0.02	0.95 ± 0.01	0.24 ± 0.01	65	-14

*Each value in the control groups represents the mean of 12 animals; the value in the experimental group is the mean of 18 animals.

TABLE 3

Effect of 6-MeO-THBC on Mouse Brain
Monoamine Oxidase (MAO) Activity

Treatment		MAO Activity (mµmoles/mg protein/hr*)
Saline Controls		49.2
6-MeO-THBC	10 mg/kg	51.4
	25 mg/kg	48.2
	50 mg/kg	46.8
	100 mg/kg	51.9

*Each value represents the mean of 2 assays.

indoleacetic acid (5-HIAA), a metabolite of 5-HT, in animals treated with 6-MeO-THBC. The observed increase, rather than decrease, in 5-HIAA levels indicated the lack of inhibition of the enzyme (Figure 5).

After the finding that the increase in brain 5-HT was not related to MAO activity, two alternative explanations remained. First, this increase in 5-HT could be due to activation of enzyme systems involved in the biosynthesis of 5-HT, such as the tryptophan hydroxylase and/or 5-HTP decarboxylase, and second, it could result from inhibition of tryptophan pyrrolase, which would then cause an increase in the catabolism of tryptophan via the 5-HT pathway (Figure 4).

At a concentration three times higher than that of the known inhibitor, allopurinol, 6-MeO-THBC caused only a slight change in the *in vitro* activity of tryptophan pyrrolase of rat liver (Table 4).

No significant change of tryptophan hydroxylase of rat brains was observed in animals treated with 6-MeO-THBC (Table 5). No evidence of activation of brain tryptophan hydroxylase by 6-MeO-THBC could be found.

5-HTP decarboxylase activities were determined in the rat brain,

TABLE 4

In vitro Effect of 6-MeO-THBC and Allopurinol
on Rat Liver Tryptophan Pyrrolase

Compound	Enzyme activity (μmole kynurenine/gm liver/hr ± S.E.*)	Percentage Diff. from Control
Controls	442.2 ± 4.2	--
Allopurinol 0.36 mM	196.5 ± 2.1	-55.6
6-MeO-THBC 1.0 mM 0.05 mM 0.005 mM	506.3 ± 16.3 434.0 ± 3.7 434.0 ± 6.1	+14.5 - 1.8 - 1.8

*Each value represents the mean of 6 assays.

TABLE 5

Effect of 6-MeO-THBC (50 mg/kg) on
Rat Brain Tryptophan Hydroxylase

Injection	Enzyme Activity (mμmole 5-HT/mg protein/hr*)	Percentage Diff. from Control
Saline	0.123	--
6-MeO-THBC	0.107	-13.0

*Each value represents the average of 2 assays.

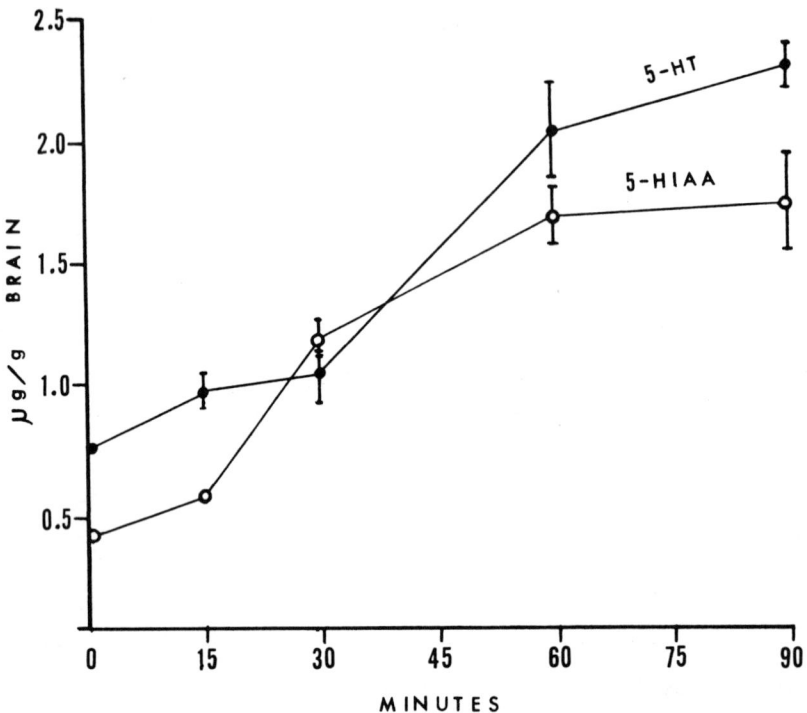

Figure 5. Levels of 5-HT and 5-HIAA in mouse brain after 6-MeO-THBC.

liver, kidney, and plasma at various time intervals after administration of 6-MeO-THBC (Table 6). A general increase in enzyme activity appeared at 30 minutes in the four tissues studied, but the increase in activity in plasma (176 percent) was much greater than that in the other three tissues (less than 40 percent).

Corresponding to the activation of 5-HTP decarboxylase in plasma and liver, there were large increases in 5-HT levels in the two tissues (Table 7). The levels of 5-HT in the platelets, however, were decreased. A parallel change of 5-HT levels in both brain and plasma was demonstrated at all time intervals, and their peak levels coincided at two hours (Figure 6). A linear relationship exists between the increase of 5-HT in brain and that in plasma, with a correction coefficient of 0.989 ($p < 0.01$) (Figure 7).

These results seem to suggest that the specific action of 6-MeO-THBC on brain 5-HT did not originate centrally but, rather, that it was mediated through an increased concentration of the amine in plasma. The accumulation of 5-HT in the plasma was apparently caused by acti-

TABLE 6

Effects of 6-MeO-THBC on 5-HTP Decarboxylase
in Various Rat Tissues

Tissue	Treatment		Enzyme Activity (mµmole 5-HT-^{14}C/gm tissue or ml plasma ± S.E.*)		Percentage Diff. from Control
Plasma	Saline controls		0.323	± 0.012	--
	6-MeO-THBC	30 min	0.847	± 0.078	+176
		1 hr	0.618	± 0.034	+ 91
		2 hr	0.551	± 0.065	+ 71
Brain	Saline controls		148.8	± 1.7	--
	6-MeO-THBC	30 min	193.5	± 4.9	+ 30
		1 hr	141.3	± 1.9	- 5
		2 hr	143.3	± 9.5	- 4
Liver	Saline controls	30 min	3,035	± 32	--
		2 hr	3,218	± 25	--
	6-MeO-THBC	30 min	3,580	± 18	+ 18
		2 hr	4,080	± 17	+ 27
Kidney	Saline controls	30 min	1,980	± 68	--
		2 hr	2,186	± 94	--
	6-MeO-THBC	30 min	2,688	± 102	+ 36
		2 hr	2,866	± 76	+ 36

*Each value represents the mean of 6 assays.

TABLE 7

Effect of 6-MeO-THBC on 5-HT Levels
in Rat Liver, Plasma, and Platelets

Tissue	Treatment	5-HT Level (µg/gm or ml S.E.†)	Percentage Diff. from Control
Liver*	Saline controls	0.40 ± 0	--
	6-MeO-THBC 2 hr	2.85 ± 0.28	+ 612
Platelets	Saline controls	0.35 ± 0	--
	6-MeO-THBC 1 hr	0.12 ± 0.01	- 66
	2 hr	0.29 ± 0.02	- 17
Plasma (platelet-rich)	Saline controls	0.37 ± 0.03	--
	6-MeO-THBC 30 min	0.78 ± 0	+ 105
	1 hr	1.13 ± 0.06	+ 205
	2 hr	1.59 ± 0.03	+ 330
	4 hr	1.32 ± 0.08	+ 257
Plasma (platelet-free)	Saline controls	0.02§	--
	6-MeO-THBC 1 hr	1.01§	+ 495
	2 hr	1.30§	+6400

*Liver homogenates were prepared in 0.01 N HCl.
†Each value represents the mean of 6 assays.
§Values obtained from the differences in 5-HT levels between platelet-rich plasma and platelets.

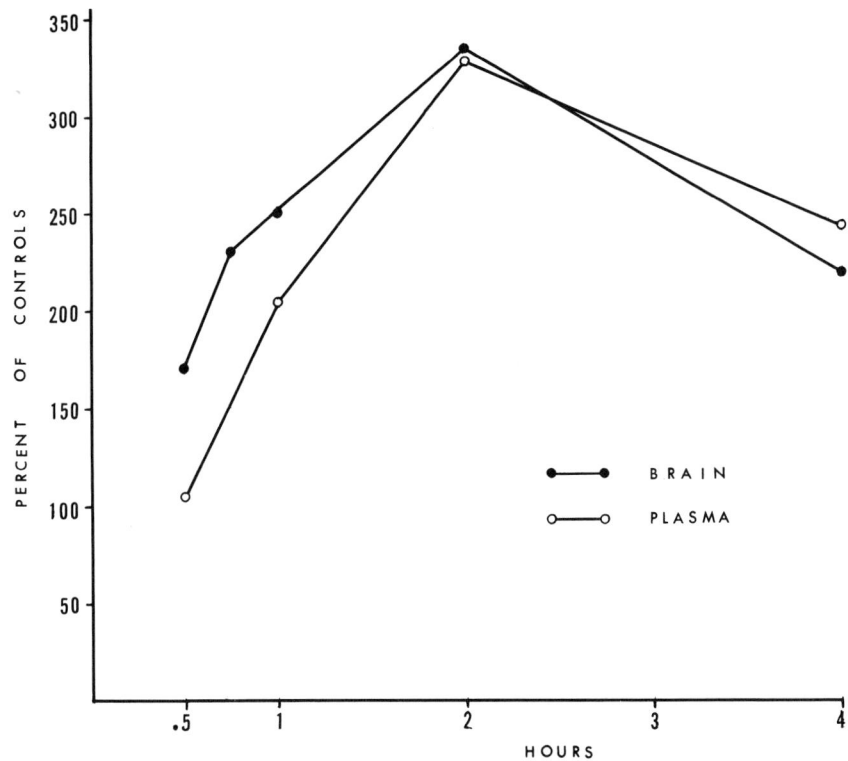

Figure 6. Effect of 6-MeO-THBC on the levels of 5-HT in rat brain and plasma.

vation of the 5-HTP decarboxylase as well as inhibition of 5-HT uptake in platelets by 6-MeO-THBC (Table 7).

If, under a special condition, the free serotonin in plasma were to increase to a sufficiently high level to cause a concentration gradient from blood to brain tissue, then influx into the CNS might occur. A great deal of controversy has arisen regarding the passage of 5-HT into the brain, and further evidence for this evaluation is required. Since our data thus far have not confirmed the origin of a central effect, elevation of the peripheral 5-HT and that in the CNS could still occur as the result of two entirely separate mechanisms.

To substantiate the postulation that the increase of brain 5-HT levels was not caused by a direct action of 6-MeO-THBC in the brain, 50 µg of the compound were injected intracerebrally into rats. If the compound in the brain was responsible for the increase of brain 5-HT, an elevation of the amine in the brain could be expected. The re-

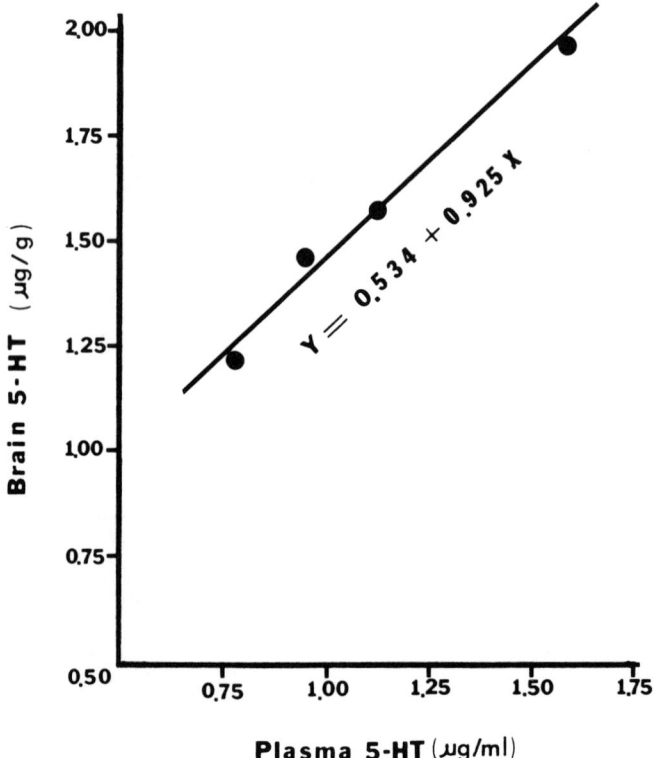

Figure 7. Linear relationship between increase of 5-HT in brain and plasma.

sults (Table 8) show that only minor changes in brain serotonin levels occurred in the animals receiving 6-MeO-THBC intracerebrally, as compared to a 336 percent increase at 2 hours when 50 mg/kg of the compound was injected intraperitoneally.

TABLE 8

Effect of Intracerebral Injection of 6-MeO-THBC
on Levels of 5-HT in Mouse Brain

Treatment	5-HT Level* (µg/gm brain)	Percentage Diff. from Controls
Saline controls	0.70	--
6-MeO-THBC 5 min 15 min 30 min	0.79 0.67 0.50	+13 - 4 -28

Animals were injected intracerebrally with 50 µg/animal of 6-MeO-THBC hydrochloride in 10 µl of saline. Control animals were injected with 10 µl of saline only. *Each value represents the mean of 2 assays.

ADDENDUM

Since the presentation of this paper, we have measured the levels of 5-HT in mouse and rat brain under the effect of 6-MeO-THBC by the o-phthaldehyde method (Curzon and Green 1970), and we have found the percentages of elevation of 5-HT to be less than those observed with the method described above. The percentages are: rat--50 mg/kg 6-MeO-THBC, 88 percent above controls; mouse--50 mg/kg, 40 percent; 100 mg/kg, 83 percent; 200 mg/kg, 135 percent above controls.

Rats were injected with tritiated 6-MeO-THBC. Following extraction of the brain for 5-HT, the aqueous phase was chromatographed on a thin layer plate. The area corresponding to the Rf value of 5-HT was found to contain no radioactivity, indicating that the elevated brain 5-HT in animals was not derived from 6-MeO-THBC by a possible demethylation and ring opening at carbon-1 of the piperidine ring.

ACKNOWLEDGMENTS

This study was supported in part by U. S. Public Health grant MH-11168. The authors wish to thank Mrs. Kay Hollenbeck and Mrs. Annie Rougeaux for their technical assistance.

REFERENCES

Bogdanski, D. F.; Pletscher, A.; Brodie, B. B.; and Udenfriend, S. 1956. The estimation of 5-hydroxytryptamine in biological tissue. *J. Pharmacol. Exp. Ther.* 117:82.

Bulat, M., and Supek, Z. 1967. The penetration of 5-hydroxytryptamine through the blood-brain barrier. *J. Neurochem.* 14:265.

Coppen, A.; Shaw, D. M.; and Farrell, J. D. 1963. Potentiation of the antidepressive effect of a monoamine oxidase inhibitor by tryptophan. *Lancet* 1:79.

Curzon, G., and Green, A. R. 1970. Rapid method for the determination of 5-hydroxytryptamine and 5-hydroxyindoleacetic acid in small regions of rat brain. *Brit. J. Pharmacol.* 39:653.

Crawford, N., and Rudd, B. T. 1962. A spectrophotofluorimetric method for the determination of serotonin in plasma. *Clin. Chim. Acta* 7:14.

Giacalone, E., and Valzelli, L. 1966. A method for the determination of 5-hydroxyindoleacetic acid in brain. *J. Neurochem.* 13:1265.

Giarman, N. J.; Freedman, D. X.; and Schanberg, S. M. 1964. In *Progress in Brain Research*, vol. 8. H. E. Himwich and W. A. Himwich (eds.). New York: Elsevier Publishing Co., p. 72.

Glassman, A. 1969. Indoleamines and affective disorders. *Psychosom. Med.* 31:107.

Ho, B. T.; McIsaac, W. M.; Walker, K. E.; and Estevez, V. 1968. Inhibitors of monoamine oxidase-influence of methyl substitution on the inhibitory activity of β-carbolines. *J. Pharm. Sci.* 57:269.

Knox, W. E. 1955. Tryptophan oxidation. In *Methods in Enzymology*, vol. 11. S. P. Colowick and N. O. Kaplan (eds.). New York: Academic Press, p. 242.

Lovenberg, W.; Jequier, E.; and Sjoerdsma, A. 1967. Tryptophan hydroxylation: Measurement in pineal gland, brainstem, and carcinoid tumor. *Science* 155:217.

Shore, P. A., and Olin, J. S. 1958. Identification and chemical assay of norepinephrine in brain and other tissues. *J. Pharmacol. Exp. Ther.* 122:295.

Snyder, S., and Axelrod, J. 1964. A sensitive assay for 5-hydroxytryptophan decarboxylase. *Biochem. Pharmacol.* 13:805.

Udenfriend, S.; Weissbach, H.; and Brodie, B. B. 1958. Assay of serotonin and related metabolites, enzymes and drugs. *Meth. Biochem. Anal.* 6:95.

Wiegland, R. G., and Perry, J. E. 1961. Effect of L-Dopa and N-methyl-N-benzyl-2-propynylamine HCl on Dopa, dopamine, norepinephrine, epinephrine and serotonin levels in mouse brain. *Biochem. Pharmacol.* 7:181.

COMPARISON OF THE EFFECTS OF ELECTRICAL STIMULATION AND

IONTOPHORETIC DOPAMINE ON NEURONS OF THE NIGRO-NEOSTRIATAL PATHWAY

John D. Connor

The Milton S. Hershey Medical Center of the Pennsylvania State University

Hershey, Pennsylvania

The dense neuropil of the caudate nucleus is notable for its content of neurohumoral substances thought to be important in synaptic transmission. High concentrations of acetylcholine (MacIntosh 1941) and the enzymes required for its synthesis (Feldberg and Vogt 1948; Hebb and Silver 1956) and catabolism (Burgen and Chipman 1951) are found in this structure. The unusually large concentration of dopamine in the caudate and other basal ganglia prompted the initial suggestion that dopamine may have a physiologic function other than as a precursor for norepinephrine in some brain areas (Carlsson, Lindqvist, and Magnusson 1957). In addition, there are also relatively large concentrations of serotonin (Bogdanski, Weissbach, and Udenfriend 1957) and gamma-amino butyric acid (Baxter and Roberts 1960), and lower levels of norepinephrine (Vogt 1954) and histamine (McGeer 1964).

The cytological distributions of cholinesterase (Shute and Lewis 1963) and dopamine (Andén et al. 1964) suggest that cholinergic and dopaminergic synapses may be operative where afferent inputs from other brain areas interact with caudate neurons. The symptoms of Parkinsonism are accompanied by a striking reduction in dopamine concentrations in the basal ganglia (Hornykiewicz 1966). Similarly, motor dysfunctions can be produced in animals by surgical procedures (Poirier and Sourkes 1965) or systemically administered compounds that markedly reduce caudate dopamine concentrations (Bertler and Rosengren 1959). These observations have served to emphasize the importance of the dopaminergic input. Changes in serotonin concentrations in basal ganglia may also be intimately involved in certain motor aberrations (Sourkes and Poirier 1965). The physiological significance of the cholinergic component is

TABLE 1

Cholinergic Agents that Elicit Tremor when
Injected into the Caudate (5 µl volumes)

	N	Dose[a] (µg)	Mean Duration (min)	Mean Tremor Time[b] (%)
Carbachol	36	7	150	76
Bethanechol	6	30	120	60
Methacholine	6	100	90	52
Acetylcholine	12	400	60	48
Oxotremorine	6	15	80	43
Arecoline	6	100	95	53
Physostigmine	6	75	60	44

[a] Quantity required for a tremor duration of one hour or more.
[b] Percentage of time spent in tremor episodes during maximal response.

more obscure. Hypotheses have been advanced, however, suggesting that caudate function, especially with regard to its participation in motor activities, may be dependent upon a critical balance of appropriate cholinergic and dopaminergic inputs (Barbeau 1962; Duvoisin 1967; Baker et al. 1969).

TREMOR AND INTRACAUDATE INJECTIONS

Several years ago my colleagues and I studied the consequences of upsetting the striatal acetylcholine-dopamine balance in unanesthetized cats prepared with chronic indwelling cannulae in their caudate nuclei. Recordings were made from an elevated hind-foot by means of a phonocartridge transducer. Intracaudate injections of acetylcholine produced conspicuous tremor of the head and limbs. Large, "pharmacologic" amounts of acetylcholine were required unless the caudates were pretreated with a cholinesterase inhibitor. However, carbachol, a cholinergic compound resistant to enzymatic hydrolysis, evoked reproducible episodes of tremor and limb rigidity when a few micrograms were injected into one caudate (Connor, Rossi, and Baker 1966a). The tremors had a frequency of about 20 Hz and a duration of about two and one-half hours. When a series of agents possessing cholinergic properties was administered, only those

compounds with muscarinic actions in the periphery (Table 1) were
effective in eliciting the motor response (Connor, Rossi, and Baker
1966b). In addition, intracaudate injections of small quantities
of anticholinergics with muscarinic blocking activity were effective
antagonists of carbachol tremor. Injections of the same amounts of
the tremorogens into the cerebral ventricles were ineffective.

Dopamine injected into the caudate during the peak of carbachol-
induced tremor rapidly suppressed the limb movements (Connor, Rossi,
and Baker 1967). The dopamine effect was reversible with time, and
tremor returned after thirty to forty minutes. Systemic pretreatment
with a monoamine oxidase inhibitor reduced the quantity of dopamine
required to antagonize the tremor and increased the duration of
dopamine effects. These chemical modifications of motor behavior
presumably involved a large population of caudate neurons.

SINGLE CAUDATE NEURON STUDIES

The effects of acetylcholine and dopamine on individual caudate
neurons have been reported by several research groups (Bloom, Costa,
and Salmoiraghi 1965; McLennan and York 1966 and 1967; Herz and
Zieglgängsberger 1966) using the technique of microiontophoresis
(microelectrophoresis). A consistent observation was that dopamine
depressed both spontaneous and/or glutamate-induced firing of responsive cells, while acetylcholine excited most spontaneously active
units to increase their firing rates.

Histofluorescence studies (Andén *et al*. 1964) indicated that
there is a close anatomical relationship between neurons of the
neostriatum (caudate and putamen) and the pars compacta of the substantia nigra. Caudate dopamine apparently occurs in fine fiber
terminals that arise from fluorescent cell bodies in the ipsilateral
nigra. The course of these uncrossed "nigroneostriatal" fibers has
been mapped by surgical intervention (Andén *et al*. 1966). Appropriate electrical stimulation of the nigra should, therefore, evoke
responses among the neurons in the ipsilateral caudate. In the last
few years, a number of research groups have reported that nigral
stimulation elicits changes in the response patterns of individual
caudate cells (Frigyesi and Purpura 1967; McLennan and York 1967;
Albe-Fessard, Raieva, and Santiago 1967; Connor 1968; Feltz and
MacKenzie 1969). The experimental conditions in these studies varied
widely, and the data were such that it is difficult to ascertain to
what extent the proposed dopaminergic pathway actually mediated the
responses.

Since neurophysiologic techniques alone seemed to yield indeci-
sive results about the specificity of the responses, a combination
of nigral stimulation and multi-barrel (iontophoretic) electrodes
was employed. Specifically, the effects produced by iontophoretic

dopamine on caudate unit firing patterns were compared to the responses of the same neuron to nigral stimuli. The working hypothesis was that electrophoretic ejection of a suspected neurotransmitter near a receptive neuron should mimic the qualitative changes in that neuron's firing pattern elicited by release of the endogenous transmitter from an afferent pathway.

Adult cats were electrolytically decerebrated and prepared for stimulation and recording by techniques described previously (Salmoiraghi and Weight 1967; Connor 1970). The nigral stimuli consisted of short trains of 10-millisecond duration, 4 pulses per train and 4 to 6 V intensity, delivered at intervals of 1.3 seconds. The effects of nigral stimuli on unit firing patterns were monitored on an oscilloscope, summed with an online computer, and read out in analog form. The responses of neurons to iontophoretically administered compounds were determined using a rate meter and polygraph system (Salmoiraghi and Weight 1967).

Few spontaneously active cells were encountered, and most recordings were obtained from neurons made to fire by iontophoretic release of d,l-homocysteic acid, an excitant amino acid. The four types of caudate unit firing patterns obtained during nigral stimulation are illustrated in Figure 1. Histograms A and B (from two different caudate cells) illustrate poststimulus firing rate depression, either simple (as in A) or complex (as in B, where the depressed period is followed by a late facilitatory episode). Histogram C was obtained from another caudate cell that was facilitated by nigral stimulation. Histogram D was obtained from a caudate unit not responding to stimulation. The incidence, latencies, and durations of these responses are given in Table 2.

The specificity of the sites of stimulation and recording was also studied. Electrical stimulation of the mesencephalic areas surrounding the nigra did not alter caudate neuronal firing patterns. Furthermore, neurons at sites other than the head of the ipsilateral caudate were either unaffected by nigral stimulation (as in the cortex) or exhibited discharge pattern changes distinctly different from those in the caudate (as in the lenticular and amygdaloid areas).

Dopamine was applied by iontophoresis near 110 caudate neurons whose responses to nigral stimulation had been determined from poststimulus histograms. The results are given in Table 3. Correlation between the effects of stimulation and iontophoretic dopamine was strongest for caudate neurons whose firing was depressed by both procedures. The absence of dopamine facilitation among neurons depressed by nigral stimuli was significantly different ($p=0.03$, Fisher Exact Probability Test; Siegel 1956) from the degree of dopamine facilitation noted in the stimulus-nonresponsive group.

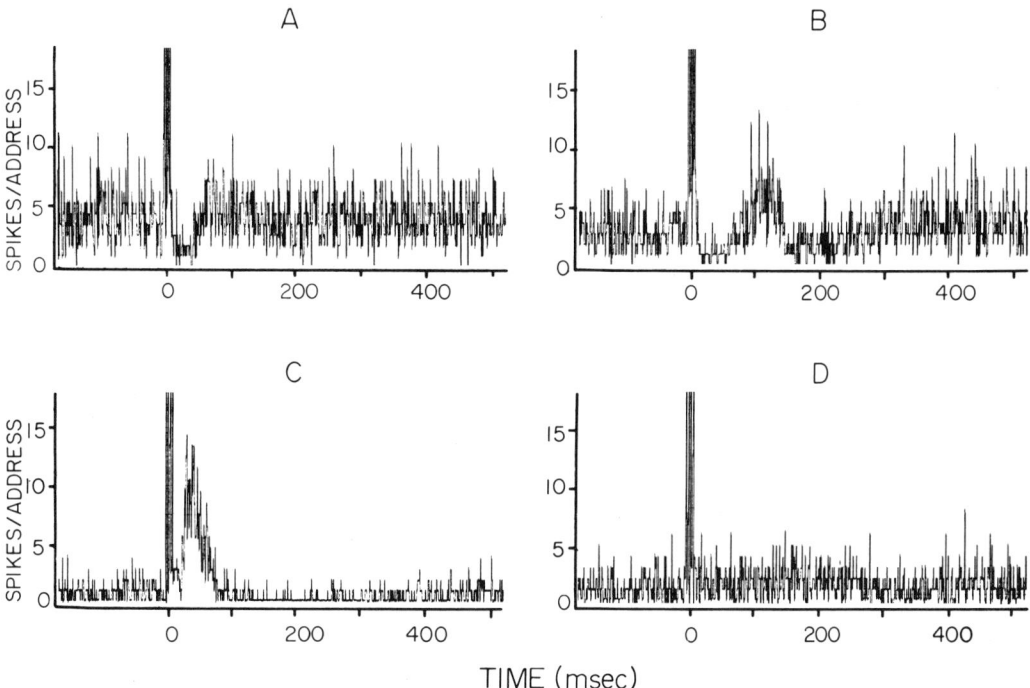

Figure 1. Types of caudate neuron action potential patterns obtained during nigral stimulation. Histograms A and B are summations of 200 stimuli; C and D, 150 stimuli. Abscissa: time after the stimulus artifact (arbitrarily labeled time zero). Ordinate: number of neuronal spikes deposited in each computer address (1-msec width). A is an example of histogram from neuron with simple poststimulus firing rate depression. B is a record of a complex response, i.e., depression followed by later facilitation. C indicates presence of simple poststimulus firing rate facilitation. Histogram D was obtained from a neuron apparently not responding to nigral stimuli.

Furthermore, continuous iontophoretic ejection of alpha-methyldopamine, a false transmitter at peripheral neuroeffector sites (Theonen et al. 1967), blocked the depressant effects of nigral stimulation and also the depressant action of dopamine. These effects are illustrated by the histograms and integrated spike rate in Figure 2.

Iontophoretic application of acetylcholine facilitated the firing of a third of the thirty-six caudate cells tested. Five units facilitated by acetylcholine were depressed by dopamine, but three were facilitated by both compounds and the remaining four cells did not respond to dopamine ejections. From this small sample there

TABLE 2

Effects of Substantia Nigra Stimulation
on Caudate Neuronal Firing Rates

	Caudate Neurons	Mean Response Latency (msec)	Mean Response Duration (msec)
Depression (simple)	64	18	59
Depression (complex)	57	17	66
Facilitation	42	14	58
No Change	97	--	--

TABLE 3

Correlation of Responses of Caudate Neurons to
Iontophoretic Dopamine and to Nigral Stimulation

Effects of Nigral Stimulation	Effects of Dopamine		
	Depression	Facilitation	No Change
Depression	31	0	9
Facilitation	3	7	5
No Change	34	6	15

does not appear to be any strong tendency for divergent or convergent effects of acetylcholine and dopamine demonstrable by the methods used. It would be difficult, however, to compare quantitatively the responses of a caudate neuron to acetylcholine and dopamine in a preparation in which an intact, largely depressant, nigral pathway may be tonically active. Kittens might serve as useful test animals for an investigation of cholinergic facilitatory mechanisms, since the caudate nuclei of newborn cats have very low concentrations of dopamine (Connor and Neff 1970), while cholinergic mechanisms are apparently functional at an early developmental stage (Kling, Finer, and Gilmour 1969).

SUMMARY

Cholinergic agents injected into the caudate nucleus of cats elicited tremor and rigidity that were suppressed by similar injections of dopamine. These observations strengthen the contention

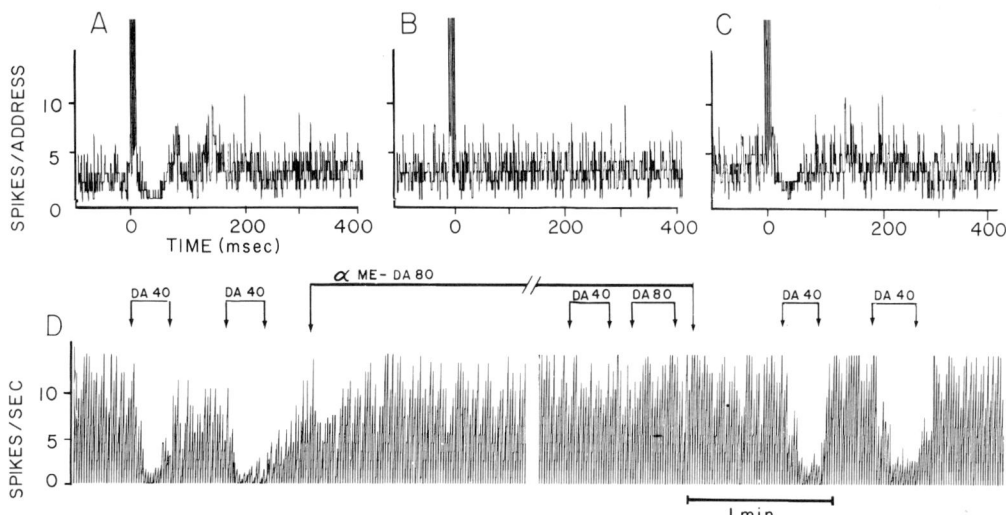

Figure 2. Blocking actions of iontophoretic alpha-methyldopamine (α-ME-DA) on the depressant effects of nigral stimulation and iontophoretic dopamine. All records from the same caudate neuron. Histogram A obtained before alpha-methyldopamine administration shows typical poststimulus firing pattern depression. This depressant effect is blocked in B which was begun after 6-minute continuous application of alpha-methyldopamine. Histogram C was begun 2 minutes after termination of alpha-methyldopamine; poststimulus depression recurs. D is the integrated spike rate running continuously from left to right. A 1.5-minute section was removed as indicated by a break in the record. Iontophoretic dopamine (DA), ejected with 40 nanoAmps of current, causes decreased firing. During alpha-methyldopamine (α-ME-DA) administration (80 nanoAmps for 4 minutes), neither 40- nor 80-nanoAmps ejections of dopamine depress neuronal spiking. After alpha-methyldopamine is turned off dopamine sensitivity returns.

that cholinergic and dopaminergic mechanisms in the caudate are critically balanced for normal motor functioning.

At the neuronal level, positive correlation was obtained between the effects of iontophoretic dopamine and nigral stimulation, especially for units depressed by both procedures. From these data it is not possible to eliminate the participation of a polysynaptic pathway originating in the nigra and influencing caudate neurons by presynaptic modulation of dopamine release. The pharmacologic correlations, however, seem to indicate that dopaminergic mechanisms are intimately involved in the depressant responses evoked by nigral stimuli. The unit responses obtained in this study, when considered in conjunction with previous biochemical and histochemical observations, support the concept that caudate neurons receive a dopaminergic input from the substantia nigra.

ACKNOWLEDGMENT

This work was supported in part by Grant NS 08884-01, National Institute of Neurologic Diseases and Stroke, United States Public Health Service. Some of the results originally published in the *Journal of Physiology* are reproduced with permission of the Physiological Society.

REFERENCES

Albe-Fessard, D.; Raieva, S.; and Santiago, W. 1967. Sur les rélations entre substance noire et noyou caudé. *J. Physiol. (Paris)* 59:324.

Andén, N. E.; Carlsson, A.; Dahlström, A.; Fuxe, K.; Hillarp, N. Å.; and Larsson, K. 1964. Demonstration and mapping out of nigro-neostriatal dopamine neurons. *Life Sci.* 3:523.

Andén, N. E.; Dahlström, A.; Fuxe, K.; Larsson, K.; Olson, L.; and Ungerstedt, U. 1966. Ascending monoamine neurons to the telencephalon and diencephalon. *Acta Physiol. Scand.* 67:313.

Baker, W. W.; Connor, J. D.; Rossi, G. V.; and Lalley, P. M. 1969. Production of tremor by intracaudate cholinergic agents and its suppression by locally administered catecholamines. In *Progress in Neuro-Genetics*, vol. 1. A. Barbeau and J. R. Brunette (eds.). Amsterdam: Excerpta Medica Foundation, p. 390.

Barbeau, A. 1962. The pathogenesis of Parkinson's disease: A new hypothesis. *Canad. Med. Assoc. J.* 87:802.

Baxter, C. F., and Roberts, E. 1960. Demonstration of thiosemicarbazide-induced convulsions in rats with elevated brain levels of gamma-aminobutyric acid. *Proc. Soc. Exp. Biol. Med.* 104:426.

Bertler, Å., and Rosengren, E. 1959. Occurrence and distribution of dopamine in brain and other tissues. *Experientia* 15:10.

Bloom, F. E.; Costa, E.; and Salmoiraghi, G. C. 1965. Anesthesia and the responsiveness of individual neurons of the caudate nucleus of the cat to acetylcholine, norepinephine and dopamine administered by microelectrophoresis. *J. Pharmacol. Exp. Ther.* 159:244.

Bogdanski, D. F.; Weissbach, H.; and Udenfriend, S. 1957. The distribution of serotonin, 5-hydroxytryptophan decarboxylase, and monoamine oxidase in brain. *J. Neurochem.* 1:272.

Burgen, A. S. V., and Chipman, L. M. 1951. Cholinesterase and succinic dehydrogenase in the central nervous system of the dog. *J. Physiol. (London)* 114:296.

Carlsson, A.; Lindqvist, M.; and Magnusson, T. 1957. 3,4-Dihydroxyphenylalanine and 5-hydroxytryptophan as reserpine antagonists. *Nature* 180:1200.

Connor, J. D. 1968. Caudate unit responses to nigral stimuli: Evidence for a possible nigro-neostriatal pathway. *Science* 160:899.
Connor, J. D. 1970. Caudate nucleus neurones: Correlation of the effects of substantia nigra stimulation with iontophoretic dopamine. *J. Physiol. (London)* 208:691.
Connor, J. D., and Neff, N. H. 1970. Dopamine concentrations in the caudate nucleus of the developing cat. *Life Sci.* 9(I):1165.
Connor, J. D.; Rossi, G. V.; and Baker, W. W. 1966a. Characteristics of tremor in cats following carbachol injections into the caudate nucleus. *Exp. Neurol.* 14:371.
Connor, J. D.; Rossi, G. V.; and Baker, W. W. 1966b. Analysis of the tremor induced by injection of cholinergic agents into the caudate nucleus. *Int. J. Neuropharmacol.* 5:207.
Connor, J. D.; Rossi, G. V.; and Baker, W. W. 1967. Antagonism of intra-caudate carbachol tremor by local injections of catecholamines. *J. Pharmacol. Exp. Ther.* 155:545.
Duvoisin, R. C. 1967. Cholinergic-anticholinergic antagonism in Parkinsonism. *Arch. Neurol.* 17:124.
Feldberg, W., and Vogt, M. 1948. Acetylcholine synthesis in different regions of the central nervous system. *J. Physiol. (London)* 107:372.
Feltz, P., and MacKenzie, J. S. 1969. Properties of caudate unitary responses to repetitive nigral stimulation. *Brain Res.* 13:612.
Frigyesi, T. L., and Purpura, D. P. 1967. Electrophysiological analysis of reciprocal caudate-nigral relations. *Brain Res.* 6:440.
Hebb, C. O., and Silver, A. 1956. Choline acetylase in the central nervous system of man and some other mammals. *J. Physiol. (London)* 134:718.
Herz, A., and Zieglgängsberger, W. 1966. Synaptic excitation in the corpus striatum inhibited by microelectrophoretically administered dopamine. *Experienta* 22:839.
Hornykiewicz, O. 1966. Dopamine (3-hydroxytyramine) and brain function. *Pharmacol. Rev.* 18:925.
Kling, A.; Finer, S.; and Gilmour, J. 1969. Regional development of acetylcholinesterase activity in the maternally reared and maternally deprived cat. *Int. J. Neuropharmacol.* 8:25.
MacIntosh, F. C. 1941. The distribution of acetylcholine in the peripheral and the central nervous system. *J. Physiol. (London)* 99:436.
McGeer, P. L. 1964. The distribution of histamine in cat and human brain. In *Comparative Neurochemistry*. D. Richter (ed.). London: Pergamon Press, p. 387.
McLennan, H., and York, D. H. 1966. Cholinergic mechanisms in the caudate nucleus. *J. Physiol. (London)* 187:163.
McLennan, H., and York, D. H. 1967. The action of dopamine on neurones of the caudate nucleus. *J. Physiol. (London)* 189:393.

Poirier, L. J., and Sourkes, T. L. 1965. Influence of the substantia nigra on the catecholamine content of the striatum. *Brain* 88:181.

Salmoiraghi, G. C., and Weight, F. 1967. Micromethods in neuropharmacology: An approach to the study of anesthetics. *Anesthesiology* 28:54.

Shute, C. C. D., and Lewis, P. R. 1963. Cholinesterase-containing systems of the brain of the rat. *Nature* 199:1160.

Siegel, S. 1956. *Nonparametric Statistics for the Behavioural Sciences*. New York: McGraw-Hill.

Sourkes, T. L., and Poirier, L. J. 1965. Influence of the substantia nigra on the concentration of 5-hydroxytryptamine and dopamine of the striatum. *Nature* 207:202.

Theonen, H.; Haefely, W.; Gey, K. F.; and Hürlimann, A. 1967. Liberation of alpha-methyldopamine as a "false" sympathetic transmitter after pretreatment of cats with alpha-methyldopa and disulfiram. *Naunyn Schmiedeberg Arch. Pharm. Exp. Path.* 258:181.

Vogt, M. 1954. The concentration of sympathin in different parts of the central nervous system under normal conditions and after the administration of drugs. *J. Physiol. (London)* 123:451.

BIOGENIC AMINES AND AFFECTIVE DISORDERS

Alec Coppen

Medical Research Council, Neuropsychiatric Research Unit
Greenbank, West Park Hospital
Epsom, Surrey, England

There is now a considerable amount of evidence suggesting that the biogenic amines are involved in the etiology of the affective disorders. This evidence consists of a growing number of investigations of the biogenic amines in patients suffering from depression and mania, and also of observations of the effect of manipulating brain amines on mood in patients and in normal subjects. This paper will examine some of the direct evidence for a disturbance in biogenic amines in patients suffering from affective disorders, to examine the etiological implications of these findings, and to consider what the implications of these findings are for treatment. I shall be dealing with the indoleamines--serotonin (5-hydroxytryptamine) and tryptamine--whose biosynthesis and metabolism are illustrated in Figure 1. I do this not because I naively think that only serotonin is important in these conditions, but because most of my own research interests have been centered in this area; in a later paper, Dr. Schildkraut will describe catecholamine metabolism in affective disorders. Moreover, I should like to stress my view that the clinical pathology of the affective disorders is probably very complex, involving not only the biogenic amines but probably other abnormalities as well.

Investigation of the chemical pathology of depression and mania is difficult because of the problems in obtaining data from the organ that is presumably most involved in the process--the brain. No one approach can give any but a limited amount of information, but by pooling the available information I believe some sort of consistent picture emerges. Direct studies of the central nervous system of depressed and manic patients must rely on investigations of the cerebrospinal fluid (CSF) of patients or on postmortem studies of the brains of depressive patients who have committed suicide. There

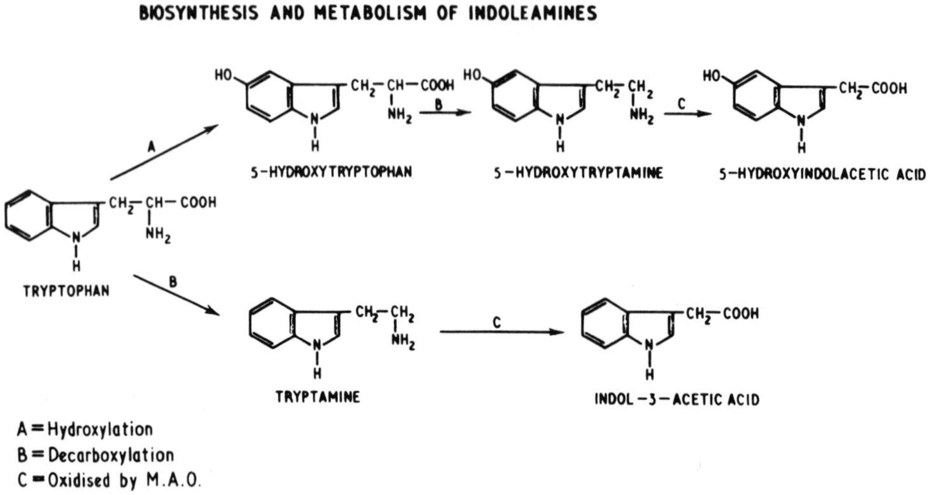

BIOSYNTHESIS AND METABOLISM OF INDOLEAMINES

A = Hydroxylation
B = Decarboxylation
C = Oxidised by M.A.O.

Figure 1. Biosynthesis and metabolism of indoleamines.

are no studies available of the brains of manic patients as suicide is relatively rare in these patients.

CEREBROSPINAL FLUID STUDIES

Although the amines that have been studied most extensively in the affective disorders--the catecholamines and serotonin--are not detectable in the CSF, the acid metabolites of these amines--5-hydroxyindoleacetic acid (5-HIAA) and homovanillic acid (HVA)--are measurable in the lumbar CSF of man. It must be emphasized that one must interpret with caution any differences one finds in lumbar CSF concentrations. Many factors are known to influence the CSF concentrations of 5-HIAA and HVA; some of these can be controlled by the experimental design and some not. For example, CSF concentration of 5-HIAA varies with age; ventricular and cisternal fluids have higher concentrations than does lumbar fluid, so that the test must be standardized and the same amount of fluid removed by the lumbar tap. Again, 5-HIAA is transported out of the CSF by an active process, and so any change of concentration of lumbar 5-HIAA may reflect changes in the transport of 5-HIAA out of the CSF rather than a change in its turnover in the central nervous system. However, if these and other limitations are borne in mind, and if the investigation is properly controlled for age of subject, amount of fluid removed, and time of day the test is performed, I believe that abnormal levels of 5-HIAA in CSF are strongly indicative of some change of serotonin activity in the central nervous system.

Early reports on the CSF concentration of 5-HIAA were in satisfying agreement (Ashcroft et al. 1966; Dencker et al. 1966). Both groups reported a decreased concentration of 5-HIAA in depressive patients. These reports were contradictory, however, as far as mania was concerned. Ashcroft's group reported normal lumbar CSF levels, but Dencker's reported decreased levels in manic patients. Subsequent reports have shown further conflicts. Bowers, Heninger and Gerbode (1969) did not find significantly lower levels in depressive patients and the Swedish group (Sjöström and Roos 1970) could not confirm their earlier findings, but van Praag, Korf, and Puite (1970) reported significantly decreased levels in depressives. We decided, therefore, to investigate the matter further, and we were particularly concerned with the following questions:

1. Is there an abnormality in CSF 5-HIAA (a) in depression and (b) in mania?

2. If so, does this abnormality revert to normal after clinical recovery?

We obtained lumbar CSF from thirty-one patients suffering from depression, from eighteen patients suffering from mania, and from twenty patients who were investigated in a neurological unit and were shown to have no conspicuous psychiatric or neurological morbidity. The test was standardized as far as possible: estimations of 5-HIAA were carried out on the first eleven milliliters of cerebrospinal fluid from the lumbar tap; patients were not treated with antidepressant drugs; the control and affective disorder groups were well-matched for age. Eight patients suffering from depression were retested after complete recovery. Some were retested while in hospital and others were retested after many months of good health out of hospital.

The results are shown in Figure 2. It will be seen that both depressive and manic patients have very significantly lower CSF 5-HIAA concentrations than do the control subjects. From this point of view, therefore, depressive and manic patients show the same deviation from normal. This is analogous to our investigations of sodium metabolism in affective disorders in which we found increased residual sodium in both mania and depression (Coppen 1967).

Some of the most significant findings in this investigation are the values obtained after clinical recovery. Most of these samples were obtained from the patients after discharge from the hospital, when they had been drug-free and clinically well for many months. If these low levels of CSF 5-HIAA are an index of abnormal serotonin activity in the central nervous system, then this abnormality per-

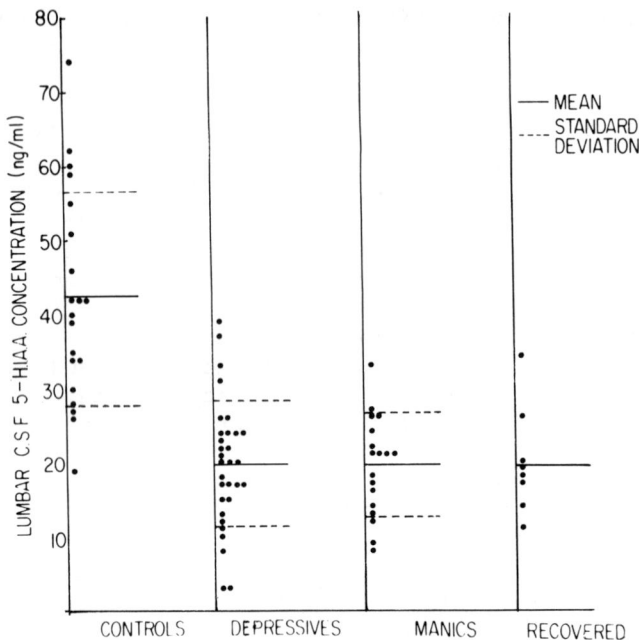
Figure 2. Lumbar CSF 5-hydroxyindoleacetic acid (5-HIAA) in control subjects, depressive patients, manic patients, and depressive patients after recovery.

sists even after apparently full recovery. This finding makes us reflect on the whole etiological role of amines in depression and mania. There is, of course, considerable evidence I shall review later that manipulating brain amines can alleviate pathological affective state, but if a patient can apparently revert to a normal affective state, with the abnormality of amines persisting, then we must conclude that there are other factors involved in the illness.

How far do these changes in lumbar CSF reflect changes in the brain? There are now three published investigations on postmortem examination of the brains of depressive subjects who committed suicide. There are all sorts of factors that cause one to interpret these results with caution. It is difficult to obtain reliable diagnostic data on these subjects: their nutritional state is uncertain; it is often difficult to be sure of the drugs they had been taking; the time of day when they committed suicide is often difficult to learn, and so on. The same drawbacks apply to the control group. Losses occurring after death and before chemical assay are also difficult to control, although Joyce (1962) has shown in animal studies that little serotonin disappeared from the brain in the first few minutes after death and that subsequent losses were small if the animals were allowed to cool slowly at room temperature. The relative stability of serotonin in the brain, however, is dependent on the brain being undisturbed. Once taken from the skull, the serotonin disappears rapidly unless deep-frozen at once, but if this is done the amine is preserved at least for a few days.

In a report from our laboratory, Shaw, Camps, and Eccleston (1967) reported significantly lower hindbrain serotonin concentration in depressive suicides than in a control group of subjects who died from other means--250 ng/gm, as compared to 307 ng/gm in the control group.

Our second investigation was done in collaboration with the National Institute of Mental Health (Bourne et al. 1968). We obtained postmortem material from a London coroner. The hindbrains were then deep-frozen and flown to Bethesda so that hindbrain concentration of serotonin, norepinephrine, and 5-HIAA could be estimated. The time between collection and assay was considerably longer than in the first investigation--174 days.

The results are shown in Table 1. It was found that the values of serotonin concentration are considerably lower than those found by Shaw et al. and we believe that this may be due to losses occasioned by the considerably longer storage time. Moreover, the control brains were stored longer (average, 184 days) than the brains from suicides (average, 159 days). If the decline in amines increased with time, this would tend to reduce differences between the groups.

The material was examined in two ways. First, mean values for all suicides were compared with the mean values for all non-suicides. There was no significant difference in norepinephrine or serotonin between the two groups; 5-HIAA was significantly reduced in the suicides. From this material two more homogeneous groups were selected: (a) a control group consisting of fifteen patients who died suddenly from a coronary infarction but who were not known to have any other medical or psychiatric problem; (b) a group who were diagnosed as having suffered from a depressive illness by a retrospective study of the information available at the Coroner's Court, and who were not alcoholic. These more homogeneous groups showed the same patterns; mean noradrenaline concentrations were slightly increased and mean serotonin concentrations slightly decreased, but not significantly so, in the depressive group. A recent publication by Pare et al. (1969) is in agreement with these findings. In a similar examination of the brains of depressed patients, serotonin was found to be significantly lower than in the control group. Pare's group only examined 5-HIAA in a small number of cases but this tended to be lower in the depressive patients than in the controls. There was no significant difference in brain norepinephrine or dopamine.

TABLE 1

Mean Norepinephrine, 5-Hydroxytryptamine, and 5-Hydroxyindoleacetic Acid Levels in Hindbrain of Suicides and Control Subjects

	All Controls (ng/gm)	N	All Suicides (ng/gm)	N	Coronary Controls (ng/gm)	N	Depressed Controls (ng/gm)	N
Norepinephrine	439	27	444	21	388	15	444	15
5-Hydroxytryptamine	234	25	213	23	218	13	211	16
5-Hydroxyindoleacetic acid	1826*	28	1315*	23	1698*	15	1271*	16

*p < 0.025
N = number of subjects

URINARY STUDIES

I should like now to discuss an investigation into tryptamine in depression that suggests, contrary to the CSF data, that there is some change with clinical recovery. In our laboratory we have examined the urinary excretion of tryptamine and its metabolite, indoleacetic acid, in thirteen patients before and after recovery from a depressive illness (Coppen et al. 1966). Diet and fluid intake were rigorously controlled. The patients were tested twice: first, a few days after admission; then the patients were treated with electroconvulsive therapy and the tests were repeated after recovery. During each period of testing two 24-hour specimens of urine were collected, and on the third day each patient was given an L-tryptophan load (50 mg/kg of body weight) and urine was collected for the following six hours. It was found that the average urinary excretion of tryptamine during the period of depression was about one-half of the normal average and one-half of the levels found in patients after recovery (Table 2). We concluded that, in the kidney, there is some change in tryptamine metabolism during depression, although one cannot decide from this experiment whether these changes are paralleled by similar changes in the central nervous system.

Taking all these findings together, I believe that they support the notion that there is a lowering of both serotonin and 5-HIAA in the brains of depressed suicides, and that the CSF findings are consistent with the view that this occurs in depressed patients both before and after clinical recovery. It would seem, therefore, that there is either a deficiency in the synthesis of serotonin in depressive patients because of a deficiency of tryptophan hydroxylase, or because of some lowering of serotonergic function in the CNS.

What is the causal relationship between this abnormality and the depressive illness? There is considerable evidence that reserpine, a drug that depletes the brain of biogenic amines, can produce depression in a significant number of patients who are given the drug for hypertension (Bunney and Davis 1965). There is also evidence that *para*-chlorophenylalanine (PCPA), which inhibits tryptophan hydroxylase and lowers the brain concentration of serotonin, can also produce symptoms of an affective nature in mentally normal subjects. It is also relevant to consider the activity of methysergide in affective disorders. This compound is a specific antagonist of serotonin, and initial reports that this drug is a specific treatment for mania were obviously of great theoretical importance (Dewhurst 1968). A carefully controlled trial showed, however, that not only was methysergide ineffective against mania but that it was significantly less effective than placebo. That is, methysergide had a deleterious effect on the course of a manic illness (Coppen et al. 1969). This is in keeping with the observation that manic patients have a deficiency of lumbar 5-HIAA similar to that of depressive patients.

TABLE 2

Urinary Excretion of Tryptamine and Indoleacetic Acid
Before and After Recovery from a Depressive Illness
(13 patients)

Clinical State	Age (years)	pH[a]	Tryptamine (µg)		Indoleacetic Acid (mg)	
			24 Hours[a]	Load[b]	24 Hours[a]	Load[b]
Depressed	56.8	6.1	39.2	53.8	3.7	4.0
Recovered		6.0	66.6	118.3	3.2	3.8
p		NS	0.001	0.05	NS	NS

[a]Average values of two 24-hour collections of urine.
[b]Six-hour collections of urine after taking L-tryptophan, 50 mg/kg of body weight.

The action of the antidepressant drugs is to increase the amount of free amines present, either by decreasing the metabolism of the amines (the monoamine oxidase inhibitors [MAOI]), or by increasing the proportion of free amine present by interfering with cellular binding (the tricyclic drugs). These two groups of drugs, however, influence both the catecholamines and serotonin. To get some idea of which amine is involved, we attempted to increase the level of brain amines selectively by administering a monoamine oxidase inhibitor together with large quantities of the amino acid precursor of the amine. From controlled trials we now have data on the therapeutic action of (a) imipramine, (b) MAOI alone, (c) tryptophan alone, and (d) tryptophan and MAOI. The results are summarized in Figure 3. We performed an analysis of co-variance and the figure shows the regression lines of Hamilton scores over time in patients suffering from depression. Our trials last 28 days. It will be seen that the regression lines for imipramine, tryptophan alone, and MAOI alone are very similar, but that the patients given tryptophan together with a MAOI show a very significantly better response ($p < 0.001$) than do the other groups. These results have been replicated by Pare (1963) and Glassman and Platman (1970). This combination of tryptophan and MAOI is presumably especially effective in increasing brain serotonin.

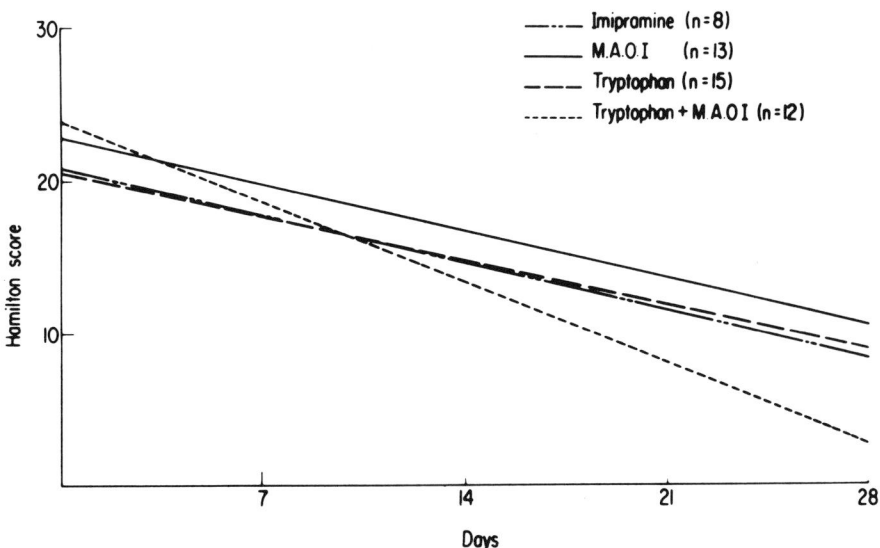

Figure 3. Regression lines of Hamilton rating scores over time in groups of depressed patients treated by (a) tryptophan, (b) monoamine oxidase inhibitor (MAOI), (c) imipramine, (d) tryptophan and MAOI.

We have no comparable data on feeding L-dopa, the precursor of the catecholamines, but initial reports by other workers were almost completely negative. Recent reports by Goodwin et al. (1970) and by Matussek et al. (1970) suggest, however, that if large doses of L-DOPA are used, with or without a peripheral decarboxylase inhibitor, then there is a therapeutic response in about one-third of the patients, although others may deteriorate. There are at the moment no therapeutic trials comparing large doses of L-DOPA and tryptophan with or without a MAOI. It may be, as several authors have suggested, that there is one group of depressive patients who will respond to L-DOPA and another group that will respond to tryptophan. This has to be demonstrated, however, and in our limited experience patients that do not respond to tryptophan do not seem to respond to L-DOPA. The possibility of combining L-DOPA and tryptophan also remains an intriguing possibility.

To summarize, it seems to me that there is good evidence of an abnormality in serotonin in both mania and depression, but it seems that clinical recovery is not accompanied by any change in this abnormality. This seems to indicate that these changes in serotonin and possibly in other amines are only part of the chemical pathology and that they may be a predisposition that requires another factor, perhaps an endocrinological one, to produce the clinical picture of depression and mania. In spite of this, the manipulation of amines seems to be useful in therapeutic intervention. Our data show that increasing amines, especially serotonin, by administering large doses of tryptophan and a MAOI is a very effective antidepressant treatment, and that certain patients may respond favorably to L-DOPA. It may be that the balance of amine activity in the brain is of particular importance in the production of affective disorders, and also in the nature of the affective disorder, whether there is a picture of retarded or agitated depression or mania. There is little evidence about this at the moment. I would also suggest that we need more studies of patients during complete remission of their illness.

REFERENCES

Ashcroft, G. W.; Crawford, T. B. B.; Eccleston, D.; Sharman, D. F.; MacDougall, E. J.; Stanton, J. B.; and Binns, J. F. 1966. 5-Hydroxyindole compounds in the cerebrospinal fluid of patients with psychiatric or neurological disease. *Lancet* 2:1049.

Bourne, H. R.; Bunney, W. E.; Colburn, R. W.; Davis, J. N.; Davis, J. M.; Shaw, D. M.; and Coppen, A. J. 1968. Noradrenaline, 5-hydroxytryptamine and 5-hydroxyindoleacetic acid in the hindbrains of suicidal patients. *Lancet* 2:805.

Bowers, M. B.; Heninger, G. R.; and Gerbode, F. 1969. Cerebrospinal fluid 5-hydroxyindoleacetic acid and homovanillic acid in psychiatric patients. *Int. J. Neuropharmacol.* 8:255.

Bunney, W. E., and Davis, J. M. 1965. Norepinephrine in depressive reactions. *Arch. Gen. Psychiat.* 13:483.

Coppen, A. 1967. Mineral metabolism in affective disorders. *Brit. J. Psychiat.* 111:1133.

Coppen, A.; Prange, A. J.; Whybrow, P. C.; Noguera, R.; and Paez, J. M. 1959. Methysergide in mania. *Lancet* 2:338.

Dencker, S. J.; Malm, V.; Roos, B.-E.; and Werdinius, B. 1966. Acid monoamine metabolites of cerebrospinal fluid in mental depression and mania. *J. Neurochem.* 13:1545.

Dewhurst, W. G. 1968. Methysergide in mania. *Nature* 219:506.

Glassman, A. H., and Platman, S. R. 1970. Potentiation of a monoamine oxidase inhibitor by tryptophan. *J. Psychiat. Res.* 7:63.

Goodwin, F. K.; Brodie, H. K. H.; Murphy, D. L.; and Bunney, W. E. 1970. Administration of a peripheral decarboxylase inhibitor with L-dopa to depressed patients. *Lancet* 1:908.

Joyce, D. 1962. Changes in the 5-hydroxytryptamine content of rat, rabbit and human brain after death. *Brit. J. Pharmacol.* 18:370.

Matussek, N.; Benkert, O.; Schneider, K.; Otten, H.; and Pohlmeier, H. 1970. L-dopa plus decarboxylase inhibitor in depression.

Lancet 2:660.
Pare, C. M. B. 1963. Potentiation of monoamine oxidase inhibitors by tryptophan. *Lancet* 2:527.
Pare, C. M. B.; Young, D. P. H.; Price, K.; and Stacey, R. S. 1969. 5-Hydroxytryptamine, noradrenaline and dopamine in brainstem, hypothalamus and caudate nucleus of controls and patients committing suicide by coal gas poisoning. *Lancet* 2:133.
Shaw, D. M.; Camps, F. E.; and Eccleston, E. 1967. 5-Hydroxytryptamine in the hindbrains of depressive suicides. *Brit. J. Psychiat.* 113:1407.
Sjöström, R., and Roos, B.-E. 1970. Measurement of 5-HIAA and HVA in CSF in manic-depressive patients after probenecid application. Seventh Congress, Collegium Internationale Neuro-Psychopharmacologicum, Prague, Czechoslovakia.
van Praag, H. M.; Korf, J.; and Puite, J. 1970. 5-Hydroxyindoleacetic acid levels in the cerebrospinal fluid of depressed patients treated with probenecid. *Nature* 225:1259.

CATECHOLAMINES AND AFFECTIVE ILLNESS: STUDIES WITH

L-DOPA AND ALPHA-METHYL-PARA-TYROSINE

Elliot S. Gershon, William E. Bunney, Jr.,
Frederick K. Goodwin, Dennis L. Murphy,
David L. Dunner, and George M. Henry

Section on Psychiatry, Laboratory of Clinical Science
National Institute of Mental Health
Bethesda, Maryland

In this paper we will review previous data and present new data on the clinical effects of L-dihydroxyphenylalanine (L-DOPA) and alpha-methyl-para-tyrosine (α-MPT) in the affective disorders and on the biochemical pharmacology of these agents in man and in the laboratory animal. These studies were prompted by the catecholamine hypothesis, which remains of central importance in current research in the affective disorders (Bunney and Davis 1965; Schildkraut 1965). This hypothesis proposes that some, if not all, depressions are associated with a deficiency of catecholamines at functionally important adrenergic sites in brain, and that mania may be associated with an excess of these amines (Schildkraut 1965). Pharmacologic agents that cause an increase in active catecholamines released by appropriate neurons should be associated with alleviation of depression or production of mania, and pharmacologic agents that cause a decrease in the amount of catecholamines available to the receptor should be associated with worsening of depression or improvement of mania.

The amount of actually functioning norepinephrine in brain (as distinguished from total brain norepinephrine) cannot now be determined, however, and the sites that may be important in the affective disorders have not been identified. In the absence of this knowledge,

---

Paper presented by Dr. Bunney. Dr. Gershon is now at Ezrath Nahim Mental Hospital, Jerusalem, Israel, Dr. Dunner at New York State Psychiatric Institute, New York City.

one strategy of research has been to study the effects of psychopharmacologic agents on the biochemistry of catecholamines in whole brain or in regions of brain, and to correlate this knowledge with the clinical effects of the drug in affective disorder. Administration of precursors of biogenic amines and inhibitors of synthesis of these amines offers an opportunity to manipulate amines in brain in man in a relatively direct and specific way, and it may enable some derivatives of the catecholamine hypothesis to be tested clinically. Such drugs have multiple biochemical effects, however, which must be considered in order to interpret the results of clinical trials of precursors or inhibitors of synthesis.

L-DOPA is the precursor of dopamine (DA) and norepinephrine (NE), bypassing tyrosine hydroxylase, the rate-limiting enzyme in catecholamine synthesis (Udenfriend 1966). In the rat, 50 mg/kg is the minimal dose required to produce catecholamine fluorescence in brain parenchyma (Bertler et al. 1966). Higher doses or combined use of L-DOPA with inhibitors of decarboxylation by oral administration are used in man (Goodwin et al. 1970a). At these higher doses in the rat, L-DOPA causes an increase in brain dopamine, but brain norepinephrine has been reported to show no change or only a slight and transient increase (Butcher and Engel 1969; Everett and Borcherding 1970; Gershon, Goodwin, and Gold 1970; Chalmers et al. to be published). Serotonin (5-HT) content of brain is decreased (Butcher and Engel 1969; Everett and Borcherding 1970). The effects of L-DOPA on turnover of central amines have been investigated by us, and our findings are presented below.

Prior to the introduction of high dosages of L-DOPA in the treatment for Parkinsonism, several studies of L-DOPA in depression were reported. In non-blind studies, in which up to 150 mg/day of DOPA was given, some improvement in depression and increased motor activity and speech were reported (Pare and Sandler 1959; Turner and Merlis 1964; Ingvarsson 1965). In a double-blind study using up to 1 gm/day of DL-DOPA with a monoamine oxidase inhibitor, Klerman et al. (1963) found no improvement in depression (Matussek, Pohlmeier, and Ruther 1966). In Parkinsonian patients treated with higher doses of L-DOPA, the reported behavioral changes included depression, hyperactivity, and hypomania (Calne et al. 1969; Goodwin-Austin et al. 1969; Yahr et al. 1969; Goodwin et al. 1970b; McDowell et al. 1970; O'Brien et al. 1971).

α-MPT is an inhibitor of the rate-limiting enzyme, tyrosine hydroxylase, and it causes marked depletion of brain norepinephrine and dopamine, but no change in 5-HT (Spector, Sjoerdsma, and Udenfriend 1965). Synthesis of norepinephrine in $vivo$ from ^{14}C-tyrosine in guinea pig brain is markedly diminished by α-MPT and this decreased synthesis correlates in time with the norepinephrine depletion. Synthesis of norepinephrine from ^{3}H-DOPA, which occurs at a later point in the pathway of synthesis, is unaffected by α-MPT (Udenfriend et al. 1966). Uptake and release of norepinephrine are not affected by α-MPT (Spector, Sjoerdsma, and Udenfriend 1965).

Behavioral effects of α-MPT have been reported in patients with pheochromocytoma, hypotension, and Raynaud's phenomenon, who were treated with 1 to 4 gm/day of this drug on a non-blind basis (Sjoerdsma et al. 1965; Engelman et al. 1968). Depression, anxiety, and agitation were seen in three of twenty hypertensive patients; all three of these had previous histories of depression. Sedation, with insomnia upon withdrawal, was seen in nearly all patients.

METHODS

Patients with moderate to severe depression or mania, requiring hospitalization, were studied on two twelve-bed research units that have been described elsewhere (Goodwin et al. 1970). Symptoms of depression included depressed mood, guilt, retardation, agitation, anorexia, loss of interest, weight loss, sleep disturbance, suicidal preoccupations, and intense feelings of helplessness, hopelessness, or worthlessness. Symptoms of mania included grandiosity, rapid incessant speech and body movement, sleeplessness, euphoria, and a type of aggressive provocativeness that has been described elsewhere (Janowsky, Leff, and Epstein 1970). The affectively ill patients were classified as bipolar (history of hospitalization for mania) or as unipolar (depression only). This division of patients into unipolar and bipolar groups has been supported by pharmacologic and genetic studies (Leonhard, Korff, and Shulz 1962; Angst 1966; Perris 1966; Winokur, Clayton, and Reich 1969; Goodwin et al. 1971). Patients with depression who had a history of hypomanic symptoms sufficient to be noticed by themselves or their families, but not resulting in hospitalization, were distinguished from the unipolar patients and are designated in this paper as "unipolar +." The classification of these patients into three groups was made independently of the drug trials (Dunner, Gershon, and Goodwin 1970).

Informed consent was obtained from all patients and from their immediate families for administration of double-blind drug protocols and for collection of blood, urine, spinal fluid, and behavioral research data. Behavioral ratings were performed by a specially trained nursing staff, using the Bunney-Hamburg scales to rate global depression, mania, anxiety, psychosis, and anger (Bunney and Hamburg 1963). Ratings on this scale range from 1 to 15, where 15 is extremely ill and 1 is normal on the symptoms being rated. Criteria for an unequivocal clinical response to a double-blind administered drug are a rating change of two or more points on the global depression scale during the drug period and an increase in ratings of 2 or more points after placebo substitution. These changes represent a significant shift in the patient's condition, as observed clinically.

L-DOPA and α-MPT were given on a non-random double-blind basis. L-DOPA was given orally in doses up to 12 gm/day. In several patients, a peripheral L-aromatic amino acid decarboxylase inhibitor was administered (alpha-methyl-DOPA-hydrazine [MK 485]). With MK 485, therapeutic amounts of DOPA reaching brain may be obtained with lower total dosage (Goodwin et al. 1970a). α-MPT was administered in doses up to 5 gm/day.

Recumbent and standing blood pressures and pulse were measured four times a day. Patients were examined regularly by a neurologist. A comprehensive battery of hematological and chemical tests was run on all patients before and during the course of drug treatment. Twenty-four-hour urine pools were collected daily, and aliquots were frozen for the determination of DOPA, dopamine, homovanillic acid (HVA), 3-methoxy-4-hydroxyphenylglycol (MHPG), 3-methoxy-4-hydroxymandelic acid (VMA), and 5-hydroxyindoleacetic acid (5-HIAA) (Udenfriend, Titus, and Weissbach 1955; Sourkes and Murphy 1961; Sato 1965; Wilk et al. 1967). Whenever possible, cerebrospinal fluid (CSF) was obtained before and during L-DOPA administration and analyzed for HVA and 5-HIAA (Gerbode and Bowers 1960; Ashcroft and Sharman 1962).

<u>Turnover measurements</u>: A recently developed technique was used to indirectly estimate changes in turnover of brain dopamine and serotonin in our patients. The principal metabolites of these amines are the organic acids, homovanillic acid and 5-hydroxyindoleacetic acid. Probenecid inhibits the active transport of 5-HIAA and HVA out of brain (Werdinius 1966; Neff, Tozer, and Brodie 1967) and CSF (Mannarino, Kirshner, and Nashold 1963; Werdinius 1967), and thus the rate of accumulation of these acid metabolites in CSF during probenecid treatment can be used as an indirect index of brain amine turnover (Guldberg, Ashcroft, and Crawford 1966; Bowers and Gerbode 1968; Roos and Sjostrum 1969).

Turnover of norepinephrine cannot now be determined by the probenecid technique. 3-Methoxy-4-hydroxyphenylglycol and its sulfate conjugate are apparently the principal metabolites of norepinephrine in brain (Mannarino, Kirshner, and Nashold 1963; Schanberg, Schildkraut, and Kopin 1967; Maas, Fawcett, and Dekirmenjian 1968; Maas et al. in press). Preliminary studies indicate that these compounds are not elevated in CSF in our patients after probenecid treatment (Kopin and Gordon, unpublished communication). Animal experiments were performed, therefore, to assess the effect of L-DOPA on turnover of norepinephrine in brain. The rate of disappearance of ^{3}H-norepinephrine after intracisternal injection was used as a measure of turnover in these experiments. Male S-D rats weighing 150 to 200 gm were injected intracisternally with 10 μc of DL-tritiated NE under light ether anesthesia. One half-hour later, they were fed 300 mg/kg of L-DOPA in cherry syrup, or cherry syrup with nothing added. Two, three, or four hours later the rats were decapitated, and the brains assayed for dopamine and norepinephrine (Anton and Sayne 1962; Weil-Malherbe, in press).

RESULTS

1. L-DOPA

Clinical studies in depression. Five of twenty-six depressed patients who received L-DOPA showed clinical improvement and demonstrated a rebound worsening during placebo substitution (Table 1) (Bunney et al. 1969, 1970, and 1971; Goodwin et al. 1970a). Three of these five patients improved on L-DOPA to the point of complete recovery and discharge. None of the bipolar patients had an unequivocal antidepressant response, while four of the five responders were in the group of unipolar depressed patients with histories of hypomania.

Manic or hypomanic responses to L-DOPA during depression occurred in nine depressed patients (Murphy et al. 1971). Of these, eight were clearly bipolar, and the ninth patient had depressions and a history of hypomania. An additional three bipolar patients did not have a hypomanic response to L-DOPA although, in one of these patients, L-DOPA was discontinued after less than one-half the average treatment time because of the development of neurological side effects. Hypomanic symptoms consisted of increased motor and verbal activity, pressured speech, increased social involvement, intrusiveness, grandiosity, increase in anger, sleeplessness, and agitated behavior. Most of these patients showed only minimal euphoria, and they remained clearly depressed during the time of hypomania, although one patient (W.L,) showed improvement while on DOPA, and had euphoria while she was hypomanic. The probability of spontaneous hypomania occurring was estimated from the duration of hospitalization and the frequency of hypomania while on placebo. In four of the patients, the probability of hypomania occurring during L-DOPA treatment was less than 0.05 (Table 2).

Two patients showed worsening in relation to L-DOPA treatment. Both patients had psychotic delusions of low self-worth and paranoid thoughts; these symptoms became worse during L-DOPA treatment and improved on withdrawal.

Urinary dopamine and the dopamine metabolite, HVA, were increased in depressed patients treated with L-DOPA (Table 3), suggesting that there was conversion of DOPA to dopamine during the administration of the drug, and that daily turnover of dopamine was elevated in these patients. The urinary NE metabolite, MHPG, was studied in only one nonmanic patient, who showed increased MHPG when L-DOPA was increased. In four patients who became hypomanic during L-DOPA treatment, urinary MHPG was increased during this period. Urinary MHPG has not been elevated during untreated hypomania as compared with controls (Greenspan et al. 1970).

TABLE 1

L-DOPA in Depressed Patients

Patient	Age	Sex	Diagnosis	History of Hypomania	Max. Dose of L-DOPA	Clinical Response	No Change Placebo
G.A.	73	M	Unipolar	+	8.1	Improvement	Worse
W.L. (2nd course)	52	F	Unipolar	+	7.0 (0.3*)	Improvement "	Worse "
W.M.	38	F	Unipolar	+	1.4*	Improvement	Worse
L.F.	62	M	Unipolar	+	0.8*	Improvement	Worse
K.F.	44	M	Unipolar	+	0.5*	Improvement	Worse
H.I.	60	F	Unipolar	−	8.0	No change	No change
W.E.	55	M	Unipolar	−	8.0	No change	No change
C.J.	47	F	Unipolar	−	8.0	No change	No change
Q.M.	24	F	Unipolar	−	7.0	No change	No change
K.S. (2nd course)	46	F	Unipolar	−	4.0 (0.3*)	No change "	No change "
T.E.	57	F	Unipolar	−	3.0	Worse	Improvement
W.T.	29	M	Unipolar	+	1.5*	No change	No change
W.A.	39	M	Unipolar	+	0.8*	No change	No change

TABLE 1 (Continued)

D.D.	66	M	Unipolar	+	0.8*	No change	No change
V.S.	49	F	Unipolar	−	1.0*	No change	No change
L.R.	43	M	Bipolar		12.5	No change	No change
M.M. (2nd course)	48	F	Bipolar		11.0 (1.6*)	No change "	No change "
A.C.	55	F	Bipolar		7.0	No change	No change
J.L.	42	M	Bipolar		6.0	Worse	Improvement
R.M.	42	F	Bipolar		5.0	No change	No change
T.J.	47	M	Bipolar		4.0	No change	No change
R.J.	36	M	Bipolar		1.3*	No change	No change
B.H.	40	F	Bipolar		1.0*	No change	No change
B.C.	32	F	Bipolar		0.6*	No change	No change
H.R.	54	F	Bipolar		0.4*	No change	No change
G.H.	27	F	Bipolar		5.0	Improvement	No change

*MK 485 plus L–DOPA

TABLE 2

Patients with Hypomanic or Manic Episodes During L-Dopa Treatment

Patient	Diagnosis	Mania Attack Frequency*	Days on L-DOPA >3.0 gm/day† prior to Hypomania	L-DOPA Dose at Time of Hypomania Onset (gm/day)	Probability of Hypomania Occurring with L-DOPA >3.0 gm/day†	Probability of Hypomania with L-DOPA >3.0 gm/day†
A.C.	Bipolar	3/203	1	3.0	1/68	.02
R.M.	Bipolar	2/156	7	4.0	7/78	.09
J.L.	Bipolar	4/76	6	6.0	6/19	.32
T.J.	Bipolar	0/113	2	4.0	--	(<.01)
L.R.	Bipolar	0/101	18	10.0	--	(<.01)
W.L.	Unipolar	0/217	13	7.0	--	(<.01)
B.C.	Bipolar	1/129	1	0.4	1/129	.01
M.M.	Bipolar	0/126	14	10.0	--	(<.01)
R.J.	Bipolar	0/76	10	1.1	--	(<.01)
					Combined Group Probability	<.001

*Episodes of mania per nonmanic days in hospital.
† or ≥ 400 mg/day with MK 485.

From Murphy, D. L., Brodie, H.K.H., Goodwin, F.K., and Bunney, W.E., Jr. Reprinted with permission of the authors and *American Journal of Psychiatry*, January 1971.

TABLE 3

Urinary Excretion of DOPA, Dopamine, Homovanillic Acid (HVA)
and 3-Methoxy-4-Hydroxy-Phenylglycol (MHPG) as Related to DOPA Dose
6 Patients

	DOPA mg/24 hrs.	Dopamine mg/24 hrs.	HVA mg/24 hrs.	MHPG mg/24 hrs.
0 gm	.13 ± .14 (28)	0.45 ± .5 (28)	8.8 ± 10 (20)	1.66 ± 1.2 (16)
2 gm	11.20 ± 7.9 (15)	62.90 ± 46.0 (12)	535.0 ± 247 (11)	1.70 ± .5 (3)
DOPA 3 gm	13.60 ± 10.0 (7)	100.20 ± 47.0 (7)	758.0 ± 101 (4)	2.05 ± 1.3 (4)
4 gm	14.90 ± 7.2 (6)	109.30 ± 59.0 (6)	1106.0 ± 152 (5)	3.70 ± 1.6 (4)
5 gm	26.80 ± 3.2 (2)	215.20 ± 107.0 (2)	1290.0 ± 145 (2)	9.96 ± 0 (1)
6 gm	41.20 ± 23.6 (12)	248.50 ± 158.0 (12)	2297.0 ± 611 (7)	- - -

From Bunney, Brodie, Murphy, and Goodwin. Reprinted with permission of the authors and *American Journal of Psychiatry*, January 1971.

TABLE 4

Cerebrospinal Fluid Metabolites

	Number of Patients	HVA ng/ml	5-HIAA ng/ml
Neurological Patients			
Off medication*	21	21 ± 4.5	35 ± 2.9
L-DOPA*	17	433 ± 70.7	31 ± 3.3
Depressed Patients			
Off medication	28	19 ± 3.4	25 ± 1.9
L-DOPA	2	419 ± 97.5	20 ± 3.0
L-DOPA +MK 485	5	174 ± 82.8	34 ± 7.70

*Data of Dr. T. N. Chase, Laboratory of Clinical Science, National Institute of Mental Health.

Studies of CNS turnover of monoamines during L-DOPA treatment.
(1) Studies of 5-HT and DA turnover in spinal fluid of man: Cerebrospinal fluid 5-HIAA levels were significantly lower in depressed patients than in the neurological patient controls (t = 3.0, p < 0.01) (Table 4). This is consistent with the results of other investigators (Ashcroft and Sharman 1960; Ashcroft et al. 1966; Dencker et al. 1966; Coppen et al. 1969; van Praag, Korff, and Puite 1970). During treatment with L-DOPA, HVA in CSF increased markedly (Table 4), while 5-HIAA decreased only slightly and nonsignificantly.

The increased concentration of 5-HIAA and HVA in CSF after probenecid treatment may be considered an index of the turnover of the amines, 5-HT and DA respectively (Bowers and Gerbode 1968). We have studied the effect of probenecid administration in five depressed patients during a placebo period and then again during treatment with L-DOPA and MK 485 (Goodwin, Dunner, and Gershon 1971). None of the patients showed clinical improvement in depression or develop-

TABLE 5

Accumulation of Monoamine Acid Metabolites During Placebo and L-DOPA Periods After Probenecid

Patient	Probenecid mg/kg	Duration hours	HVA Accumulation ng/ml		5-HIAA Accumulation ng/ml	
			Placebo	L-DOPA	Placebo	L-DOPA
B.C.	92	18	286	585	126	87
B.H.	104	9	161	297	90	52
D.D.	104	20	174	554	70	48
V.S.	138	8	113	376	107	65
W.T.	66	9	73	568	50	55
Mean Accumulation			161.4 ± 35.9	476.0 ± 58.5*	88.6 ± 13.4	61.4 ± 7.0†

*p < .01, paired t-test.
†p < .05, paired t-test.

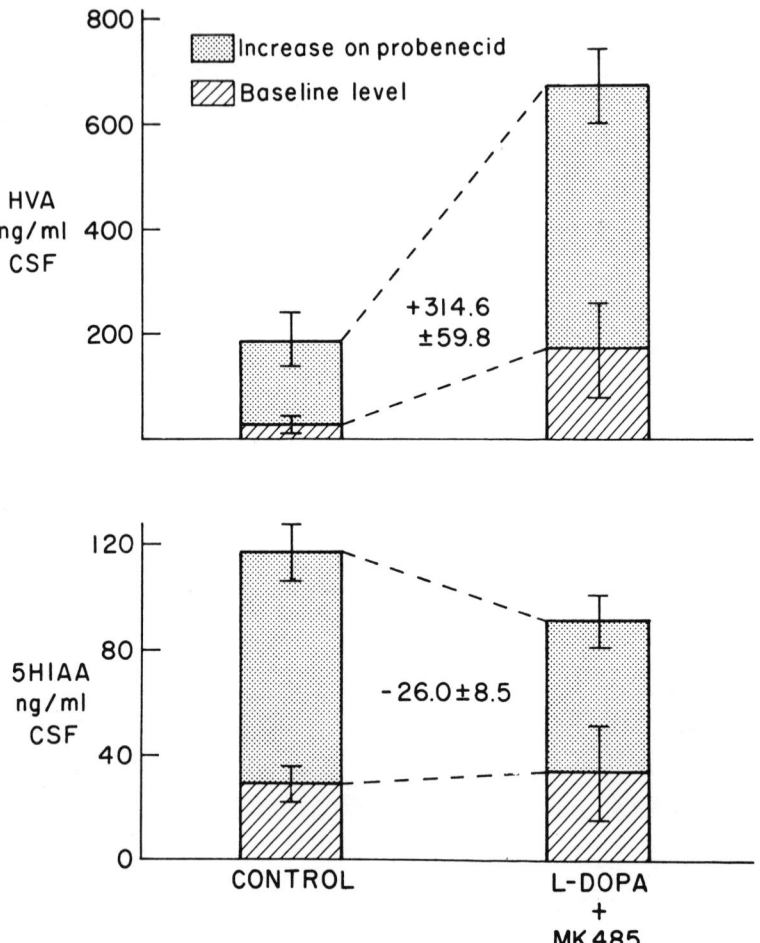

Figure 1. Changes in HVA and 5-HIAA accumulation in CSF with probenecid during treatment with L-DOPA and MK 485.

ment of hypomanic symptoms during the period of treatment with L-DOPA.

Comparison of the changes in cerebrospinal HVA and 5-HIAA produced by probenecid revealed an increase in HVA accumulation and a decrease in 5-HIAA accumulation during the L-DOPA treatment period, in comparison to the placebo period (Table 5, Figure 1). The difference between changes was statistically significant for HVA ($p <$

0.01) and for 5-HIAA (p < 0.05). Because the time of the lumbar punctures and the dose of probenecid varied somewhat from patient to patient, we attempted to correct for these variations by dividing the change in HVA and 5-HIAA by probenecid dose (mg/kg) and by time. The difference between the L-DOPA and placebo periods remained significant after this correction.

These results suggest that turnover of brain dopamine is increased and that turnover of brain serotonin is decreased during treatment with L-DOPA.

(2) Studies of NE turnover in rat brain *in vivo*: The rate of disappearance of labeled ^{3}H-NE after intracisternal injection was used as a measure of turnover. The rate of disappearance was faster in the L-DOPA-treated rats (Figure 2). The rate constants were significantly different from each other (control rats = 0.092 hr^{-1}, L-DOPA = 0.131 hr^{-1}, t = 2.14, p < 0.05, method of McNemar [1969]). There was less ^{3}H-NE remaining in brain in the L-DOPA-fed rats at each point in time. The brain dopamine was elevated in the L-DOPA-fed rats as compared with controls (1.21 ± 0.23 µg/gm versus 0.71 ± 0.03 µg/gm, t = 4.04, p < 0.001). Brain norepinephrine was not significantly different in the two groups of rats (0.65 ± 0.04 µg/gm versus 0.67 ± 0.03 µg/gm, t = 0.04, N.S.).

These data indicate that, although the level of norepinephrine in brain was not affected by L-DOPA, the rate of turnover of this amine was significantly increased. This is consistent with the view that tyrosine hydroxylase limits the rate of formation of NE, and that bypassing the rate-limiting step by the administration of L-DOPA results in increased NE formation and turnover.

2. Alpha-Methyl-Para-Tyrosine

Clinical effects of α-MPT *in mania and in depression.* In mania, the clinical changes seen during α-MPT treatment have not been consistent improvement or worsening, although all patients treated have shown marked changes (Bunney *et al.* 1971; Brodie *et al.*, in press): Of eight patients, two have had unequivocal improvement, and one has had unequivocal worsening while on the drug (Table 6). Three other patients improved and one became worse while being treated with α-MPT, but they did not show changes in the opposite direction when the drug was discontinued. The behavioral changes seen in these manic patients included sedation, increased sleep time, excessive salivation with drooling, some rigidity of movement, and long periods of quiescence with very little body movement, even though the patient was clearly awake and responsive.

The psychiatric improvement, when it was present, could be distinguished from the sedative effects of α-MPT. There were decreases in demanding and provocative behavior, and less euphoria and grand-

TABLE 6

Behavioral Effects of α-MPT in Mania

Patient	Total Days on α-MPT	Maximum Daily Dose	Number of Courses	Clinical Response	Change on Placebo
R.E.	35	4 gm	3	Improved	Worse x 3
M.J.	48	4 gm	3	Improved	Worse x 1 No change x 2
N.R.	15	2 gm	1	Improved	No change
R.J.	5	3 gm	1	Improved	No change
R.M.	8	4 gm	1	Improved	No change
K.M.	9	3.75 gm	1	Worse	Improved
W.F.	29	5 gm	1	Worse over 4 gm	No data

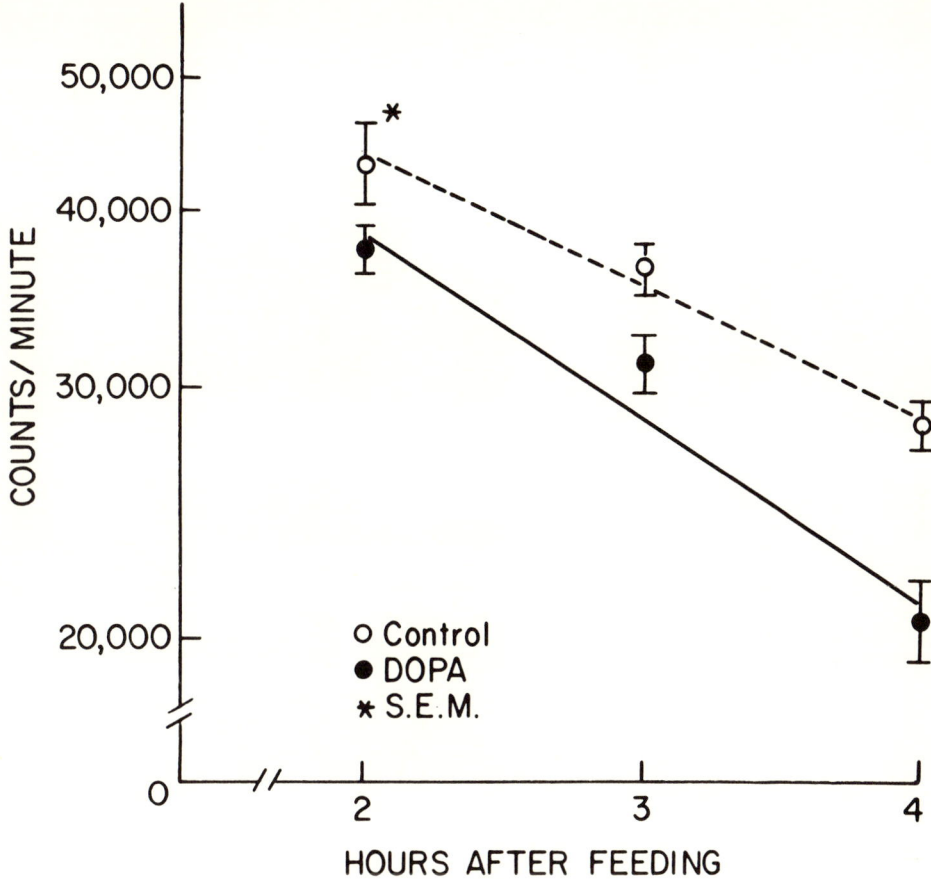

Figure 2. Disappearance of ^{3}H-norepinephrine from rat brain.

iosity. However, the improvement did not extend to complete remission of manic symptoms in most of the patients treated, as illustrated in Figure 3. Some patients improved on the drug and then showed relapse despite continued high dosage. For example, in one patient (Figure 3) manic symptoms were clearly present even after 14 days of treatment. These symptoms, however, were milder than those she had when the drug administration was begun. A rebound insomnia, which occurred within 48 hours after discontinuation of the drug, was a constant behavioral change produced in all of the patients treated with α-MPT.

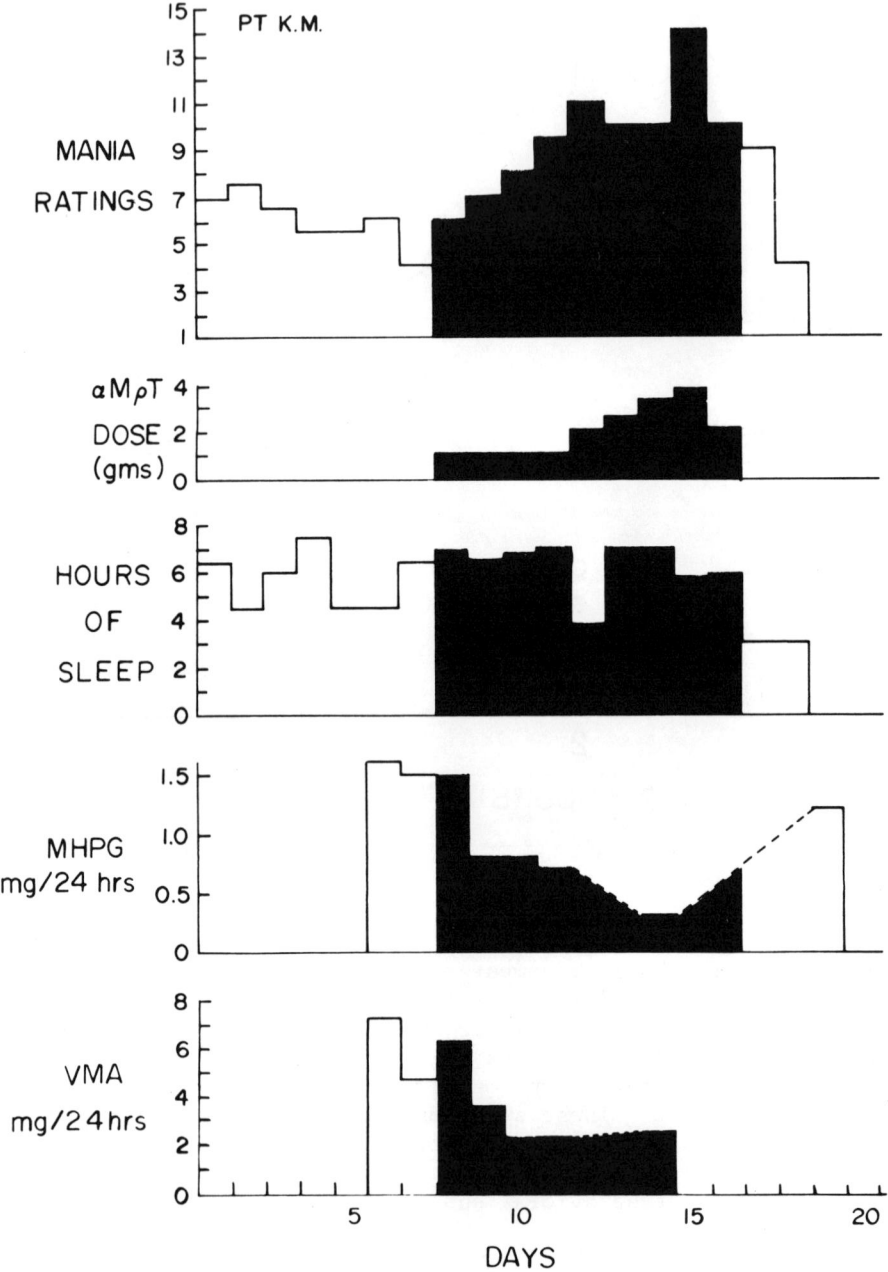

Figure 3. Increase in mania on α-MPT.

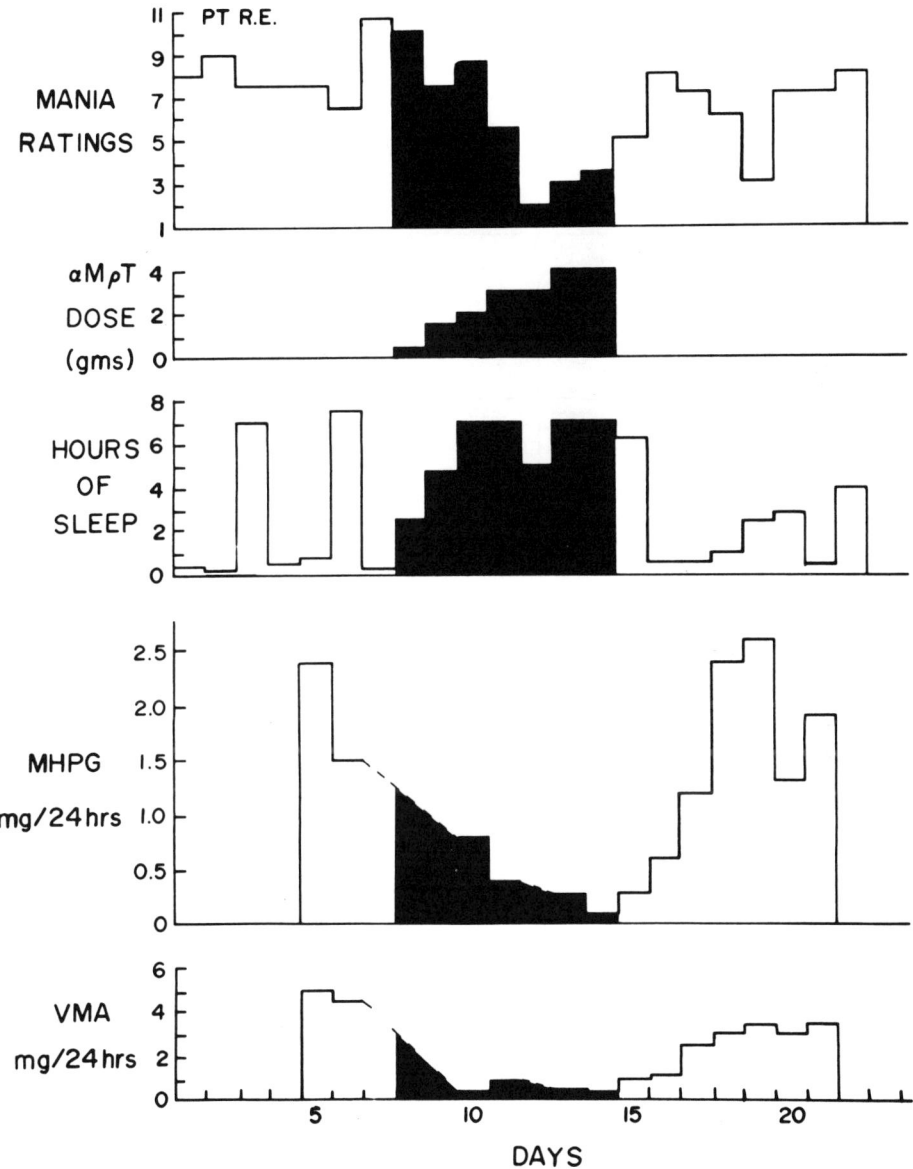

Figure 4. Decrease in mania on α-MPT.

TABLE 7

Behavioral Effects of Alpha-Methyl-Tyrosine in Depression

Patient	Clinical Subgroup	History of Hypomanic Episodes	Total Days on α-MT	Maximum Daily Dose	Number of Courses	Clinical Response	Change on Placebo
W.G.	Unipolar	−	6	3 gm	1	Worse	Improved
C.J.	Unipolar	−	6	3 gm	1	Worse	Improved
D.D.	Unipolar	+	12	3 gm	1	Worse	No change
B.G.	Unipolar	+	6	3 gm	1	No change	No change
G.T.	Bipolar		6	2 gm	1	Worse	Improved
B.B.	Bipolar		19	4 gm	1	No change	No change

Six patients were treated with α-MPT during depression. Three showed unequivocal worsening of their depression, with improvement upon withdrawal of the drug, and one patient became worse on the drug and showed no change upon withdrawal. The remaining two patients showed no clinical change in relation to administration or withdrawal of the drug (Table 7). Rebound insomnia, however, was observed in all patients after α-MPT was discontinued, regardless of the clinical response.

Clinical biochemical findings. Decreased urinary metabolites of norepinephrine were consistently observed in the patients treated with α-MPT, even when the clinical responses were quite opposite (Figures 3 and 4). MHPG, the urinary metabolite of NE which may be related to CNS NE turnover, was decreased to progressively lower levels as the dose of α-MPT was increased. Similar changes occurred in VMA excretion (Table 8).

Spinal fluid data are available for three manic patients and two depressed patients treated with α-MPT. Mean HVA was 19.0 ± 8.6 ng/ml during the placebo period, and 4.0 ± 3.5 ng/ml during α-MPT treatment. This difference was not statistically significant. However, HVA values of this low magnitude may be unreliable with the determination used. Spinal fluid 5-HIAA was unchanged by α-MPT; the means were 30.8 ± 7.2 ng/ml and 28.8 ± 4.4 ng/ml for these five patients.

DISCUSSION

This series of investigations is concerned with the clinical effectiveness of L-DOPA and α-MPT in stimulating or inhibiting catecholamine synthesis and activity in CNS, and with the changes in affective state that result when these substances are used as psychopharmacologic agents. As a therapeutic agent in depression, L-DOPA was not associated with improvement in most of the patients treated. Hypomanic behavioral changes, however, were provoked by L-DOPA in depressed patients with bipolar affective illness. α-MPT was associated with improvement in mania in five patients, and with worsening in two patients. In depressed patients, treatment with α-MPT was associated with worsening in three patients, and with no change in the remaining three. In virtually all the patients with bipolar affective illness, hypomania was apparently provoked by treatment with L-DOPA during depressive illness, and marked clinical changes in mania appeared in relation to α-MPT administration.

These changes in mania or hypomania produced by either drug are in contrast to the less frequent changes in depression. More than half the patients treated with L-DOPA, and half the patients treated with α-MPT, showed no unequivocal changes in depression in relation to the drug trials. These results suggest that biochemical changes

TABLE 8

Urinary Excretion of Catecholamine Metabolites and
Dopamine as Related to α-MPT Administration
N = 5

	VMA µg/24 hrs.	MHPG µg/24 hrs.	Dopamine µg/24 hrs.
Before α-MPT	4.26 ± 1.2	1.82 ± .50	387.6 ± 108.8
On >2 gm α-MPT per day	1.00 ± 0.7†	0.59 ± .36†	95.6 ± 30.6*
After α-MPT stopped	3.04 ± 0.4*	1.86 ± .52*	222.3 ± 40.0*

*Significantly different from previous level at $p < .01$ by Student's t test.
†Significantly different from previous level at $p < .05$ by Student's t test.

From Bunney, Brodie, Murphy and Goodwin. Reprinted with permission of the authors and *American Journal of Psychiatry*, January 1971.

associated with these pharmacologic agents may be more consistently related to the pathophysiology of mania and hypomania than to depression. Among the notable biochemical changes produced by α-MPT and L-DOPA are alterations in turnover and level of CNS monoamines.

Effects of L-DOPA on turnover of biogenic monoamines. In depressed patients treated with L-DOPA, we found that the CNS turnover of dopamine is increased and the turnover of 5-HT may be decreased, as indicated by the accumulation of acid metabolites of monoamines in CSF after probenecid treatment. Turnover of brain NE could not be measured in these patients by this method. Turnover of NE during L-DOPA administration was therefore studied in rat brain *in vivo*. The rate of disappearance of ^{3}H-NE was increased by L-DOPA treatment, although the total NE was unchanged. These results suggest that synthesis of NE in brain may be increased by L-DOPA treatment. Increased urinary excretion of HVA and MHPG during treatment with DOPA is also compatible with increased turnover of their amine precursors, DA and NE.

These findings are compatible with the known pharmacology of L-DOPA and α-MPT. In guinea pig heart *in vitro*, L-DOPA has been demonstrated to bypass the rate-limiting step in NE synthesis, so that over a wide range of concentrations, increasing L-DOPA in the perfusate is associated with proportionally increased NE synthesis (Udenfriend 1966). In rat brain *in vivo*, our findings of increased turnover are consistent with these findings in heart and with recent studies in rat brain using a similar design to ours (Chalmers, Baldessarini, and Wurtman, to be published).

Increases in turnover of brain DA and decreased turnover of 5-HT, which are implied by our studies of CSF in depression, are also suggested by recent studies of brain slices. Ng and co-workers (1971) have found that L-DOPA causes efflux of labeled 5-HT or DA from rat striatal slices, suggesting that L-DOPA is displacing the already present amines from their storage sites by the formation of dopamine, and that DA may be acting as a false transmitter at serotonergic neurons. Competition of L-DOPA with 5-hydroxytryptophan for L-aromatic amino acid decarboxylase may also be occurring (Johnson, Kim, and Boukma 1968), as well as competition for shared uptake mechanisms.

Other metabolic effects of L-DOPA. L-DOPA is largely O-methylated shortly after it is administered to the rat. Brain levels of the methyl donor, S-adenosylmethionine, are rapidly reduced by this reaction (Wurtman *et al.* 1970; Rose, Chou, and Wurtman 1970). Since S-adenosylmethionine is the methyl donor in the O-methylation of catecholamines by catechol-O-methyltransferase (COMT), there may be a reduction in the methylation of catecholamines due to competition with L-DOPA for S-adenosylmethionine. Relatively decreased O-methylated metabolites of ^{3}H-NE have been reported after L-DOPA administration (Chalmers, Baldessarini, and Wurtman, to be published), which is consistent with this formulation.

The principal O-methylated derivative of L-DOPA, 3-methoxytyrosine, is greatly increased in brain after L-DOPA administration (Kuruma, Bartholini, and Pletscher 1970). The predominant metabolic fate of O-methylated DOPA may be demethylation to DOPA, since it is a poor substrate for L-aromatic amino acid decarboxylase (Bouhon 1970). Since this substance is not an amine, it seems unlikely that it is acting as a false transmitter.

Pathophysiologic implications of clinical studies with L-DOPA and α-MPT. The effects of L-DOPA and α-MPT on norepinephrine and dopamine at "functionally important adrenergic receptor sites" in brain may be considered in the light of this biochemical knowledge. Although brain norepinephrine activity cannot be detected in man, the activity of dopamine can be; the therapeutic effect of L-DOPA in Parkinsonism is presumably due to increased dopamine activity at functionally important receptor sites. This implies that the doses of L-DOPA used in our depressed patients are adequate to produce increased dopamine activity in the central nervous system. Two mechanisms may be operating: First, it has been suggested that decreased O-methylation may potentiate the action of released norepinephrine and dopamine in brain (Wurtman *et al.* 1970). Second, increased synthesis may be associated with increased release of active amine (newly synthesized norepinephrine is preferentially released by nerve stimulation in cat spleen *in vitro*) (Kopin *et al.* 1968).

The mechanisms whereby L-DOPA may be producing increased dopamine activity are applicable to norepinephrine activity as well, suggesting that norepinephrine as well as dopamine activity may be increased in CNS in patients treated with L-DOPA. In view of this possibility, our clinical findings are of much interest. There was no consistent change in the symptoms of depressive illness. Psychomotor stimulation seemed a more widely applicable descriptive term to these patients than improvement in depression. Hypomania, however, was a consistent finding in bipolar patients treated with L-DOPA. These results are compatible with the hypothesis that increasing activity of dopamine and possibly also norepinephrine in brain was not generally associated with reversal of already established depressive illness in our patients. Increasing activity of catecholamines at adrenergic receptors may be associated with provocation of hypomania in patients with bipolar affective disorder. The multiple biochemical actions of L-DOPA, however, allow other possible explanations of the clinical results, such as that the changes in brain 5-HT or S-adenosylmethionine are responsible for the lack of clinical change in depression during L-DOPA treatment.

In comparison with L-DOPA, α-MPT has an opposite effect on catecholamine turnover in the central nervous system. Decreased catecholamine turnover is associated, presumably, with decreased release of the catecholamines, dopamine and norepinephrine, at the nerve ending. Unlike L-DOPA, α-MPT does not affect brain or cerebrospinal fluid levels of 5-HT and, since it is metabolized slowly and is not a substrate for COMT, one would not expect it to have an effect on S-adenosylmethionine or methylation reactions. α-MPT, then, is a more specific pharmacological tool for studying the effect of changes in catecholamine activity on the clinical state in affective illness.

α-MPT treatment, like L-DOPA treatment, was consistently associated with changes in mania in bipolar patients, but it did not produce any change in depression in two of six patients treated. In the manic state, although clinical change was consistently present, the direction of change (improvement or worsening) was very variable. The most consistent behavioral effect of α-MPT was sedation while on the drug, and rebound insomnia upon withdrawal.

During depression, it was the bipolar patients who had hypomanic episodes in response to L-DOPA, and the patients with cyclothymic histories (unipolar +) who showed clinical improvement. Unipolar patients without a hypomanic history generally did not show these changes in response to L-DOPA. The response to α-MPT in depression, however, did not follow the unipolar-bipolar division in the six patients studied.

As we have noted, one interpretation compatible with our current level of understanding is that the clinical effects of L-DOPA and α-MPT represent opposite pharmacological effects of stimulating or reducing functionally active dopamine and norepinephrine at receptor sites in the central nervous system. The clinical and biochemical findings with these agents could then be understood in a formulation such as this: In persons subject to mania, manipulation of catecholamine activity at the nerve ending is consistently associated with change in clinical state. There is not a simple relationship between the direction of change in catecholamines and the direction of change in clinical state. The direction of clinical change is a function of current clinical status, and possibly also of interindividual variations in the response to catecholamines. Depression represents a more heterogeneous set of disorders with regard to response to changes in CNS catecholamines. Although some patients show improvement after L-DOPA or worsening after α-MPT, others show no change in response to either agent; one possible interpretation of these data is that pharmacologic manipulations affecting the amount of available dopamine and norepinephrine at nerve endings in central nervous system may have no effect on clinical status in a significant proportion of patients with depression. This provocative hypothesis cannot be satisfactorily tested, however, until further investigation is performed on pharmacologic agents affecting central nervous system amines, and until a satisfactory yardstick is developed for activity of noradrenergic receptor sites in the central nervous system.

REFERENCES

Angst, J. 1966. Zur Atiologie und Nosologie endogener depressiver Psychosen. *Monographien aus dem Gesamtgebiete der Neurologie und Psychiatrie*, No. 112. Berlin: Springer-Verlag.

Anton, A. H., and Sayne, D. F. 1962. A study of the factors affecting the aluminum oxidethihydroxyindole procedure for the analysis of catecholamines. *J. Pharmacol. Exp. Ther.* 138:360.

Ashcroft, G. W.; Crawford, T. B. B.; Eccleston, D.; Sharman, D. F.; MacDougall, E. J.; Stanton, J. B.; and Binns, J. K. 1966. 5-Hydroxyindole compounds in the cerebrospinal fluid of patients with psychiatric or neurological diseases. *Lancet* 2:1049.

Ashcroft, G. W., and Sharman, D. F. 1960. 5-Hydroxyindoles in human cerebrospinal fluids. *Nature* 186:1050.

Ashcroft, G., and Sharman, D. F. 1962. Changes in the concentration of 5-OR indolyl compounds in cerebrospinal fluid and caudate nucleus. *Brit. J. Pharmacol.* 19:153.

Bertler, A.; Falck, B.; Owman, C.; and Rosengreen, E. 1966. The localization of monoaminergic blood-brain barrier mechanisms. *Pharmacol. Rev.* 18:369.

Bouhon, C. 1970. Pharmacological and immunological studies of catechol-O-methyltransferase. Seminar given at Laboratory of Clinical Science. National Institute of Mental Health.

Bowers, M. B., Jr., and Gerbode, F. 1968. CSF 5HIAA: Effects of probenecid and parachlorophenylalanine. *Life Sci.* 7:773.

Brodie, H. K. H.; Murphy, D. L.; Goodwin, F. K.; and Bunney, W. E., Jr. Catecholamines and mania: the effect of alpha-methyl-para-tyrosine on manic behavior and catecholamine metabolism. *Clin. Pharmacol. Ther.*, in press.

Bunney, W. E., Jr.; Brodie, H. K. H.; Murphy, D. L.; and Goodwin, F. K. 1971. Studies of alpha-methyl-para-tyrosine, L-DOPA, and L-tryptophan in depression and mania. *Amer. J. Psychiat.* 127:872.

Bunney, W. E., Jr., and Davis, J. M. 1965. Norepinephrine in depressive reactions. *Arch. Gen. Psychiat.* 13:483.

Bunney, W. E., Jr., and Hamburg, D. A. 1963. Methods for reliable longitudinal observation of behavior. *Arch. Gen. Psychiat.* 9:280.

Bunney, W. E., Jr.; Janowsky, D. S.; Goodwin, F. K.; Davis, J. M.; Brodie, H. K. H.; Murphy, D. L.; and Chase, T. N. 1969. Effect of L-DOPA on depression. *Lancet* 1:885.

Bunney, W. E., Jr.; Murphy, D. L.; Brodie, H. K. H.; and Goodwin, F. K. 1970. L-DOPA in depressed patients. *Lancet* 1:352.

Butcher, L. L., and Engel, J. 1969. Behavioral and biochemical effects of L-DOPA after peripheral decarboxylase inhibition. *Brain Res.* 15:233.

Calne, D. B.; Stern, G. M.; Laurence, D. R.; Sharkey, J.; and Armitage, P. 1969. L-DOPA in postencephalitic parkinsonism. *Lancet* 1:744.

Chalmers, J. P.; Baldessarini, R. J.; and Wurtman, R. J. Effects of L-DOPA on brain norepinephrine metabolism. To be published.

Coppen, A.; Prange, A. J.; Whybrow, P. C.; Noguera, R.; and Paez, J. M. 1969. Methysergide in mania: a controlled trial. *Lancet* 2:338.

Dencker, S. J.; Malm, U.; Roos, B. E.; and Werdinius, B. 1966. Acid monoamine metabolites of cerebrospinal fluid in mental depression and mania. *J. Neurochem.* 13:1545.

Dunner, D. L.; Gershon, E. S.; and Goodwin, F. K. 1970. Heritable factors in the severity of affective illness. Presented to annual meeting American Psychiatric Association, San Francisco.

Engelman, K; Horwitz, D.; Jequier, E.; and Sjoerdsma, A. 1968. Biochemical and pharmacologic effects of α-methyltyrosine in man. *J. Clin. Invest.* 47:577.

Everett, G. M., and Borcherding, J. W. 1970. L-DOPA: Effect on concentrations of dopamine, norepinephrine and serotonin in brains of mice. *Science* 168:849.

Gerbode, F., and Bowers, W. 1960. Measurement of acid monoamine metabolites in human and animal cerebrospinal fluid. *J. Neurochem.* 15:1053.

Gershon, E. S.; Goodwin, F. K; and Gold, P. 1970. Effect of L-tyrosine and L-DOPA on norepinephrine turnover in rat brain in vivo. *Pharmacologist* 12:268.

Goodwin-Austen, R. B.; Tomlinson, E. B.; Frears, C. C.; and Kok, H.W.L. 1969. Effects of L-DOPA in Parkinson's disease. *Lancet* 2:165.

Goodwin, F. K.; Brodie, H. K. H.; Murphy, D. L.; and Bunney, W. E., Jr. 1970a. Administration of a peripheral decarboxylase inhibitor with L-DOPA to depressed patients. *Lancet* 1:908.

Goodwin, F. K.; Dunner, D. L.; and Gershon, E. S. Turnover estimates of brain amines in depressed patients treated with L-DOPA. In preparation, 1971.

Goodwin, F. K.; Murphy, D. L.; Brodie, H. K. H.; and Bunney, W. E., Jr. 1970b. L-DOPA, catecholamines, and behavior: a clinical and biochemical study in depressed patients. *Biol. Psychiat.* 2:341.

Goodwin, F. K.; Murphy, D. L.; Dunner, D. L.; Bunney, W. E., Jr. 1971. Lithium response in unipolar vs. bipolar depression. Presentation to annual meeting, American Psychiatric Association, Washington, D. C.

Greenspan, K.; Schildkraut, J. J.; Gordon, E. K.; Baer, L.; Aronoff, M. S.; and Durell, J. 1970. Catecholamine metabolism in affective disorders -- III: MHPG and other catecholamine metabolites in patients treated with lithium carbonate. *J. Psychiat. Res.* 7:171.

Guldberg, H. C.; Ashcroft, G. W.; and Crawford, T. B. B. 1966. Concentrations of 5-hydroxyindoleacetic acid and homovanillic acid in the cerebrospinal fluid of the dog before and during treatment with probenecid. *Life Sci.* 5:1571.

Ingvarsson, V. C. G. 1965. Orientierende klinische Versuche zur Wirkung des Dioxyphenylalanins (L-DOPA) bei endogener Depression. *Arzneimittelforschung* 15:849.

Janowsky, D. S.; Leff, M.; and Epstein, R. S. 1970. Playing the manic game. *Arch. Gen. Psychiat.* 22:252.

Johnson, G. A.; Kim, E. G.; and Boukma, S. J. 1968. Mechanism of NE depletion by 5-hydroxytryptophan. *Proc. Soc. Exp. Biol. Med.* (Pharmacol.) 128:509.

Klerman, G. L.; Schildkraut, J. J.; Hasenbush, L. L.; Greenblatt, M.; and Friend, D. G. 1963. Clinical experience with dihydroxyphenylalanine (Dopa) in depression. *J. Psychiat. Res.* 1:289.

Kopin, I. J.; Breese, G. R.; Krauss, R. R.; and Weise, V. K. 1968. Selective release of newly synthesized norepinephrine from the cat spleen during sympathetic nerve stimulation. *J. Pharmacol. Exp. Ther.* 161:271.

Kopin, I. J., and Gordon, E. Unpublished communication.

Kuruma, I.; Bartholini, G.; and Pletscher, A. 1970. L-DOPA induced accumulation of 3-O-methyl-DOPA in brain and heart. *Europ. J. Pharmacol.* 10:189.

Leonhard, K.; Korff, I.; and Shulz, H. 1962. Die Temperamente in den Familien der monopolaren und bipolaren phasischen Psychosen. *Psychiat. Neurol.* 143:416.

Maas, J. W.; Fawcett, J.; and Dekirmenjian, H. 1968. 3-Methoxy-4-hydroxy phenylglycol (MHPG) excretion in depressive states. *Arch.*

Gen. Psychiat. 18:129.

Maas, J. W.; Fawcett, J.; Dekirmenjian, H.; and Landis, D. H. Catecholamine metabolism and depressive states: current studies, in NIMH workshop, recent advances in the psychobiology of depressive illnesses, held in Williamsburg, Virginia, April 1969. U. S. Govt. Printing Office, in press.

Mannarino, E.; 'Kirshner, N.; and Nashold, B. S. 1963. The metabolism of [C^{14}] noradrenaline by cat brain in vivo. J. Neurochem. 10:373.

Matussek, N.; Pohlmeier, H.; and Ruther, E. 1966. Die Wirkung von Dopa auf gehemmte Depressionen. Klin. Wschr. 44:727.

McDowell, F.; Lee, J. E.; Swift, T.; Sweet, R. D.; Ogsbury, J. S.; and Kessler, J. T. 1970. Treatment of Parkinson's syndrome with 1-dihydroxyphenylalanine (levodopa). Ann. Intern. Med. 72:29.

McNemar, Q. 1969. Psychological Statistics. 4th Ed. New York: Wiley.

Murphy, D. L.; Brodie, H. K. H.; Goodwin, F. K.; and Bunney, W. E., Jr. 1971. Regular induction of hypomania by L-DOPA in "bipolár" manic-depressive patients. Nature 229:135.

Neff, N. H.; Tozer, T. N.; and Brodie, B. B. 1967. Application of steady-state kinetics to studies of the transfer of 5-hydroxyindoleacetic acid from brain to plasma. J. Pharmacol. Exp. Ther. 158:214.

Ng, K. Y.; Chase, T. N.; Colburn, R. W.; and Kopin, I. J. 1971. L-DOPA induced release of cerebral monoamines. Science 170:76.

O'Brien, C. P.; DiGiacomo, J. N.; Fahn, S.; and Schwarz, G. A. 1971. Mental effects of high-dosage levodopa. Arch. Gen. Psychiat. 24:61.

Pare, C. M. B., and Sandler, M. J. 1959. A clinical and biochemical study of a trial of iproniazid in the treatment of depression. J. Neurol. Neurosurg. Psychiat. 22:247.

Perris, C. 1966. A study of bipolar (manic-depressive) and unipolar recurrent depressive psychoses. Acta Psychiat. Scand. 42:suppl. 194.

Roos, B. E.; and Sjostrum, R. 1969. 5-Hydroxyindoleacetic acid (and homovanillic acid) levels in the cerebrospinal fluid after probenecid application in patients with manic-depressive psychosis. Pharmacologia Clinica 1:153.

Rose, C. M.; Chou, C.; and Wurtman, R. J. 1970. The metabolism of ^{14}C-DOPA in the whole mouse. Fed. Proc. 29:511.

Sato, T. L. 1965. The quantitative determination of 3-methoxy-4-hydroxyphenylacetic acid (homovanillic acid) in urine. J. Lab. Clin. Med. 66:517.

Schanberg, S. M.; Schildkraut, J. J.; and Kopin, I. J. 1967. Normetanephrine H^3 (NMN-H^3) turnover and conversion to a deaminated conjugate as a major metabolite in rat brain. Fed. Proc. 26:464.

Schildkraut, J. J. 1965. The catecholamine hypothesis of affective disorders: A review of supporting evidence. Amer. J. Psychiat. 122:509.

Sjoerdsma, A.; Engelman, K.; Spector, S.; and Udenfriend, S. 1965. Inhibition of catecholamine synthesis in man with alphamethyltyrosine, an inhibitor of tyrosine hydroxylase. Lancet 2:1092.

Sourkes, T. L., and Murphy, G. F. 1961. Determination of catecholamines and catecholamino acids by differential spectrophotofluorimetry. *Meth. Med. Res.* 9:147.
Spector, S.; Sjoerdsma, A.; and Udenfriend, S. 1965. Blockade of endogenous norepinephrine synthesis by α-methyl-tyrosine, an inhibitor of tyrosine hydroxylase. *J. Pharmacol. Exp. Ther.* 147:86.
Turner, W., and Merlis, S. 1964. A clinical trial of pargyline and Dopa in psychotic subjects. *Dis. Nerv. Syst.* 25:538.
Udenfriend, S. 1966. Tyrosine hydroxylase. *Pharmacol. Rev.* 18:43.
Udenfriend, S.; Titus, E.; and Weissbach, H. 1955. The identification of 5-hydroxy-3-indoleacetic acid in normal urine and a method for its assay. *J. Biol. Chem.* 216:499.
Udenfriend, S.; Zaltzman-Nirenberg, P.; Gordon, R.; and Spector, S. 1966. Evaluation of the biochemical effects produced in vivo by inhibitors of the three enzymes involved in norepinephrine biosynthesis. *Molec. Pharmacol.* 2:95.
van Praag, H. M.; Korff, J.; and Puite, J. 1970. 5-Hydroxyindoleacetic acid levels in the cerebrospinal fluid of depressive patients treated with probenecid. *Nature* 225:1259.
Weil-Malherbe, H. The estimation of total (free and conjugated) catecholamines and some catecholamine metabolites in human urine. In *Methods of Biochemical Analysis*. D. Glick (ed.). 16:293. Interscience Publishers, in press.
Werdinius, B. 1966. Effect of probenecid on the level of homovanillic acid in the corpus striatum. *J. Pharmacol. Exp. Ther.* 18:546.
Werdinius, B. 1967. Effect of probenecid on the levels of monoamine metabolites in the rat brain. *Acta Pharmacol.* 25:18.
Wilk, S.; Gitlow, S. E.; Clarke, D. D.; and Paley, D. H. 1967. Determination of urinary 3-methoxy-4-hydroxy-phenylethylene glycol by gas-liquid chromatography and electron capture detection. *Clin. Chim. Acta* 16:403.
Winokur, G.; Clayton, P. J.; and Reich, T. 1969. *Manic-Depressive Illness*. St. Louis: C. V. Mosby.
Wurtman, R. J.; Rose, C. M.; Matthysse, S.; Stephenson, J.; and Baldessarini, R. 1970. L-Dihydroxyphenylalanine: effect on S-adenosylmethionine in brain. *Science* 169:395.
Yahr, M. D.; Duvoisin, R. C.; Schear, J. J.; Barrett, R. E.; and Hoehn, M. M. 1969. Treatment of Parkinsonism with levodopa. *Arch. Neurol.* 21:343.

RELATIONSHIPS BETWEEN STRESS AND BRAIN 5-HYDROXYTRYPTAMINE

AND THEIR POSSIBLE SIGNIFICANCE IN AFFECTIVE DISORDERS

G. Curzon

Institute of Neurology

London, England

The work I will describe was prompted by the hope of eventually developing an animal model relevant to depressive illness. It is a truism that any animal model of a human affective disturbance suffers from a limitation imposed by the relative inability of animals to communicate with us, and this is compounded by our own tendency to anthropomorphize. Such limitations do not apply to the partial and less ambitious models in which biochemical abnormalities reported in the disturbance are simulated in animals. Here, however, the questions arise whether these abnormalities in man are in any way responsible for the disturbed mood or behavior, and whether the way in which the biochemical model is generated in the animal has etiological relevance.

Using rats we have investigated a relationship between two biochemical parameters for which there is some evidence of abnormality in depressive illness--defective brain 5-hydroxytryptamine (5-HT) metabolism and high levels of plasma cortisol. There is fairly good evidence consistent with abnormal brain amine metabolism in depression (Bunney and Davis 1965; Maclean *et al*. 1965), and in particular with a functional deficiency of 5-HT (Coppen *et al*. 1967; van Praag and Leijnse 1963; van Praag, Korf, and Puite 1970; Shaw, Camps, and Eccleston 1967). The relationship between depression and cortisol levels, however, is more controversial. Although high corticoid levels have been found by many workers (Hullin *et al*. 1967; Bridges and Jones 1966; Doig *et al*. 1966), the significance of these findings has been questioned (Brooksbank and Coppen 1967; Sachar 1967). Earlier studies of the relationship between pituitary adrenal function and depression have been reviewed in some detail by Fawcett and Bunney (1967). A particularly well-planned investi-

TABLE 1

Urinary Excretion of Tryptophan Metabolites by
Female Subjects after 30 mg/kg L-Tryptophan

	Kynurenine	3-Hydroxy-kynurenine	3-Hydroxy-anthranilic acid
Endogenous Depression			
Ill	148±153 (9)[1]	151±133 (9)	75±61 (9)
Recovered	135±126 (9)	159±108 (9)[2]	100±49 (9)
Mean	143± 95 (9)[3]	155± 50 (9)[4]	82±21 (9)
Not with Endogenous Depression			
Ill	29± 14 (9)[1]	65± 40 (9)	86±51 (9)
Recovered	40± 26 (7)	62± 31 (7)[2]	97±51 (7)
Mean	35± 17 (7)[3]	65± 29 (7)[4]	92±46 (7)

All determinations are in μmoles. Numbers of subjects in parentheses.

1, 2, 3 -- pairs of values significantly different $p < 0.05$ to 0.01.

4 -- $p < 0.01$

All other relevant pairs are not significantly different.

gation in which high levels were found in depression was described by Fullerton *et al.* (1968a and b).

In view of these findings, we wondered whether a biochemical relationship occurring in depression might involve provocation of elevated adrenocortical secretion by various mechanisms or combinations of mechanisms--environmental stimulus, for example, or hypersensitivity to environmental stimulus, or defective regulation of secretion--and that this adrenocortical charge might result in defective brain 5-HT synthesis, possibly with behavioral consequences. It seemed reasonable and, indeed, it had often been suggested that brain 5-HT synthesis might be decreased by a mechanism involving the well-known induction of the liver enzyme, tryptophan pyrrolase, by adrenocortical hormones, this causing diversion of tryptophan from the pathway of 5-HT synthesis. This possibility is strengthened by the finding that female patients classified as endogenous depressives converted significantly more of a tryptophan load to metabolites formed subsequent to pyrrolase action than did mental hospital patients classified otherwise (Table 1) (Curzon and Bridges 1970).

Evidence has now been obtained that adrenocortical activity may result in decreased brain 5-HT in the rat. Whether this occurs through a change of pyrrolase activity or whether decreased brain 5-HT and increased liver pyrrolase are two separate, unrelated effects of adrenocortical activity is less certain.

Summarizing our recent findings, cortisol was shown to cause a significant fall of both brain 5-HT and its metabolite, 5-hydroxyindoleacetic acid (5-HIAA) (Curzon and Green 1968). The maximum falls after 5 mg/kg Solu-Cortef (cortisol) intraperitoneally were about 30 percent and they occurred six to seven hours after injection. Since both 5-HT and 5-HIAA fell, results probably indicated decreased 5-HT synthesis (Figure 1). Higher doses of cortisol did not result in larger falls of 5-HT. This suggests perhaps, that not all pools of brain 5-HT are susceptible or that these higher dosages have other effects that oppose the 5-HT fall. The rather long interval between injection and maximum change of brain 5-HT suggests that the mechanism responsible is an indirect one, and the fact that a rise of liver pyrrolase preceded the 5-HT change was consistent with a causal relationship between these two effects of cortisol. A stronger indication of such a relationship was that drugs reported to decrease rat liver pyrrolase activity also prevented the fall of 5-HT after cortisol. Allopurinol and yohimbine had this effect (Green and Curzon 1968).

Not only cortisol but corticosterone and the synthetic corticoid, betamethasone (Scapagnini, De Schaepdryver, and Preziosi 1969), and the oral contraceptive, norethynodrel plus mestranol (Nistico and Preziosi 1970), all cause both a fall in brain 5-HT and an increase in liver pyrrolase. The mechanism by which 5-HT falls is not known. Three possibilities have been suggested, all of them involving increased pyrrolase activity. The first, most obvious, and most frequent speculation is that a decrease in brain tryptophan levels results in decreased brain 5-HT synthesis. This seems unlikely; although cortisol caused plasma tryptophan to fall transiently, total brain tryptophan did not change significantly (Green, Joseph, and Curzon 1970). A second suggestion is that induction of pyrrolase results in increased tryptophan metabolism on the pyrrolase pathway and that, since many steps subsequent to kynurenine formation require pyridoxal, there are increased demands for this sub-

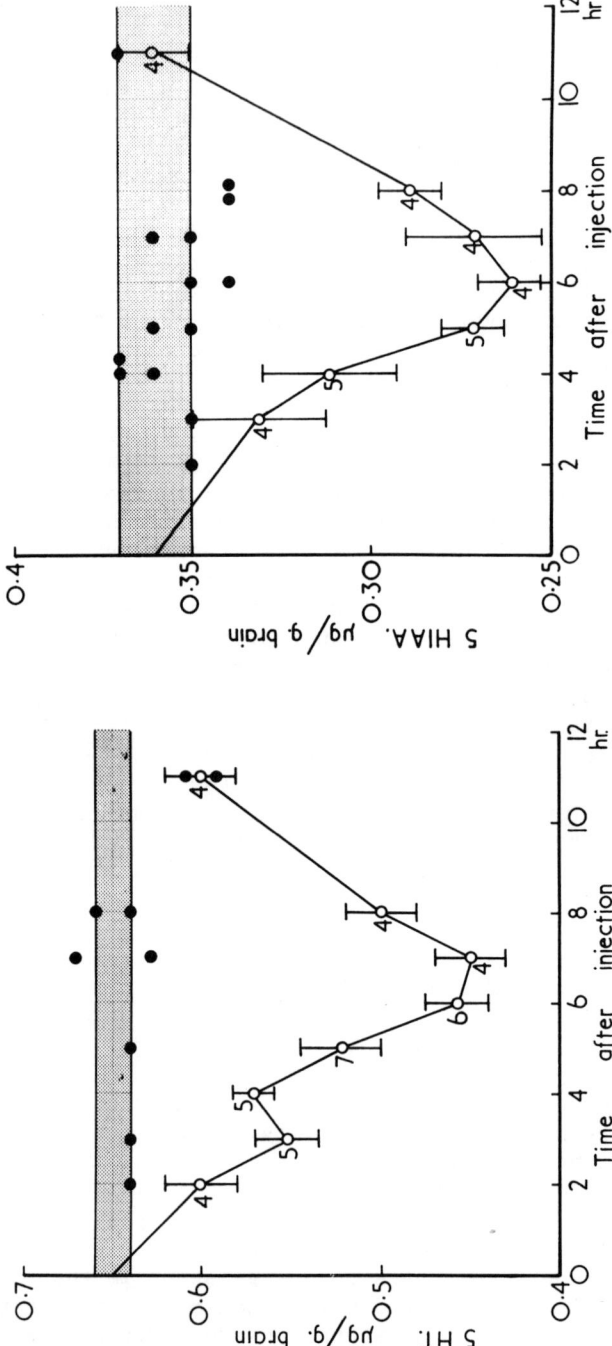

Figure 1. Effects of 5 mg/kg cortisol on rat brain 5-HT and 5-HIAA. Open circles: cortisol injected. Number of rats on which determinations were done is shown. Closed circles: saline injected. Shaded areas: mean determinations on uninjected rats ± 1 S.D. Differences between cortisol-injected and -uninjected rats are significant ($p < 0.01$) for 5-HT (2 to 8 hours inclusive, after injection) and for 5-HIAA (4 to 8 hours inclusive, after injection).

stance. A functional deficiency of pyridoxal in the brain then leads to low 5-hydroxytryptophan decarboxylase activity and thus to low brain 5-HT. This mechanism has been discussed specifically in relation to depression in women taking oral contraceptives. Evidence is against its being responsible for the fall of rat brain 5-HT after cortisol because this was not prevented by pyridoxine (Table 2). One cannot exclude the possibility, however, that 5-HT synthesis in human brain may be more sensitive to pyridoxal changes than in rat brain. A third possibility is that elevated levels of tryptophan metabolites formed on the pyrrolase pathway result in decreased brain 5-HT synthesis. It has been shown that kynurenine, hydroxykynurenine, and hydroxyanthranilic acid injected into rats cause a fall of brain 5-HT (Green and Curzon 1970). The likelihood that these substances are responsible for the fall after cortisol is difficult to assess, however, because we know almost nothing about their *in vivo* levels.

Whether increased pyrrolase activity is in fact responsible for the fall and pyrrolase inhibition responsible for its prevention is also debatable. Although allopurinol markedly inhibits pyrrolase activity when a standard *in vitro* pyrrolase assay of liver homogenate and high concentration of added tryptophan is used, Kim and Miller (1969) showed that this assay system may grossly exaggerate *in vivo* changes of pyrrolase activity. This is probably so because the ratio of active to inactive forms is influenced by tryptophan concentration.

TABLE 2

Effect of Cortisol on
Tryptophan Metabolism in the Rat

Treatment	Hours after Injection	Plasma Tryptophan (μg/ml plasma)	Brain Tryptophan (μg/gm brain wet wt.)
Saline	3	19.7±0.9 (5)	3.31±0.31 (5)
Hydrocortisone	3	14.6±2.2 (6)*	3.13±0.21 (6)

Number of determinations shown in parentheses.
*Different from control $p < 0.01$.

TABLE 3

Effect of Allopurinol on Cortisol-Provoked
Increase of $^{14}CO_2$ (Counts/Min.) from DL-Tryptophan-2-^{14}C

	Time after 0.65 µCi tryptophan (hours)		
Injected*	0.5	1.0	1.5
Saline	215 (4)	510 (4)	965 (4)
Cortisol 5 mg/kg	555 (4)	1485 (4)	2300 (4)
Allopurinol 20 mg/kg plus Cortisol 5 mg/kg	565 (3)	1880 (3)	3000 (3)

*2.5 hr. before injection of tracer amount of tryptophan.
Number of rats in parentheses.

From Green, A. R. 1969.

It was important, therefore, to investigate the effect of allopurinol on *in vivo* pyrrolase activity. This was done by measuring labeled CO_2 output after injecting a tracer amount of D,L-tryptophan labeled in the 2-position of the pyrrole ring. Allopurinol did not oppose the increase of CO_2 output caused by previous cortisol injection and, thus, evidence of inhibition *in vivo* could not be obtained (Table 3). In a similar *in vivo* assay, however, Sourkes and Missala (1969) were able to show that yohimbine which, like allopurinol, prevents the decrease of brain 5-HT after cortisol, did inhibit pyrrolase.

Whatever the mechanism by which cortisol causes brain 5-HT to fall may be, this finding--though of pharmacological interest--would be without much physiological or pathological interest if the adrenal gland *in vivo* were not also capable of secreting sufficient corticoid material to cause such a change. We were able to show, however, that when rats were placed under stress by being immobilized, their brain 5-HT fell (Table 4). This has now been confirmed by Nistico and Preziosi (1969). The change seemed to be mediated through the adrenal gland since it did not occur in adrenalectomized animals (Curzon and Green 1969). Unlike the findings of the cortisol experiments, 5-HIAA did not fall, but rose, and this increase occurred in both intact and adrenalectomized animals. Allopurinol partly prevented the fall of 5-HT in the intact animals, but it had no effect on the adrenalectomized ones. These results point to

TABLE 4

Effects of Immobilization and Allopurinol on Liver
Tryptophan Pyrrolase and Brain 5-HT and 5-HIAA

Treatment	Injected	Pyrrolase Activity (μmoles kynurenine/ hr/gm liver dry wt.)	5-HT (μg/gm brain wet wt.)	5-HIAA
Control	--	5.17±1.73 (4)		
Immobilized 3 hr.	--	19.52±4.00 (4)[1]		
Immobilized 3 hr.	allopurinol 20 mg/kg	4.09±0.09 (4)		
Control	--	5.52±0.98 (11)	0.64±0.02 (10)	0.35±0.02 (8)
Immobilized 5 hr.	saline	21.20±9.06 (7)[1]	0.47±0.04 (8)[1]	0.51±0.04 (7)[1]
Immobilized 5 hr.	allopurinol 20 mg/kg	13.80±6.42 (9)	0.56±0.03 (10)[1,2]	0.47±0.04 (8)[1]
Adrenalectomized rats				
Control	saline	5.60±1.84 (9)	0.71±0.03 (9)	0.36±0.01 (6)
Immobilized 5 hr.	saline	6.96±3.76 (4)	0.65±0.02 (4)[1]	0.56±0.04 (4)[1]
Immobilized 5 hr.	allopurinol 20 mg/kg	3.08±0.40 (4)	0.64±0.02 (4)[1]	0.55±0.03 (4)[1]

Number of animals in parentheses. [1]Different from control $p < 0.01$. [2]Different from immobilized saline-treated $p < 0.01$. From Curzon, G., and Green, A. R. 1969. Reprinted with permission from *Brit. J. Pharmacol.* 37:689.

immobilization as causing the fall of 5-HT through the influence of the adrenal gland, possibly via an increase in pyrrolase, and to an increase in 5-HT turnover, as shown by the 5-HIAA rise. The latter seems to occur through a more direct central effect.

These findings point to one factor that may influence brain 5-HT metabolism. There are, of course, many other important influences, and we cannot infer that, normally, brain 5-HT metabolism is entirely at the mercy of the adrenal gland. It may be significant that brain 5-HT and 5-HIAA values both rose back toward control values when immobilization was prolonged (Curzon and Green 1969) (Figure 2). Moreover, when cortisol was injected once a day, brain 5-HT was low six hours after injection on the first and second days, but when injections were continued for five days or more, brain 5-HT no longer fell (Curzon and Green 1968). In both of these experiments, pyrrolase activity remained high throughout. Somewhat similar results were obtained by Nistico and Preziosi (1970) who found that rats injected for ten days with the oral contraceptive mixture, norethynodrel plus mestranol, showed a significant fall of brain 5-HT, though not of 5-HIAA, and high liver pyrrolase, whereas both 5-HT and pyrrolase returned to normal upon more prolonged treatment. These findings suggest the existence of regulatory mechanisms that oppose the falls of 5-HT. It is worth noting that Azmitia and McEwen (1969) found that the activity of tryptophan hydroxylase, an enzyme required by the rat for the rate-determining step in brain 5-HT synthesis, is dependent on adrenal activity. Another significant point is that both cortisol injection and the imposition of immobilization are sudden changes. It may be that more gradual changes in corticoid levels or less suddenly imposed stresses lead less readily to detectable changes of 5-HT level, because regulatory mechanisms may be able to compensate for them more effectively. One is led to the possibility that inefficient mechanisms for brain amine regulation may have a role in the genesis and persistence of depressive states or other affective disorders. Interesting evidence already exists for a defect in feedback control in severe depression, that is, in the inhibition of ACTH output by adrenocortical secretion (Butler and Besser 1968; Carroll 1969; McLeod, Carroll, and Davies 1970), although this abnormality is not restricted solely to depression; it also follows surgical shock (Liddle, Island, and Meador 1962) and occurs in Cushing's disease.

If one looks at the proposed model for relationships between biochemical changes in endogenous depression from a wider point of view, one might think that a stress situation such as immobilization--though it may provide an analogy to reactive depression--bears little relationship to endogenous depression in which precipitating stressful circumstances are usually thought not to have a major role.

However, the judgment by either doctor or patient of circum-

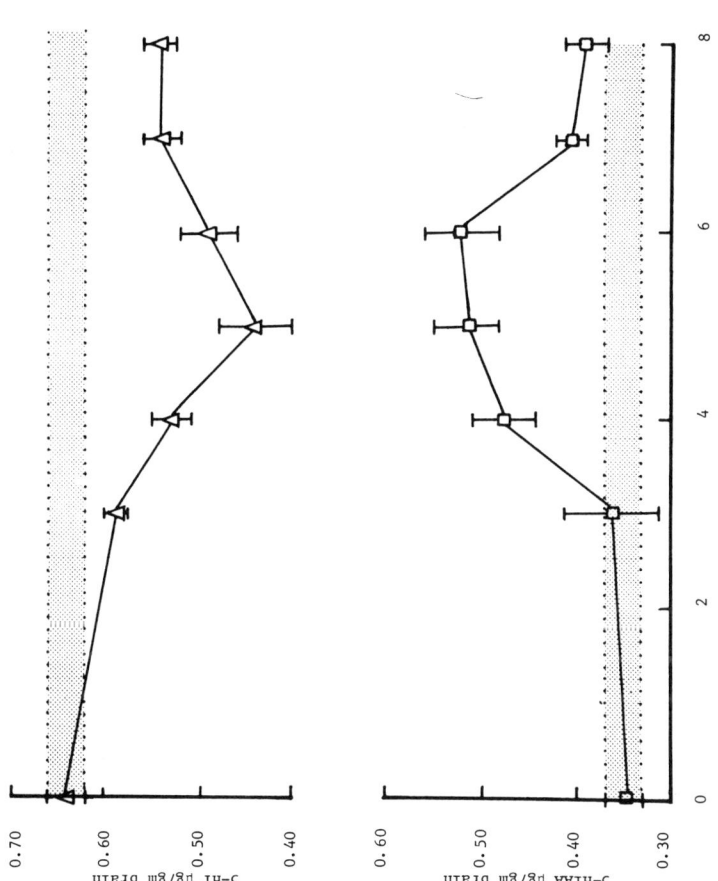

Figure 2. Effect of duration of immobilization on rat brain 5-hydroxytryptamine (5-HT) and 5-hydroxyindoleacetic acid (5-HIAA). △ : 5-HT; □ : 5-HIAA. Points represent means (± S.D.) of determinations on at least four rats. Shaded areas indicate mean (± S.D.) of determinations on uninjected control animals.

stance as being precipitant involves subjective decisions and is
dependent upon depth of enquiry and introspective ability. Lewis
(1938) has commented that "the more thorough the analysis that can
be made of the life of the patient and of his response to circumstances the stronger is our inclination" to consider his disease as
reactive. Even when precipitating circumstances are not discover-
able, there may be a physiologically determined inability to adjust
to changes in environment or state that, being small or part of the
normal pattern of life, may easily be disregarded. Thus, absence
of precipitants may be more apparent than real. Furthermore, metabolic response to stress situation may be very variable. Some evidence that endogenous depressives may be particularly responsive to
stresses is provided by Elithorn *et al.* (1969) who determined the
rise in plasma cortisol in depressive patients upon initial electroconvulsive treatment, and showed that this increase was much greater than in a similarly treated schizophrenic group. It is, of
course, debatable whether this in fact indicates the response of
depressives to be abnormally large, or that of schizophrenics to be
abnormally small.

Recent work with rats of different ages (Green and Curzon,
unpublished) shows that the response to the same dose per kilogram
of injected cortisol is very different, significant falls of brain
5-HT and 5-HIAA occurring only in the younger animals (65 days and
younger), while the increase in pyrrolase activity per gram of liver
is greater in the younger than in the older animals. Furthermore,
while younger rats responded to immobilization with a large increase
in pyrrolase activity and a fall of brain 5-HT, older animals showed
a much smaller pyrrolase and no 5-HT change. Rather similarly,
Schapiro, Geller, and Yuwiler (1965/66) found that infant rats respond to 30-minute shocking with large increases of liver aromatic
amino acid transaminase activities, while adult rats do not. These
findings point to defective maturation of metabolic response to
adrenocortical change as a factor to be studied in affective illness.
There was no obvious difference between the responses of male and
female rats to cortisol. It would be worthwhile, however, to look
at the responses of female rats at different stages of the menstrual
cycle.

It is necessary to discuss whatever evidence there may be to
suggest, not merely that increased adrenocortical activity or low
brain 5-HT occurs in endogenous depression, but that these changes
have a role in the causation of symptoms. Depression occurs fairly
frequently in association with the adrenal hyperactivity of Cushing's
disease (Trethowan and Cobb 1952), and also in association with the
hypoactivity of Addison's disease (Cleghorn 1951). In addition,
euphoria has been reported more frequently than depression following
corticoid administration (see Rubin and Mandell 1966 for references).
Perhaps it would be naive to expect one specific mood or behavioral

response when substances with manifold metabolic effects are given to patients at varying dosage and duration and for a therapeutic purpose.

In view of the often reported early-morning waking in depression, it is of interest that patients on high dosage of cortisone or ACTH are said often to have difficulty in sleeping (Clark, Bauer, and Cobb 1952). The frequently found abnormal diurnal variation of plasma cortisol in endogenous depression (Bridges and Jones 1966; Doig et al. 1966; McClure 1966; Knapp, Keane, and Wright 1967; but not Fullerton et al. 1969a and b), the plasma cortisol peak being displaced to an earlier time, might possibly cause a similar displacement of a brain 5-HT minimum. Animal experiments suggest this could result in early waking. For example, Weitzmann et al. (1968) found increased wakefulness in monkeys when they were given sufficient amounts of the inhibitor of 5-HT synthesis, p-chlorophenylalanine, to cause a moderate decrease of brain 5-HT. The best defined behavioral change associated with low 5-HT in rat brain obtained either by midbrain raphe lesions (Kostowski et al. 1968), or by inhibition of synthesis (Brody 1970) is an increased sensitivity to external stimulation. Brody, however, also found slightly decreased activity when external stimulation was absent. One can only speculate about the analogy these changes may bear to depression or to such other affective states as anxiety.

ACKNOWLEDGMENT

I thank the Medical Research Council, the Mental Health Research Fund, and the Research Advisory Committee of the Institute of Neurology for financial support.

REFERENCES

Azmitia, E. C., and McEwen, B. S. 1969. Corticosterone regulation of tryptophan hydroxylase in mid-brain of the rat. *Science* 166:1274.

Bridges, P. K.; and Jones, M. T. 1966. The diurnal rhythm of plasma cortisol concentration in depression. *Brit. J. Psychiat.* 112:1157.

Brody, J. F. 1970. Behavioural effects of serotonin depletion and of p-chlorophenylalanine (a serotonin depletor) in rats. *Psychopharmacologia* 17:14.

Brooksbank, B. W. L., and Coppen, A. 1967. Plasma 11-hydroxycorticoids in affective disorders. *Brit. J. Psychiat.* 113:395.

Bunney, W. E., and Davis, J. M. 1965. Norepinephrine in depressive reactions: A review. *Arch. Gen. Psychiat.* 13:483.

Butler, P. W. P., and Besser, G. M. 1968. Pituitary-adrenal function in severe depressive disease. *Lancet* 1:1234.

Carroll, B. J. 1969. Hypothalamic-pituitary function in depressive illness: Insensitivity to hypoglycaemia. *Brit. Med. J.* 3:27.

Clark, L. D.; Bauer, W.; and Cobb, S. 1952. Preliminary observations on mental disturbances occurring in patients under therapy with cortisone and ACTH. *New Eng. J. Med.* 246:205.

Cleghorn, R. A. 1951. Adrenal cortical insufficiency: psychological and neurological observations. *Canad. Med. Assoc. J.* 65:449.

Coppen, A.; Shaw, D. M.; Herzberg, B; and Maggs, R. 1967. Tryptophan in the treatment of depression. *Lancet* 2:1178.

Curzon, G.; and Bridges, P. K. 1970. Tryptophan metabolism in depression. *J. Neurol. Neurosurg. Psychiat.* 33:698.

Curzon, G., and Green, A. R. 1968. Effect of hydrocortisone on rat brain 5-hydroxytryptamine. *Life Sci.* 7:657.

Curzon, G.; and Green, A. R. 1969. Effects of immobilization on rat liver tryptophan pyrrolase and brain 5-hydroxytryptamine metabolism. *Brit. J. Pharmacol.* 37:689.

Doig, R. J.; Mummery, R. V.; Wills, M. R., and Elkes, A. 1966. Plasma cortisol levels in depression. *Brit. J. Psychiat.* 112:1263.

Elithorn, A.; Bridges, P. K.; Hodges, J. R.; and Jones, M. T. 1969. Adrenocortical responsiveness during courses of electro-convulsive therapy. *Brit. J. Psychiat.* 115:575.

Fawcett, J. A., and Bunney, W. E. 1967. Pituitary adrenal function and depression. *Arch. Gen. Psychiat.* 16:517.

Fullerton, D. T.; Wenzel, F. J.; Lohrenz, F. N.; and Fahs, H. 1968a. Circadian rhythm of adrenal cortical activity in depression. I. A comparison of depressed patients with normal subjects. *Arch. Gen. Psychiat.* 19:674.

Fullerton, D. T.; Wenzel, F. J.; Lohrenz, F. N., and Fahs, H. 1968b. Circadian rhythm of adrenal cortical activity in depression. II. A comparison of types in depression. *Arch. Gen. Psychiat.* 19:682.

Green, A. R. 1969. Effects of hydrocortisone and stress on tryptophan metabolism. Ph.D. Thesis, University of London.

Green, A. R.; and Curzon, G. 1968. Decrease of 5-hydroxytryptamine in the brain provoked by hydrocortisone and its prevention by allopurinol. *Nature* 220:1095.

Green, A. R., and Curzon, G. 1970. The effect of tryptophan metabolites on brain 5-hydroxytryptamine metabolism. *Biochem. Pharmacol.* 19:2061.

Green, A. R.; Joseph, M. G.; and Curzon, G. 1970. Oral contraceptives, depression and amino acid metabolism. *Lancet* 1:1288.

Hullin, R. P.; Bailey, A. D.; McDonald, R.; Dransfield, G. A.; and Milne, H. B. 1967. Variations in 11-hydroxycorticosteroids in depression and manic-depressive psychosis. *Brit. J. Psychiat.* 113:593.

Kim, J. H., and Miller, L. L. 1969. The functional significance of changes in activity of the enzymes, tryptophan pyrrolase and tyrosine transaminase, after induction in intact rats and in the isolated, perfused rat liver. *J. Biol. Chem.* 244:1410.

Knapp, M. S.; Keane, P. M.; and Wright, J. G. 1967. Circadian rhythm of plasma 11-hydroxycorticoids in depressive illness, congestive heart failure, and Cushing's syndrome. *Brit. Med. J.* 2:27.

Kostowski, W.; Giacalone, E.; Garattini, S.; and Valzelli, L. 1968. Studies on behavioural and biochemical changes in rats after lesion of mid-brain raphe. *Europ. J. Pharmacol.* 4:37.

Lewis, A. 1938. States of depression: their clinical and aetiological differentiation. *Brit. Med. J.* 2:875.

Liddle, G. W.; Island, D.; and Meador, C. K. 1962. Normal and abnormal regulation of corticotrophin secretion in man. *Recent Progr. Hormone Res.* 18:125.

Maclean, R.; Nicholson, W. J.; Pare, C. M. B.; and Stacey, R. S. 1965. Effect of monoamine oxidase inhibitors on the concentration of 5-hydroxy-tryptamine in the human brain. *Lancet* 2:205.

McClure, D. J. 1966. The diurnal variation of plasma cortisol levels in depression. *J. Psychosom. Res.* 10:189.

McLeod, W. R.; Carroll, B. J.; and Davies, B. 1970. Hypothalamic dysfunction and antidepressant drugs. *Brit. Med. J.* 2:480.

Nistico, G., and Preziosi, P. 1969. Brain and liver tryptophan pathways and adrenocortical activation during restraint stress. *Pharmacol. Res. Commun.* 1:363.

Nistico, G., and Preziosi, P. 1970. Contraceptives, brain serotonin and liver tryptophan pyrrolase. *Lancet* 2:213.

Rubin, R. T., and Mandell, A. J. 1966. Adrenal cortical activity in pathological emotional states. *Amer. J. Psychiat.* 123:387.

Sachar, E. J. 1967. Corticosteroids in depressive illness. I. A reevaluation of control issues and the literature. *Arch. Gen. Psychiat.* 17:544.

Scapagnini, U.; De Schaepdryver, A. F.; and Preziosi, P. 1969. Influence of restraint stress, corticosterone and betamethasone on brain amine levels. *Pharmacol. Res. Commun.* 1:63.

Schapiro, S.; Geller, E.; and Yuwiler, A. 1965/66. Differential effects of a stress on liver enzymes in adult and infant rats. *Neuroendocrinology* 1:138.

Shaw, D. M.; Camps, F. E.; and Eccleston, E. G. 1967. 5-Hydroxytryptamine in the hind-brain of depressive suicides. *Brit. J. Psychiat.* 113:1407.

Sourkes, T. L.; and Missala, K. 1969. Effect of yohimbine on $^{14}CO_2$ production from ^{14}C-pyrrole-ring-labeled DL-tryptophan in rats treated with L-tryptophan, DL-α-methyltryptophan and cortisol. *Canad. J. Biochem.* 47:1049.

Trethowan, W. H.; and Cobb, S. 1952. Neuropsychiatric aspects of Cushing's syndrome. *Arch. Neurol. Psychiat.* 67:283.

van Praag, H. M.; Korf, J.; and Puite, J. 1970. 5-Hydroxyindoleacetic acid levels in the cerebrospinal fluid of depressive patients treated with probenecid. *Nature* 225:1259.

van Praag, H. M., and Leijnse, B. 1963. Die Bedeutung der Monoaminoxydasehemmung als antidepressives Prinzip-I. *Psychopharmacologia* 4:1.

Weitzmann, E. D; Rapport, M. M.; McGregor, P.; and Jacoby, J. 1968. Sleep patterns of the monkey and brain serotonin concentration: effect of p-chlorophenylalanine. *Science* 160:1361.

INTERACTIONS BETWEEN ADRENOCORTICAL STEROID HORMONES, ELECTROLYTES, AND THE CATECHOLAMINES

James W. Maas

Illinois State Psychiatric Institute and
University of Illinois College of Medicine
Chicago, Illinois

> *"In biology the purpose of the hypothesis is the generation of experiments."*
>
> Anon.

Adrenocortical steroid hormones, electrolytes, and catecholamines have all been implicated as being associated with alterations in mood and behavior, particularly mania and depression, and each of these areas has been the focus of a great deal of investigative effort (Bunney and Davis 1965; Schildkraut 1965; Schildkraut and Kety 1967; Fawcett and Bunney 1967; Maas, Fawcett, and Dekirmenjian 1968; Williams, Katz, and Shield 1969; Coppen 1967; Gibbons 1963). In general, however, each group of investigators have pursued their "own thing," and there have been only a limited number of attempts at establishing interrelationships (Baer et al. 1969). This paper will review some of the evidence in the biological literature that suggests processes by which the steroid hormones, electrolytes, and catecholamines are interrelated. There seems to be ample evidence that adrenocortical steroid hormones have an important role in the regulation of the disposition of the catecholamines, and that Na^+ and K^+ concentrations as well as cation transport are intimately associated with transport and biosynthesis of the catecholamines. It is suggested that the steroid hormones via their action on electrolytes and/or Mg^{2+}-Na^+-K^+ adenosine triphosphatase (ATPase) regulate transport and perhaps synthesis of the catecholamines. Whatever the ultimate fate of this proposal, it is hoped that it will have the heuristic value of stimulating substantive thought about interrelationships of steroid hormones, electrolytes, and catecholamines in the affective disorders.

THE ADRENAL CORTEX AND THE DISPOSITION OF CATECHOLAMINES

Organs and tissues other than brain. Ramey and Goldstein (1957) reviewed the physiological studies on the relationship between the adrenal cortex and the sympathetic nervous system and they concluded that the adrenocortical steroids and catecholamines operate as a physiologically functional unit. Although the evidence for such a relationship was impressive, mechanisms or processes by which the functional relationship between the two systems could be understood were not clearly apparent. Hokfelt (1951) found that adrenalectomy did not appreciably alter the endogenous content of norepinephrine (NE) in heart, whereas hypophysectomy and ACTH treatment altered these levels in heart, but the changes were sometimes small and seemed related to time. Numerous subsequent studies, some of which are cited later, confirmed the finding that endogenous concentrations of norepinephrine in tissue were not altered by adrenalectomy. In recent years, however, several techniques have become available for assaying the turnover of the catecholamines, and with their use a rather different picture as to the interrelationship between endocrine hormones and norepinephrine has emerged. Landsberg and Axelrod (1968a and b) and Landsberg, DeChamplain, and Axelrod (1969) reported that hypophysectomized rats had an increased turnover of cardiac norepinephrine and that treatment of the hypophysectomized rats with ACTH restored the turnover time to about 40 percent of normal, treatment with thyroxine to about 60 percent of normal, and ACTH plus thyroxine resulted in turnover times that were comparable to those seen in intact rats. Thyroidectomy and adrenalectomy, but not ovariectomy, also resulted in an increased turnover of norepinephrine in heart. Westfall and Osada (1969) and Dailey and Westfall (1970) showed that adrenalectomized rats had an increased turnover of norepinephrine in heart and that this change could be prevented by desoxycorticosterone acetate (DOCA) but not by hydrocortisone or corticosterone. They suggested that DOCA prevented a reflexly mediated increase in sympathetic nervous system activity by maintaining normotension, thereby preventing the increase in norepinephrine turnover. It has also been noted that totally adrenalectomized rats have an increased excretion of norepinephrine and that this is abolished by treatment with corticosterone (Imms and Jones 1967), while medulloadrenalectomized animals do not have elevated levels of urinary norepinephrine (DeSchaepdryver, Preziosi, and Van DerStricht 1958; Sakai 1967). Caesar, Collins, and Sandler (1970) found a highly significant increase in 3-methoxy-4-hydroxyphenylglycol (MHPG), and to a lesser degree in homovanillic acid (HVA) in urine of adrenalectomized rats, and they noted that this effect was abolished by treatment with hydrocortisone for seven days (Caesar, Collins, and Sandler 1970).

Other systems known to be involved in the disposition of catecholamines in tissues outside the central nervous system have also been found to be altered by adrenalectomy. Monoamine oxidase activity is significantly increased in heart, brain, and vas deferens, but not in liver, by adrenalectomy (Avakian and Callingham 1968; Landsberg, DeChamplain, and Axelrod 1969; Caesar, Collins, and Sandler 1970). Cardiac norepinephrine stores are more sensitive to depletion by β-tetrahydronaphthylamine in the adrenalectomized rat, but not in the adrenal-demedullated rat (Avakian and Vogt 1966), and it has been reported that there is a significant reduction in the uptake of norepinephrine at high concentrations of the amine (5 µg/ml-uptake$_2$) by isolated perfused heart obtained from adrenalectomized rats (Avakian and Callingham 1968), and that this effect is completely prevented by treatment with hydrocortisone (10 mg/kg). No effect upon uptake by adrenalectomy was noted at a norepinephrine concentration of 10 ng/ml. Interpretation of data as to uptake of catecholamines by tissues obtained from hypophysectomized or adrenalectomized animals is difficult since these operations lead to significant changes in organ size, and hence the usual methods of expressing results may not be valid (Landsberg and Axelrod 1968a).

Brain. In contrast to studies in which heart tissue has been used, the relationship between adrenal steroid hormones and the disposition of catecholamines in brain is less clear, perhaps for reasons that will emerge from this review. One line of investigation has involved the possibility that adrenocorticosteroids might induce enzymes involved in the synthesis of brain catecholamines or alter the production of the enzymes that might shunt tyrosine away from the catecholamine pathway [see Richter (1967) and Mandell and Rubin (1966) for a similar model involving tryptophan pyrrolase]. However, tyrosine transaminase in brain is principally, if not solely, associated with mitochondria and is not induced by hydrocortisone as it is in liver (Miller and Litwack 1969; Jones and Maas, unpublished observations). Further, Litwack (1969) has noted that the K_m's of tyrosine hydroxylase and tyrosine aminotransaminase are such that a shunt away from the hydroxylation of tyrosine is an unlikely mechanism for the regulation of the synthesis of catecholamines.

Landsberg and Axelrod (1968a and b) have reported that hypophysectomy does not affect the turnover time of norepinephrine in the brain of the rat, whereas Javoy, Glowinski, and Kordon (1968) found that brain norepinephrine turnover in adrenalectomized and control animals was the same two or three days after the operation and slightly increased (specific activity of norepinephrine was decreased by 21 percent) on the sixth day. Maas and Mednieks (1971) found that slices of adult rat cerebral cortex, when preincubated with hydrocortisone, took up more norepinephrine from the media than did control preparations. The enhanced uptake of norepinephrine that occurred in the presence of cortisol was blocked by ouabain and was temperature-dependent. It was concluded that the hydrocortisone-mediated increase in norepinephrine uptake occurred as a result of an action of the steroid hormone on the amine "pump" or transport system. Because of the relationship between the uptake of catecholamines and the regulation of their synthesis (see later portion of this review), the steroid effect noted above prompted our laboratory to reinvestigate the question of the turnover of brain norepinephrine in sham-operated and adrenalectomized animals. In reviewing earlier work on brain norepinephrine turnover, it was noted that the adrenalectomized animals were maintained solely on isotonic saline or were given a choice of isotonic saline or water, whereas the sham-operated or control animals were maintained on tap water. It is known that the adrenalectomized animal maintained on saline, unless stressed, is in many ways similar to the intact animal (Ramey and Goldstein 1957; Brodie et al. 1966); electrolytes are importantly involved in catecholamine disposition in neural tissues ($q.v.$); and, by definition, brain function might be expected to be particularly sensitive to the ionic environment. Crane (1965) notes that a controversy over the mechanism of intestinal absorption of sugars began with the observation that glucose absorption was decreased in adrenalectomized animals and was resolved when it was demonstrated that this decrease was prevented by maintaining the adrenalectomized animals on saline. For these reasons, it seemed possible that the differential maintenance (water vs. saline) of control and adrenalectomized animals, as noted above, might be a significant variable to be examined. When this was done, it was found that adrenalectomized rats maintained for two or three days on tap water have a significantly ($p < .01$) greater depletion of brain norepinephrine following an injection of α-methyltyrosine (α-MT) than do sham-operated animals. Adrenalectomized animals maintained on saline have lower levels of brain norepinephrine after α-MT than do sham-operated tap water-maintained animals, but the difference between the two groups is not as marked and does not reach the usually accepted level of statistical significance ($p \simeq 0.1$). Without pretreatment with α-MT no difference in brain norepinephrine concentration between sham-operated tap water-maintained, adrenalectomized salt water-maintained, or adrenalectomized tap water-maintained animals was found. Some of the data from these studies, which will be presented in detail elsewhere, are shown in Table 1. These data indicate that adrenocortical hormones have an important role in regulating norepinephrine disposition in brain, and they suggest that this effect is exerted via a mechanism related in some way to the role these hormones have in regulating salt metabolism.

In summary, there is a good deal of evidence from *in vivo* and *in vitro* studies indicating that hypophysectomy or adrenalectomy is associated with an increase in the synthesis of catecholamines in tissues other than brain. This increment in synthesis can be reversed by the appropriate replacement treatment. In contrast to studies of peripheral tissues, reports dealing with the relationship between adrenocortical steroid hormones and brain norepinephrine are less congruent. In these latter studies, the maintenance of the adrenalectomized animals on water vs. saline is an important variable, however, and adrenalectomy is most clearly associated with an alteration in the disposition of norepinephrine in brain when the adrenalectomized animal is maintained on water rather than on saline.

TABLE 1

Type of Operation	Sham	Adrenal-ectomized	Sham	Adrenal-ectomized
Maintenance	Water	NaCl	Water	Water
Pretreatment	0	0	Hydro-cortisone	Hydro-cortisone
Controls	.318 ± .012	.341 ± .012	.331 ± .022	.317 ± .028
MT Treatment	.243 ± .006	.179 ± .022	.207 ± .016	.141 ± .004
	$p \approx 0.10$		$p < .01$	

Table 1. A comparison of brain NE levels in sham-operated and adrenalectomized rats sacrificed four hours following an injection i.p. of water (control) or alpha-methyl-para-tyrosine (200 mg/kg). Animals were maintained on either tap water or saline, as indicated, for two days preceding a given experiment. Two of the groups were pretreated with a single i.p. injection of hydrocortisone succinate (25 mg/kg) two hours preceding the indicated experiment, as this prevented an increased mortality in the adrenalectomized animals and is without effect upon NE turnover in the hearts of adrenalectomized rats (Dailey and Westfall 1970). Values are expressed as mean µg NE/gm brain ± S.E.M., and the N for each cell varied from 10 to 12.

ELECTROLYTES, DISPOSITION OF CATECHOLAMINES, AND Mg^{2+}-DEPENDENT Na^+-K^+-ACTIVATED ATPase*

Because of the noted importance of NaCl maintenance of the adrenalectomized animal in studies of the disposition of brain norepinephrine, I will review some of the relevant reports on the relationship between electrolytes, cation transport, and catecholamines. The role of electrolytes in the disposition of catecholamines has been

---

*The term ATPase as used in this paper means the Mg^{2+}-dependent Na^+-K^+-activated adenosine triphosphatase. Where other ATPases are discussed they are so designated.

TABLE 2

Experimental Variable	Type of Preparation	Effect upon Synthesis of Catecholamines	Effect upon Uptake of Catecholamines	Effect upon Efflux of Catecholamines	Expected Action of Experimental Variable on Mg^{2+}-Na^+-K^+ ATPase Activity (20,21,22,23)
Electrical stimulation	Submax glands Heart Vas deferens Pulmonary artery Spleen	Increase (3)	Decrease (8,9) No effect (10) Increase (10,11)	Increase (18)	See text
Ouabain	Brain slices	Increase (1)	Decrease (6,7)	Increase (1)	Inhibition
High concentration of K^+ in media	Vas deferens Brain slices	Increase (4,5)	Decrease (12,13)	Increase (4,14)	Decrease
Rb treatment	Brain stem	Increase (2)	Unknown	Unknown	? Decrease
Absence of Na^+	Heart slices Perfused heart	Unknown	Decrease (14,15,16,17)	Increase (14,16,17,19)	Decrease
Absence of K^+	Heart slices	Unknown	Decrease (12) Little effect (16)	Increase (12)	Decrease

Table 2. Relationships between cations, cation transport, and the disposition of the catecholamines. The known or predicted effect of the experimental variable on Mg^{2+}-Na^+-K^+ ATPase activity is noted in the last column. The numbers refer to the study cited and the references are as follows:

1. Goldstein, Ohi, and Backstrom 1970.
2. Stolk, Barchas, and Vernikas-Danellis 1970.
3. Kupferman, Gillis, and Roth 1970.
4. Harris and Roth 1970.
5. Boadle-Biber and Hughes 1970.
6. Maas and Mednieks 1971.
7. Dengler, Spiegel, and Titus 1961.
8. Palaic and Panisset 1969.
9. Blakely and Brown 1964.
10. Gillis 1963.
11. Chang and Chiueh 1968.
12. Gillis and Paton 1967.
13. Bogdanski and Brodie 1969.
14. Bogdanski and Brodie 1966.
15. Iverson and Kravitz 1966.
16. Dorst, Kopin, and Ramey 1968.
17. Nash and Tu 1969.
18. Katz and Kopin 1969.
19. Keen 1967.
20. Skou 1957.
21. Skou 1960.
22. Skou 1962.
23. Neufield and Levy 1969.

well studied, and data from a wide variety of experimental preparations have been published. Some representative data are presented in Table 2. The emphasis in this tabulation is on the effects of sodium and potassium (and neural processes intimately related to these cations) on synthesis, uptake, and efflux of catecholamines. In general, it may be seen that experimental conditions that alter cation transport have important consequences for the disposition of catecholamines. More specifically, if the membrane is depolarized by electrical stimulation, high concentrations of potassium, or ouabain, there is a decrease in uptake and an increased efflux of the amine associated with an increase in synthesis. If sodium or potassium is omitted from the incubation or perfusion media, there is a marked decline in uptake and an increased efflux of norepinephrine from the tissue. In the presence of sodium, low concentrations of K^+ added to the media result in a marked stimulation of norepinephrine uptake, but higher concentrations of K^+ lead to a decrease in uptake (Gillis and Paton 1967; Bogdanski and Brodie 1966 and 1969).

The expected effects of the tabulated experimental conditions upon ATPase are noted in the last column of Table 2. For some of the experimental variables, the noted and expected effect upon ATPase activity in whole tissue preparations, such as those used for the catecholamine experiments, are fairly certain, whereas for others they are inferential in that the ATPase data were obtained from experiments with partially purified enzyme (Skou 1957, 1960, and 1962; Neufield and Levy 1969). Comments on the experimental conditions, ATPase activity, and catecholamine disposition, as summarized in Table 2, are as follows:

1. <u>The action of ouabain</u>: When brain slices are incubated with ouabain, there is a decrease in the activity of ATPase (which is subsequently isolated from the tissue) and a remarkably good correlation between the degree of this enzyme inhibition and of inhibition of Na^+ extrusion and K^+ maintenance (Yoshida, Nukada, and Fujisowa 1961; Bonting, Caravaggio, and Hawkins 1962; Albers, Fohn, and Koval 1963; Swanson and McIlwain 1965) [a 50 percent inhibition of Na^+ extrusion from brain slices occurs at a ouabain concentration of $\simeq 1 \times 10^{-6}$ M, and this is close to the amount giving one-half maximal inhibition of brain ATPase (Bourke and Tower 1966)]. The work of Akera, Larsen, and Brody (1970) is of particular interest for this review; they found that, following the infusion of dogs with ouabain, cardiac contractile force was progressively increased, atrioventricular conductivity inhibited, and the degree of ATPase inhibition and the inotropic action of the glycoside were correlated, that is, the greater the enzyme inhibition, the greater the inotropic action. Similar results were obtained by Besch *et al.* (1970).

2. <u>The absence of Na^+ or K^+</u>: In the presence of Mg^{2+}, but the absence of either Na^+ or K^+, the activity of the ATPase is by definition markedly less than under optimal conditions (Skou 1957, 1960,

and 1962). Since tissue contains a significant quantity of intracellular K^+, the absence of Na^+ would probably be more crucial in terms of ATPase activity, and it is almost certain that, in the absence of Na^+, ATPase activity would be decreased. It is problematical whether the remarkable degree of correlation between norepinephrine uptake and Na^+ concentration found by Iverson and Kravitz (1966) can be explained on the basis of ATPase activity alone.

3. <u>High concentrations of K^+ or Rb^+ and Na^+-K^+ interactions</u>: In his early work, Skou (1957) concluded that "in high concentrations K^+ ions inhibit that part of the activity (of crab nerve ATPase) which is due to sodium," and he noted in a later paper (1960) that at higher concentrations K^+ inhibits competitively, the K_i being 9 mM. Neufield's data indicate that there are two sites for Na^+ on the ATPase, and that the second site is inhibited by K^+, the K_i being 10^{-2} M (Neufield and Levy 1969). Bogdanski and Brodie (1969) noted that the transport of norepinephrine is decreased by high concentrations of K^+ and in the presence of Na^+, indicating that the inhibition is a competitive one, but suggesting that K^+ acts by displacing Na^+ from a norepinephrine carrier molecule, rather than from ATPase. Rb^+ can substitute for K^+ (Skou 1962), and in the high quantities given by Stolk, Barchas, and Vernikas-Danellis (1970), it is possible that the effects on ATPase activity mimicked those seen with high concentrations of K^+ and in the presence of Na^+. In the presence of Na^+ and Mg^{2+}, K^+ at low concentrations markedly stimulates the activity of ATPase (Skou 1957, 1960, and 1962); Gillis and Paton (1967) and Bogdanski and Brodie (1969) showed that, in the presence of Na^+, small amounts of K^+ added to the medium result in a remarkable increase in the uptake of norepinephrine by tissue preparations. Gillis and Paton varied the relative concentrations of Na^+ and K^+ to each other, keeping the total $Na^+ + K^+$ concentration constant at 150 mM, and they examined the effect upon norepinephrine uptake by slices of rat ventricle. Skou (1962) examined the activity of partially purified ATPase enzyme from brain and kidney as a function of the relative concentrations of Na^+ and K^+ with the total concentration of the two cations also being 150 mM. Data from these two separate reports are plotted in Figure 1. As may be seen, the effects of varying the Na^+ and K^+ concentrations have somewhat similar effects upon catecholamine transport and ATPase activity.

In summary, ouabain inhibits ATPase, decreases the rate of uptake of catecholamines, and increases their turnover; absence of Na^+ or K^+ is associated with decreased ATPase activity and decreased uptake of norepinephrine by tissues. In the presence of higher concentrations of Na^+ ($\simeq$ 100 mM), the addition of small amounts of K^+ (3 to 6 mM) leads to a marked increase in both ATPase activity and the rate of uptake of catecholamines. High concentrations of K^+ in the presence of Na^+ are associated with a decrease in ATPase activity and a decrease in the uptake of catecholamines.

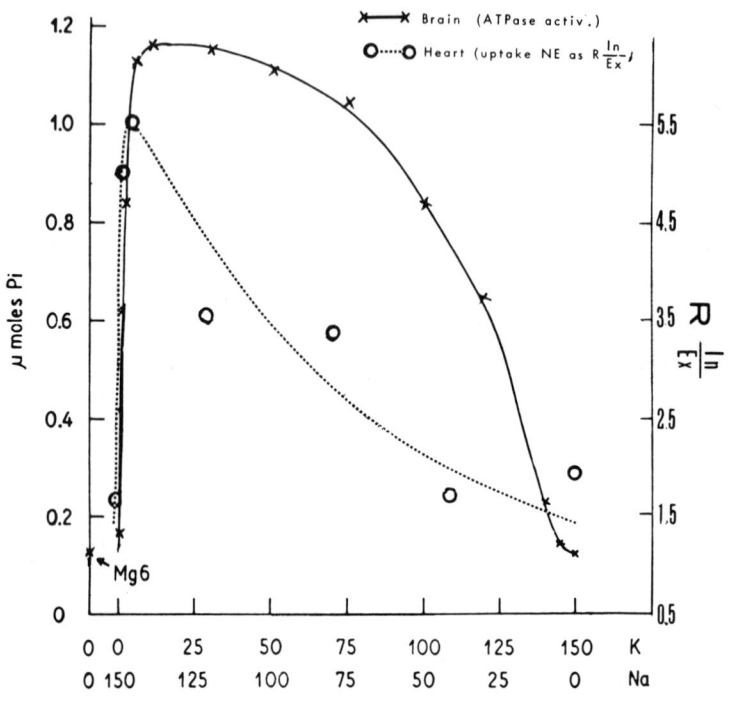

Figure 1. Comparison between the effects of varying concentrations of Na^+ and K^+ on the activity of Mg^{2+}-Na^+-K^+ ATPase obtained from brain (Skou 1962) and the uptake of norepinephrine (NE) by heart (Gillis and Paton 1967). Norepinephrine uptake is expressed as the ratio of the NE concentration in tissue to that in the media, i.e., $R \frac{In}{Ex}$. A ratio significantly greater than 1.0 indicates transport against a gradient.

These results suggest that the transport of catecholamines is regulated by ATPase activity that is, in turn, regulated by Na^+ and K^+ concentrations. Since the transport of the catecholamines seems to be intimately associated with the rate of their synthesis, this latter process (synthesis) would also be expected to be dependent upon shifts in Na^+ and K^+ concentrations.

ADRENOCORTICAL HORMONES, ATPase ACTIVITY, AND ELECTROLYTES

Aldosterone and corticosterone have been shown to regulate ATPase activity in the kidney. Chignell and Titus (1966) found that, following adrenalectomy, the ATPase activity in rat kidney decreased without an appreciable change in the affinity of the enzyme for ATP or Na^+ or K^+. This led them to suggest that the effect was due to a decrease in enzyme level. They found that the administration of aldosterone was without effect, whereas corticosterone administration returned activity to normal levels within two to three days. Joergensen (1969) also found that adrenalectomy resulted in a 37 to 44 percent decrease in ATPase activity, that corticosterone restored the activity after twenty-four to thirty hours, but that repeated injections of aldosterone, that is, every four and one-half hours, also induced a return of enzyme activity toward normal values during the first twenty-four hours of treatment. Suzuki and Ogawa (1969) found decreased enzyme activity in microsomes obtained from the kidneys of adrenalectomized rats. They noted that aldosterone, DOCA, corticosterone, and cortisol all resulted in a return of the enzyme activity to nearly normal levels. In contrast to the results found with rats, the ATPase activity was increased in the kidneys of adrenalectomized mice, and this effect was reversed by DOCA and cortisol, but not by aldosterone. Revetto, Murphy, and Lefer (1970) found a decrease of ATPase activity of myocardial contractile proteins in adrenalectomized cats. Gallagher and Glaser (1968) found no effects of adrenalectomy on the ATPase of brain, but they used a subtraction method rather than a purification step for separating Mg^{2+}-ATPase from the Na^+-K^+ activated enzyme, and the number of animals used was small.

The literature dealing with the established relationship between the adrenocortical hormones and salt metabolism is immense and will not be reviewed here. However, the review by Woodbury (1958) dealing with the relationship between the adrenal cortex and the central nervous system is particularly relevant. He notes abundant evidence supporting the concept that the adrenal steroid hormones regulate the distribution of Na^+ and K^+ in brain. Unfortunately, the picture that emerges is not clear in that seemingly opposite treatments may produce the same results. As an example, it is noted that the brain of the adrenalectomized animal has an increased concentration of intracellular sodium, and that acute administration of cortisol also results in an increase in the intracellular level of sodium. Chronic treatment with ACTH, cortisone, cortisol, corticosterone, dehydrocorticosterone, and 11-desoxy-17-hydroxycorticosterone was without demonstrable effect on brain Na^+ or K^+. Woodbury notes, however, that in experiments in which animals are adrenalectomized or administered steroids chronically, profound metabolic effects occur that may obscure the actual distribution of electrolytes. In summary, ATPase activity in the kidney, and perhaps the heart, is dependent upon adrenocortical steroid hormones. Aldosterone and corticosterone seem to be particularly important. Many reports have been reviewed elsewhere indicating that the concentration and distribution of Na^+ and K^+ within the central nervous system are altered by the adrenocortical steroid hormones.

A PROPOSED MODEL FOR THE REGULATION OF CATECHOLAMINE TRANSPORT
AND SYNTHESIS BY ADRENOCORTICAL HORMONES AND ELECTROLYTES

From the data reviewed here it is suggested that, by regulating ATPase concentrations and/or Na^+ and K^+ concentrations (which, in turn, change ATPase activity), the adrenocortical steroid hormones control the amount of energy available for transporting the catecholamines. This transport rate (in and out) has been implicated in many studies as being intimately related to the regulation of the rate of catecholamine synthesis. The suggested series of steps connecting adrenocortical hormones, electrolytes, ATPase activity, and catecholamine transport and synthesis are shown in Figure 2. In this model, adrenalectomy is associated with a reduction in ATPase activity due to Na^+ loss and/or a decrease in the enzyme concentration leading, in turn, to a decreased rate of uptake of catecholamines (and perhaps increased efflux), resulting in increased synthesis. That the published experimental data agree with this series of events is hardly surprising since the schemata shown in Figure 2 were derived from these experiments. However, this model has heuristic value in that it also suggests the possibility of a sequence of events leading to opposite results, that is, an increase in ATPase activity should be associated with accelerated norepinephrine uptake and perhaps a <u>decreased</u> rate of catecholamine synthesis. The finding that hydrocortisone enhances norepinephrine uptake by brain slices (Maas and Mednieks 1971) suggests experimental approaches for the investigation of this predicted sequence. Further, it will be interesting to see whether increased adrenocortical hormone secretion and/or an increased concentration of Na^+ are associated with increased ATPase activity and the predicted effects on catecholamines. Goldstein *et al*. (1967) found, after treating guinea pigs with aldosterone (18 µg/twice a week) for three to six months, that ^{14}C-norepinephrine increased and ^{14}C-dopamine decreased following the administration of labeled dopamine. They believed this suggested that the aldosterone treatment produced an effect on dopamine-β-hydroxylase activity or that it increased transport to the β-hydroxylating site. Some of the apparently contradictory data on norepinephrine uptake with electrical stimulation, as noted in Table 1, are also relevant to ATPase activity and catecholamine transport. In their review, Harvey and McIlwain (1969) note that, during the first six minutes of supramaximal stimulation of brain slices, there is a marked increase of sodium influx into the non-inulin space, balanced by a loss of K^+. Upon cessation of stimulation there is a rapid return to normal non-inulin content of Na^+ and K^+ that is complete within ten minutes. The events during the time of stimulation are probably extremely complex, both in terms of ATPase activity and transmitter (norepinephrine) release, but it seems quite likely that, during the recovery period following cessation of electrical stimulation, there is an increase in ATPase activity. Gillis (1963) found that electrical stimulation of the cardioaccelerator nerve <u>preceding</u> administration of a labeled norepinephrine pulse was associated with an in-

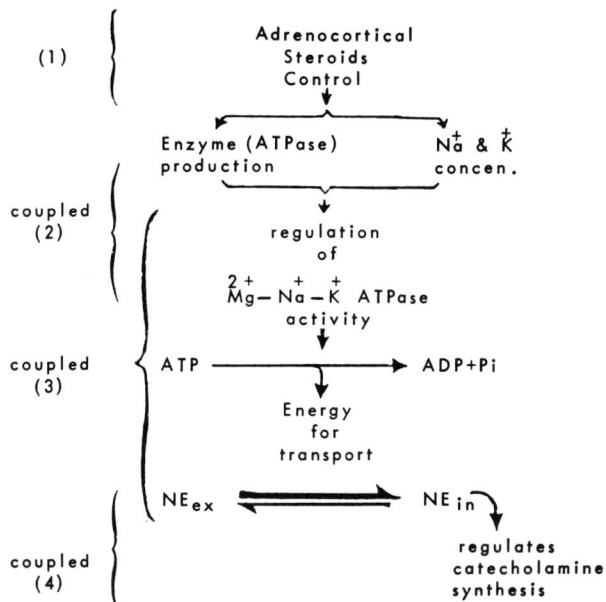

Figure 2. Proposed model for the regulation of catecholamine disposition by adrenocortical steroid hormones. In this schema, these hormones regulate tissue Mg^{2+}-Na^+-K^+ ATPase activity by a direct effect on enzyme concentration and/or indirectly by an effect upon Na^+ and K^+ concentrations and distribution. A decrease in ATPase activity is associated with a decrease in the amount of energy available for active transport, whereas an increase in ATPase activity is seen as resulting in an increase in uptake. The rate of transport of norepinephrine into the tissue regulates catecholamine synthesis (see text for details).

crease in total ^3H and ^3H-norepinephrine in the atria (not the ventricle), but that, if the pulse of norepinephrine was given first, there was no increase in norepinephrine uptake. Chang and Chiueh (1968) infused norepinephrine for a thirty-minute period concomitant with sympathetic nerve stimulation, waited another thirty minutes (no stimulation, then removed the submaxillary gland, and found an increase in norepinephrine content, that is, increased uptake. Blakely and Brown (1964) found that norepinephrine uptake by spleen was decreased during stimulation of the splenic nerve. Although there are many variables in these experiments, it is tentatively suggested that, following cessation of electrical stimulation, there is an increase in ATPase activity associated with an increase in norepinephrine uptake. (Uptake during electrical stimulation is difficult to assess because of the concomitant activation of mechanisms causing increased efflux.)

The focus in the sequence presented in Figure 2 is on catecholamine disposition, but it is well known that Na^+ and K^+ concentrations have a regulatory effect upon the rate of transport of sugars and amino acids (Crane 1965) and of acetyl choline (Liang and Quastel 1969). It was these earlier observations, in fact, that led to the cited studies on cation concentrations and catecholamine uptake. Crane's model for the Na^+-K^+ control of sugar transport involves a carrier that is itself altered by cations (Crane 1965). Since the Bogdanski and Brodie (1969) model for the cationic regulation of norepinephrine uptake is a direct adaptation of Crane's, they also posit that Na^+ and K^+ exert their effects via an action on a carrier molecule. The model suggested here is different in that Na^+ and K^+ are seen as acting via the regulation of ATPase. Which of the schemes is correct cannot be stated with certainty but most, if not all, of the data are consistent with the cationic regulation occurring via ATPase (in particular, the stimulations of norepinephrine uptake by low concentrations of K^+ in the presence of Na^+ cannot be easily explained in terms of the action of Na^+ on a carrier molecule).

The scheme presented in Figure 2 is believed to have general applicability to catecholamine disposition, but it may be that norepinephrine systems in brain have special characteristics. It has been noted, for example, that while there is an increase in norepinephrine synthesis in the heart of adrenalectomized saline-maintained animals, a change in the disposition of brain norepinephrine does not become clearly manifest unless the adrenalectomized animal is taken off saline and maintained on water. Aldosterone and corticosterone probably control the level of the ATPase enzyme in kidney (Chignell and Titus 1966; Joergensen 1969; Suzuki and Ogawa 1969) and perhaps heart (Revetto, Murphy, and Lefer 1970), but this has not been demonstrated for brain. In fact, the only available evidence is negative (Gallagher and Glaser 1968). From the review of Woodbury (1958), however, it is clear that the Na^+ and K^+ intra-and extra-cellular concentrations in the central nervous system are regulated by the adrenocortical hormones. So it seems possible that, even if these steroid hormones do not influence the ATPase enzyme levels in brain per se, they may affect the activity of this enzyme in brain indirectly via their effects upon Na^+ and K^+ excretion.

SUMMARY

Adrenocortical steroid hormones, electrolytes, and catecholamines have each been suggested as having a role in the psychobiology of the affective disorders. In this paper some of the literature relevant to interactions between these systems has been reviewed and the following noted:

1. There is ample evidence to indicate that adrenalectomy is associated with an increased turnover of norepinephrine in heart. In contrast to studies of peripheral tissue, reports dealing with the relationship between adrenocortical steroid hormones and brain norepinephrine are less congruent. It is noted that the maintenance of the adrenalectomized animal on water vs. saline is an important variable in that adrenalectomy is associated with an alteration in the disposition of norepinephrine in brain when the adrenalectomized animals are maintained on water rather than on saline.

2. There is an intimate relationship between cation concentrations, cation transport, and catecholamine transport and synthesis. The adrenocortical steroid hormones regulate $Mg^{2+}-Na^+-K^+$ ATPase activity and cation concentrations and distribution.

3. It is suggested that the adrenocortical steroid hormones regulate catecholamine transport and synthesis via a direct effect upon $Mg^{2+}-Na^+-K^+$ ATPase, or indirectly by regulating cations upon which ATPase activity depends.

4. The abundant evidence indicating that the adrenocortical steroid hormones, electrolytes, and catecholamines are biologically interconnected has relevance to studies of the affective disorders since each of these systems has been associated with alterations in mood and behavior.

ACKNOWLEDGMENT

This study was supported in part by National Institute of Mental Health grant No. 15954-02.

REFERENCES

Akera, T.; Larsen, F. S.; and Brody, T. M. 1970. Correlation of cardiac Na^+ and K^+ activated ATPase activity with ouabain-induced inotropic stimulation. *J. Pharmacol. Exp. Ther.* 173:145.

Albers, R. W.; Fohn, S.; and Koval, G. J. 1963. The role of sodium ions in the activity of electrophorus electric organ adenosine triphosphatase. *Proc. Nat. Acad. Sci.* 50:474.

Avakian, V. M., and Callingham, B. A. 1968. An effect of adrenalectomy on catecholamine metabolism. *Brit. J. Pharmacol.* 33:211.

Avakian, V. M., and Vogt, M. 1966. Role of adrenal hormones in maintaining tissue stores of noradrenaline during increased sympathetic activity. *Brit. J. Pharmacol. Chemother.* 27:532.

Baer, L.; Durell, J.; Bunney, W. E.; Levy, B.; and Cardon, P. V. 1969. Sodium-22 retention and 17-hydroxycorticosteroid excretion in affective disorders: A preliminary report. *J. Psychiat. Res.* 6:289.

Besch, H. R.; Allen, J. C.; Glich, G.; and Schwartz, A. 1970. Correlation between the inotropic action of ouabain and its effects on subcellular enzyme systems from canine myocardium. *J. Pharmacol. Exp. Ther.* 171:1.

Blakely, H. G. H., and Brown, G. L. 1964. The effect of nerve stimulation on the uptake of infused noradrenaline by perfused spleen. *J. Physiol. (London)* 172:19.

Boadle-Biber, M. C., and Hughes, J. 1970. Acceleration by potassium of catecholamine biosynthesis in the isolated guinea pig vas deferens. *Fed. Proc.* 29:413.

Bogdanski, D. F., and Brodie, B. B. 1966. Role of sodium and K^+ ions in storage of norepinephrine by sympathetic nerve endings. *Life Sci.* 5:1563.

Bogdanski, D. F., and Brodie, B. B. 1969. The effects of inorganic ions on the storage and uptake of ^{3}H-norepinephrine by rat heart slices. *J. Pharmacol. Exp. Ther.* 165:181.

Bonting, S. L.; Caravaggio, L. L.; and Hawkins, N. M. 1962. Studies on sodium potassium-activated adenosine triphosphatase. IV. Correlation with cation transport sensitive to cardiac glycosides. *Arch. Biochem. Biophys.* 98:413.

Bourke, R. S., and Tower, B. B. 1966. Fluid compartmentation and electrolytes of cat cerebral cortex in vitro. *J. Neurochem.* 13:1099.

Brodie, B. B.; Davie, J. I.; Hynie, S.; Krishner, G.; and Weiss, B. 1966. Interrelationships of catecholamines with other systems. *Pharmacol. Rev.* 18:273.

Bunney, W. E., Jr., and Davis, J. M. 1965. Norepinephrine in depressive reactions. *Arch. Gen. Psychiat.* 13:483.

Caesar, P. M.; Collins, G. G. S.; and Sandler, M. 1970. Catecholamine metabolism and monoamine oxidase activity in adrenalectomized rats. *Biochem. Pharmacol.* 19:921.

Chang, C. C., and Chiueh, C. C. 1968. Increased uptake of noradrenaline in the rat submaxillary gland during sympathetic nerve stimulation. *J. Pharm. Pharmacol.* 20:157.

Chignell, C. F., and Titus, E. 1966. Effect of adrenal steroids on a Na^+ and K^+ requiring ATPase from rat kidney. *J. Biol. Chem.* 241:5083.

Coppen, A. 1967. The biochemistry of affective disorders. *Brit. J. Psychiat.* 113:1237.

Crane, R. T. 1965. Sodium-dependent transport in the intestine and other animal tissues. *Fed. Proc.* 24:1000.

Dailey, J. W., and Westfall, T. C. 1970. Effect of adrenal steroids on the turnover of ^{3}H-NE in the rat heart. *Fed. Proc.* 29:413.

Dengler, H. J.; Spiegel, H. E.; and Titus, E. 1961. Uptake of tritium-labeled norepinephrine in brain and other tissues of cat in vitro. *Science* 133:1072.

DeSchaepdryver, A. F.; Preziosi, P.; and Van DerStricht, J. 1958. Urinary adrenaline and noradrenaline output after medulloadrenalectomy in the dog. *Arch. Int. Pharmacodyn.* 121:464.

Dorst, W. D.; Kopin, I. J.; and Ramey, E. R. 1968. Influence of sodium and calcium on norepinephrine uptake by isolated perfused rat hearts. *Amer. J. Physiol.* 215:817.

Fawcett, J. A., and Bunney, W. E., Jr. 1967. Pituitary adrenal function and depression. *Arch. Gen. Psychiat.* 16:517.

Gallagher, B. B., and Glaser, G. H. 1968. Seizure threshold, adrenalectomy and sodium-potassium stimulated ATPase in rat brain. *J. Neurochem.* 15:525.

Gibbons, J. L. 1963. Electrolytes and depressive illness. *Postgrad. Med. J.* 39:19.

Gillis, C. N. 1963. Increased retention of exogenous norepinephrine by cat atria after electrical stimulation of the cardioacceleration nerves. *Biochem. Pharmacol.* 12:593.

Gillis, C. N., and Paton, D. M. 1967. Cation dependence of sympathetic transmitter retention by slices of rat ventricle. *Brit. J. Pharmacol. Chemother.* 29:309.

Goldstein, M.; Anagnoste, B.; and Dashkoff, A. 1967. The effect of aldosterone on the catecholamine biosynthesis. *Fed. Proc.* 26:463.

Goldstein, M.; Ohi, Y.; and Backstrom, T. 1970. The effect of ouabain on catecholamine biosynthesis in rat brain cortex slices. *J. Pharmacol. Exp. Ther.* 174:77.

Harris, J. E., and Roth, R. H. 1970. The effect of potassium on catecholamine biosynthesis and release in rat brain cortical slices. *Fed. Proc.* 29:413.

Harvey, J. A., and McIlwain, H. 1969. Electrical phenomena and isolated tissues from the brain. In *Handbook of Neurochemistry.* A. Lajtha (ed.). New York: Plenum Press, p. 115.

Hokfelt, B. 1951. Noradrenaline and adrenaline in mammalian tissues. *Acta Physiol. Scand.* 25:1.

Imms, F. J., and Jones, M. T. 1967. Catecholamine excretion and adrenocortical hormones. *J. Endocr.* 38:17.

Iverson, L. L., and Kravitz, E. A. 1966. Sodium dependence of transmitter uptake at adrenergic nerve terminals. *Molec. Pharmacol.* 2:360.

Javoy, F.; Glowinski, J.; and Kordon, C. 1968. Effects of adrenalectomy on turnover of norepinephrine in the rat brain. *Europ. J. Pharmacol.* 4:103.

Joergensen, P. L. 1969. Regulation of the sodium-potassium activated ATP-hydrolyzing enzyme system in rat kidney. II: Effect of aldosterone on the activity in kidneys of adrenalectomized rats. *Biochem. Biophys. Acta* 192:326.

Jones, F., and Maas, J. W. Unpublished observations.

Katz, R. I., and Kopin, I. J. 1969. Electrical field-stimulated release of ^{3}H-NE from rat atrium: Effects of ions and drugs. *J. Pharmacol. Exp. Ther.* 169:229.

Keen, P. 1967. Release of d,l-^{3}H-NE from rat heart slices. *Fed. Proc.* 26:570.

Kupferman, A.; Gillis, C. N.; and Roth, R. H. 1970. Influence of sympathetic nerve stimulation on conversion of ^{3}H-tyrosine to ^{3}H-catecholamine and on ^{3}H-norepinephrine disposition in rabbit pulmonary artery. *J. Pharmacol. Exp. Ther.* 171:214.

Landsberg, L., and Axelrod, J. 1968a. Influence of pituitary, thyroid and adrenal hormones on norepinephrine turnover and metabolism in the rat heart. *Circ. Res.* 22:559.

Landsberg, L., and Axelrod, J. 1968b. Increased turnover of cardiac norepinephrine following hypophysectomy. *Fed. Proc.* 27:602.

Landsberg, L.; DeChamplain, J.; and Axelrod, J. 1969. Increased biosynthesis of cardiac norepinephrine after hypophysectomy. *J. Pharmacol. Exp. Ther.* 165:102.

Liang, C. C., and Quastel, J. H. 1969. Uptake of acetylcholine in rat brain cortex slices. *Biochem. Pharmacol.* 18:1169.

Maas, J. W.; Fawcett, J. A.; and Dekirmenjian, H. 1968. 3-Methoxy-4-hydroxyphenylglycol (MHPG) excretion in depressive states - a pilot study. *Arch. Gen. Psychiat.* 19:129.

Maas, J. W., and Mednieks, M. 1971. Hydrocortisone effected increase of norepinephrine uptake by brain slices. *Science* 171:178.

Mandell, A. J., and Rubin, R. T. 1966. ACTH induced changes in tryptophan turnover along inducible pathways in man. *Life Sci.* 5:1153.

Miller, J. E., and Litwack, G. 1969. Subcellular distribution of tyrosine aminotransferase in rat brain. *Arch. Biochem.* 134:149.

Nash, C. W., and Tu, T. 1969. The influence of sodium and chloride ions on the uptake and retention of ^{3}H-noradrenaline by perfused rat hearts. *Fed. Proc.* 28:673.

Neufield, A. H., and Levy, H. M. 1969. Second ouabain-sensitive sodium-dependent ATPase in brain microsomes. *J. Biol. Chem.* 244:6493.

Palaic, D., and Panisset, J. 1969. Effect of nerve stimulation and angiotension on the accumulation of ^{3}H-norepinephrine and the endogenous norepinephrine level in guinea pig vas deferens. *Biochem. Pharmacol.* 18:2693.

Ramey, E. R., and Goldstein, M. S. 1957. The adrenal cortex and the sympathetic nervous system. *Physiol. Rev.* 37:155.

Revetto, M. J.; Murphy, R. A.; and Lefer, A. M. 1970. Cardiac impairment in adrenal insufficiency in the cat. Reduced ATPase activity of myocardial contractile proteins. *Circ. Res.* 26:419.

Richter, D. 1967. Tryptophan metabolism in mental illness. In *Amines and Schizophrenia.* H. E. Himwich, S. S. Kety, and J. R. Smythies (eds.). New York: Pergamon Press, p. 167.

Sakai, Y. 1967. Effect of medullo-adrenalectomy upon urinary excretion of adrenaline and noradrenaline in cats. *Tohoku J. Exp. Med.* 93:279.

Schildkraut, J. J. 1965. The catecholamine hypothesis of affective disorders: A review of supporting evidence. *Amer. J. Psychiat.* 122:509.

Schildkraut, J. J., and Kety, S. S. 1967. Biogenic amines and emotion. *Science* 156:21.

Skou, J. C. 1957. The influence of some cations on an adenosine triphosphatase from peripheral nerve. *Biochim. Biophys. Acta* 23: 394.

Skou, J. C. 1960. Further investigations on a $Mg^{2+} + Na^+$ - activated ATPase possibly related to the active, linked transport of Na^+ and K^+ across the nerve membrane. *Biochim. Biophys. Acta* 42:6.

Skou, J. C. 1962. Preparation from mammalian brain and kidney of the enzyme system involved in active transport of Na^+ and K^+. *Biochim. Biophys. Acta* 58:314.

Stolk, J. M.; Barchas, J. D.; and Vernikas-Danellis, J. 1970. Increased turnover of rat brain norepinephrine during Rb^+ treatment. *Fed. Proc.* 29:511.

Suzuki, S., and Ogawa, E. 1969. Experimental studies on the carbonic anhydrase activity - XII. *Biochem. Pharmacol.* 18:993.

Swanson, P. D., and McIlwain, H. 1965. Inhibition of the sodium-ion-stimulated adenosine triphosphatase after treatment of isolated guinea pig cerebral cortex with ouabain and other agents. *J. Neurochem.* 12:877.

Westfall, T. C., and Osada, H. 1969. Influence of adrenalectomy on the synthesis of norepinephrine in rat heart. *J. Pharmacol. Exp. Ther.* 167:300.

Williams, T. A.; Katz, M.; and Shield, J. A. 1969. *Recent Advances in the Psychobiology of the Depressive Illnesses*. Williamsburg Conference NIMH Workshop. Washington, D. C.: U. S. Government Printing Office, in press.

Woodbury, D. M. 1958. Relation between the adrenal cortex and the central nervous system. *Pharmacol. Rev.* 10:275.

Yoshida, T.; Nukada, A.; and Fujisowa, H. 1961. The effects of ouabain on ion transport and metabolic turnover of phospholipids on brain slices. *Biochim. Biophys. Acta* 48:614.

THYROID-IMIPRAMINE INTERACTION:

CLINICAL RESULTS AND BASIC MECHANISM

Arthur J. Prange, Jr.*, Ian C. Wilson**, Angelina E. Knox, Thomas K. McClane, George R. Breese*, Billy R. Martin*, Lacoe B. Alltop**, and Morris A. Lipton*

*University of North Carolina School of Medicine and
**North Carolina Department of Mental Health

Chapel Hill, North Carolina

In recent years, our group has drawn attention to a new phenomenon that can be described quite simply. Patients with primary depression recover more quickly if, to a usual regimen of imipramine, one adds a small dose of thyroid hormone, L-triiodothyronine (T3) (Prange et al. 1968; Prange et al. 1969; Wilson et al. 1970; Prange et al. 1970). Since then we have worked in two directions in both our clinic and our laboratory. We have explored the clinical dimensions of our finding and have tried simultaneously to elucidate the mechanisms that underlie it. This paper will outline the phenomenon briefly and then discuss one of our attempts to understand it. In another paper (Prange, Wilson, and Lipton, in preparation) we shall publish data that verify the following qualifications:
 1. When imipramine alone is given, men respond much faster than women.
 2. When T3 is added to imipramine, women benefit enormously and men benefit little, if at all.
 3. Whether patients are retarded or agitated has no influence on the T3 phenomenon, though it has some influence on basic response to imipramine.

We have learned other things about the tricyclic-T3 interaction. It is not limited to imipramine. In a double-blind study of

---

Dr. Knox is Unit Director at Dorothea Dix Hospital, Raleigh, North Carolina, and Dr. McClane is in private practice, Lakeland, Florida.

outpatients, Wheatley (manuscript in preparation) showed that it pertains to amitriptyline, and Earle (1970) showed in an open trial that it pertains to other tricyclic drugs as well, including demethylated tricyclics. T3 potentiation even extends to some aspects of phenothiazine action in animals, as Park, Prange, and Happy (manuscript in preparation) have discovered in our laboratories.

Clearly, more than one drug may interact with T3. In addition, hormones other than T3 may interact with imipramine. McClure and Cleghorn (1968) believe that imipramine action in depression can be potentiated by the synthetic adrenal steroid, dexamethasone. Thyroid-stimulating hormone (TSH) will serve the purpose, as Figure 1 shows.

We have published a complete report of the clinical aspects of this study (Prange et al. 1970). Here it is necessary to note only that patients who received TSH improved very rapidly, and that the week of maximum improvement correlated well with the week of maximum thyroid stimulation.

Figure 2 shows that on Hamilton's retardation factor and his agitation factor (Hamilton 1960) patients are benefited equally by TSH.

Regarding possible mechanisms, we have an embarrassment of potential riches. In our view, the first question to be answered is whether depressed patients are truly euthyroid, that is, whether for each patient the balance between tissue need and tissue supply is ideal. We have a variety of evidence (Prange et al. 1969; Wilson et al. 1970; Prange et al. 1970), all of it unfortunately indirect, that in depressed women there is less thyroid hormone delivered than is required. But whatever the thyroid state of depressed patients, one must still ask what it is that a small dose of thyroid hormone does in the presence of imipramine that is antidepressant.

Thyroid hormone could have an effect on imipramine metabolism. The hormone could affect the uptake, distribution, or removal of the drug. We have some weak inferential evidence that this occurs in animals (Prange and Lipton 1962; Prange, Lipton, and Love 1963 and 1964), but somewhat stronger evidence in animals and in man that, in the dose range that interests us, a hormone effect on drug metabolism is unimportant.

There are a number of reasons to examine thyroid-amine interactions. Interactions between catecholamines and thyroid hormones are not only numerous but venerable. Goetsch showed in 1918 that an epinephrine infusion could be used to diagnose hyperthyroidism. The interactions of indoleamines with thyroid hormones are less well

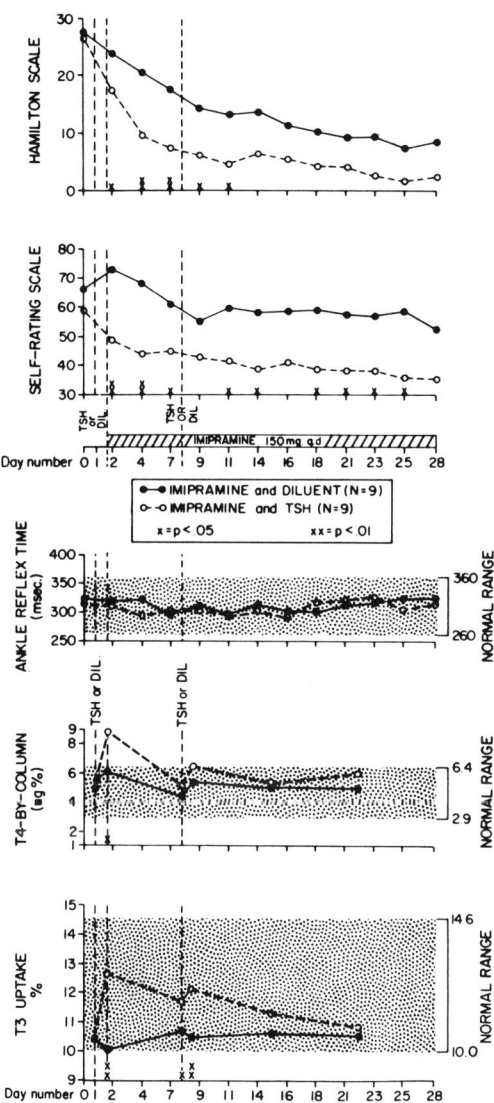

Figure 1. Diminishing scores on both Hamilton scale and self-rating scale (Zung 1970) indicate clinical improvement. Slow reflexes (higher ART scores) correlate with hypothyroidism, fast reflexes with hyperthyroidism. T4-by-column is a standard chemical measure of thyroid state and is comparable to the protein-bound iodine (PBI) test. T3 uptake test is an index of residual protein binding space for thyroid hormones.

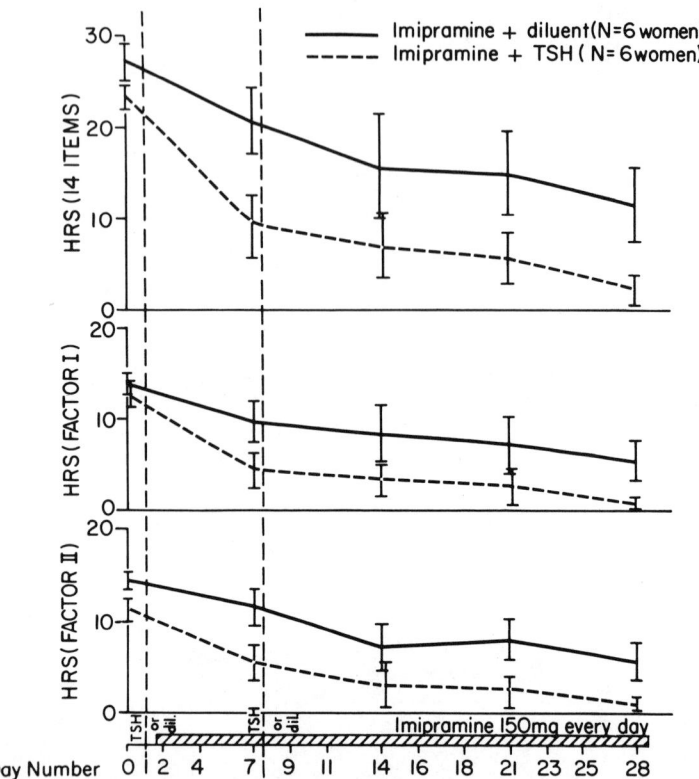

Figure 2. Presents the Hamilton rating scale results (14 items) pertaining to the 12 women whose 24-hour urine was assayed weekly. Patients in each group improved about equally on Factor I (retardation) and Factor II (agitation). The advantage of having received TSH was equally apparent for both factors.

studied but some do exist (Spencer and West 1961; Toth and Csaba 1966), and it is of some interest that thyroid gland is a source of serotonin (Williams 1968). We had, then, an abundance of reasons to examine amine metabolism while manipulating thyroid state.

METHOD

During our TSH study, whose main clinical results are shown in Figure 1, we collected 24-hour urine samples from our patients initially and weekly. The urine was collected over acid, chilled, mixed, divided into aliquots, and deep-frozen. Unfortunately, we were not able to impose a special diet on our patients. They were offered a standard hospital diet and were allowed nothing else to

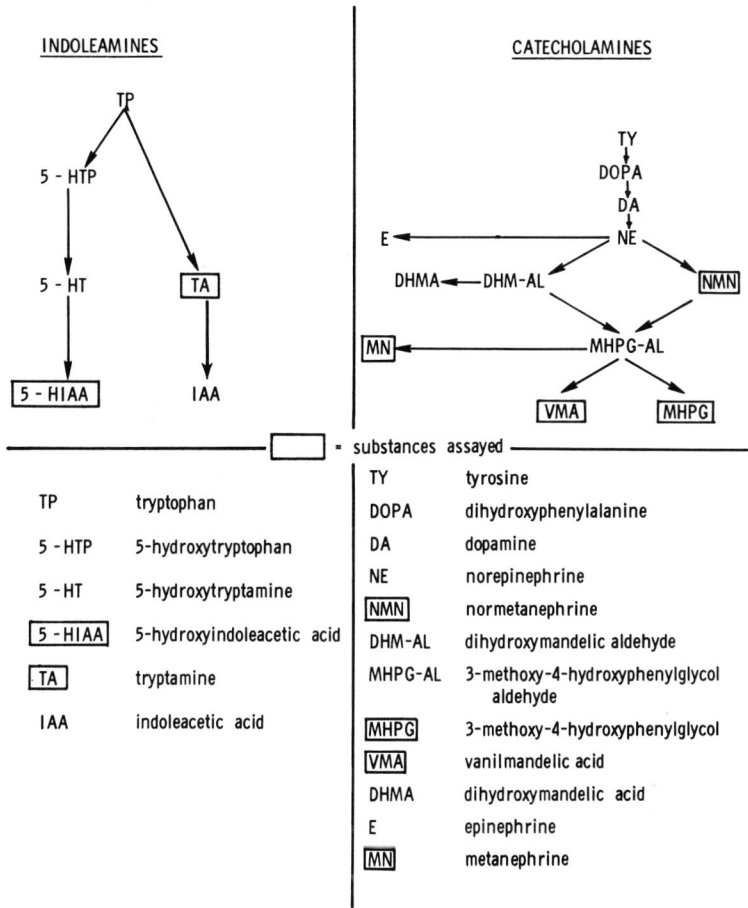

Figure 3. Shows in abbreviated form the sources and metabolic fates of certain indoleamines and catecholamines.

eat or drink except water. The diet was nutritionally adequate but rather bland. Patients tended to eat less early in treatment than they did later, but it is not possible to understand our data comprehensively simply by reference to increased food intake.

Figure 3 shows in abbreviated form the sources and fates of norepinephrine (NE), epinephrine, serotonin (5-HT), and tryptamine (TA). The boxes identify the substances for which we assayed urine. 3-Methoxy-4-hydroxyphenylglycol (MHPG) may be of special importance since a relatively high proportion of what appears in human urine is thought to come from brain (Maas, Fawcett, and Dekirmenjian 1968).

Metanephrine (MN) and normetanephrine (NMN) were analyzed by the method of Taniguchi, Kakimoto, and Armstrong (1964), MHPG by the method of Wilk et al. (1967), vanillylmandelic acid (VMA) by the method of Wilk et al. (1965), TA as recommended by a standard text (Long 1968), and 5-hydroxyindoleacetic acid (5-HIAA) by the method of Udenfriend, Titus, and Weissbach (1955).

All urine was assayed at least in triplicate. All urine aliquots were coded. Each assay dealt with all urine from a given patient at one laboratory session. Thus, variations that may have entered our technique would not have affected changes over time for a given patient but they could have affected differences between different patients. Since they showed sex differences in clinical response, we decided to exclude our few male patients. We also excluded women if they produced one or more 24-hour specimens that were of doubtful volume or doubtful creatinine content. These exclusions were done in ignorance of chemical results. As it happened, we were left with six women out of nine patients who had received TSH and six women out of nine patients who had received placebo. Both groups, of course, received imipramine throughout. The clinical responses of these women are shown in Figure 2. They were typical of the responses of their respective larger groups (Figure 1).

Before examining results it is necessary to consult a study performed in our clinic under the leadership of McClane (McClane, Wilson, and Prange, manuscript in preparation). McClane matched our patients in age with ten normal women who worked in our hospital. On one occasion he gave them imipramine, 150 mg daily, for two weeks along with 25 µg of T3 daily. On another occasion, a month later, he gave them imipramine plus placebo. Among many other tests they performed or underwent, these women collected 24-hour urine samples before treatment and two weeks later at its conclusion, both before and after imipramine-T3, and before and after imipramine-placebo. Urinary assays were performed exactly as specified for our patients.

RESULTS

The results of urinary assays are shown in Table 1. One can see that the chemical variables were similar in response to both treatments; that is, if a variable rose or fell with one treatment, it rose or fell with the other. Variance was small and there was a high degree of intrasubject reliability, not shown in the table. The fall in MHPG in response to imipramine was statistically significant under the imipramine-placebo condition. The fall in VMA in response to imipramine-T3 was significant, as was the rise in 5-HIAA. It is interesting to note that both treatments caused a small, consistent fall in NMN. This is in contrast to what has been reported in imipramine-treated patients (Schildkraut, Gordon, and Durrell 1965), and in contrast to what we found in our patients as

TABLE 1

Effect of Treatments on 24-Hour Secretion of
Urinary Metabolites in Ten Normal Women
(Means ± standard error)

	Imipramine plus Placebo		Imipramine plus T3	
	Before	After	Before	After
MN µg	135±20	160±47	164±32	189±59
NMN µg	250±23	228±41	280±34	232±26
MHPG mg	2.09±0.30	1.00±0.11*	1.89±0.16	1.60±0.38
VMA mg	3.16±0.42	2.34±0.57	3.60±0.29	2.81±0.39*
TA µg	156±28.3	163±21.1	164±21.8	196±14.1
5-HIAA mg	5.20±0.62	5.59±0.72	5.73±0.71	7.52±66*

* $p < .05$, compared to respective "before" values. Student's *t* test.

well. In the case of all chemicals, the resting values McClane determined are quite similar to those reported by other authors.

Table 2 shows the effects of treatments on the same chemical variables in patients. In proceeding from normals to patients we changed hormones--TSH replaced T3--but, of course, TSH can only stimulate thyroid hormone secretion. At the dose of TSH we used, 10 international units initially and a week later, the gain in thyroid state was probably somewhat greater than that produced by T3, 25 µg daily (Prange *et al.* 1969 and 1970).

Patients showed a large variance in resting values for all chemical parameters. For evaluation of treatment-induced changes, the proper comparisons to normals are the two-week values. In the two-week columns one finds a rise in TA for the imipramine-alone group, a rise in 5-HIAA for the TSH patients, and a rise in TA when the patients are considered together. At four weeks, one finds a drop in MHPG for the placebo patients and for all patients, and a rise in TA for all patients. Statistically reliable findings are supported by nonsignificant trends in comparison groups.

In the patients receiving imipramine alone, there was no important change in MN. NMN was elevated at the outset and showed a

TABLE 2

Effect of Treatments on 24-Hour Secretion of
Urinary Metabolites in Depressed Women

(Units as in Table 1)
(Means ± standard error)

	Imipramine plus Placebo (n = 6)			Imipramine plus TSH (n = 6)			All Patients (n = 12)		
	Before	After 2 Weeks	After 4 Weeks	Before	After 2 Weeks	After 4 Weeks	Before	After 2 Weeks	After 4 Weeks
MN	113±27.0	126±22.9	109±21.3	177±43.3	192±46.3	155±22.1	148±27.3	162±28.1	134±16.4
NMN	397±121	357±62.9	541±137	236±67.5	258±65.3	307±96.5	316±70.5	308±45.7	307±68.3
MHPG	2.17±0.50	1.51±0.37	1.12±0.29*	1.46±0.32	1.27±0.36	0.99±0.22	1.84±0.32	1.39±0.26	1.05±0.18**
VMA	5.49±0.44	4.74±0.62	4.38±0.59	3.86±0.74	4.46±0.37	4.30±0.72	4.68±0.47	4.60±0.34	4.34±0.45
TA	102±32.0	209±52.5**	214±64.0	178±56.8	217±36.4	250±51.0	140±35.3	213±31.1**	232±40.5**
5-HIAA	9.85±1.13	10.1±1.67	11.7±3.48	10.8±2.39	18.8±4.81*	15.2±3.25	10.3±1.27	14.5±2.88	13.5±2.44

*p <.05, compared to respective "before" values. Student's t test.
**p <.025

sharp rise by the fourth week. MHPG was slightly elevated and then fell quickly. VMA was high throughout but fell slightly. TA was low normal and rose steadily to high normal. 5-HIAA was high and remained high.

In the women who received TSH as well as imipramine, MN was not remarkable. NMN again rose, earlier than in the placebo group. MHPG was a bit low at the outset and fell slightly. VMA was not remarkable. A slow steady rise for TA was apparent. 5-HIAA was high and variable.

Table 3 shows the results of our attempt to find statistical correlations week by week between clinical change and chemical change. It was a matter of interest to break the total Hamilton scores down into a factor for retardation and a factor for agitation, using Hamilton's criteria (Figure 2, Table 3). Neither factor, however, yielded information that could not be learned from the total Hamilton scale. When all twelve patients were considered together, we found a constant relationship between falling Hamilton scores and falling MHPG secretion. The same was true of VMA. In the imipramine-alone patients, VMA fell step by step with Hamilton scores. In the TSH patients TA rose as Hamilton scores fell, that is, as improvement occurred. The effect did not reach statistical significance in the patients who received imipramine alone.

We believe that a positive result obtained with this statistical technique is quite meaningful but that the technique may obscure as much as it reveals. For example, the significance of consistent changes at crucial times could be washed out by small random variations earlier or later. It was necessary, therefore, to look at the sequence of change in individual patients.

In Figure 4 we have indicated graphically the week in which maximum change occurred. The TSH patients' greatest clinical improvement occurred very early (see also Figure 2). In the imipramine-alone patients, maximum clinical improvement was later. Patient 3 improved equally in weeks one and four, and more than in weeks two and three. In a similar way patient 5 improved equally and maximally in weeks three and four.

In the TSH patients, NMN showed maximum rise the week after maximum clinical improvement (patients 1, 2, 3 and 4) or with it (patient 5). The rise was delayed more than a week only in patient 6. In the placebo patients, the NMN rise tended to be later, as was clinical improvement. The lag was about the same. In only one of twelve patients (placebo patient 4) did the maximum NMN rise precede maximum clinical improvement. It is also worth emphasizing that in normals we found these treatments to diminish NMN secretion, not increase it.

TABLE 3

Correlation Coefficients Between Clinical Change and
24-Hour Secretion of Urinary Metabolites

	Clinical Improvement Hamilton Scale 16 (or 14) Items			Clinical Improvement Hamilton Scale Factor I, Retardation			Clinical Improvement Hamilton Scale Factor II, Agitation		
	All Patients	Placebo Patients	TSH Patients	All Patients	Placebo Patients	TSH Patients	All Patients	Placebo Patients	TSH Patients
MHPG	neg.*	n.s.	n.s.	neg.*	n.s.	n.s.	n.s.	n.s.	n.s.
VMA	neg.**	neg.**	n.s.	neg.*	neg.**	n.s.	neg.**	neg.**	n.s.
TA	n.s.	n.s.	pos.*	n.s.	n.s.	n.s.	n.s.	n.s.	n.s.

* $p < .05$
** $p < .01$

No significant correlations, positive or negative, occurred between MN, NMN, or 5-HIAA and any clinical measure.

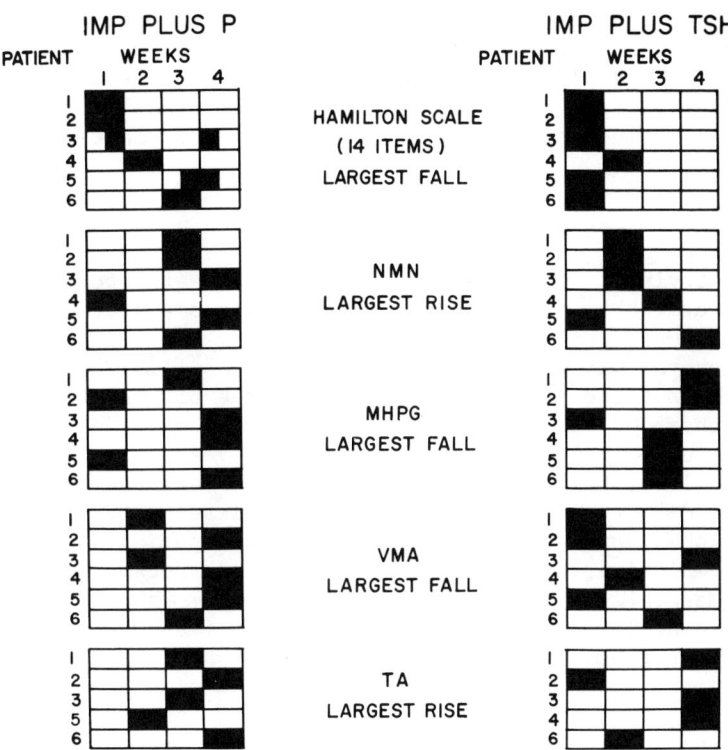

Figure 4. Solid boxes show weeks in which each patient in each treatment group showed maximum change in the parameter and direction indicated. Patient 4 (IMP plus placebo [P]) and patient 5 (IMP plus TSH) each produced one urine sample in which tryptamine could not be assayed because of technical difficulty.

Although we found a consistent negative relationship between clinical improvement and MHPG secretion (Table 3), the relationship of maximum changes is less clear than with NMN. It is true that maximum MHPG fall coincided with or followed maximum clinical improvement eleven of twelve times--the exception was placebo patient 5--but the lag was quite variable. In a similar way, maximum VMA fall never preceded maximum clinical improvement, but again the lag between the two events varied considerably.

As regards TA, one imipramine-alone patient (patient 5) showed a maximum rise before maximum improvement. Otherwise the chemical change followed the clinical change, but the interval was variable.

One of the striking generalizations one can make is that

chemical change usually followed and rarely preceded clinical change. Our measure of clinical change, of course, was what a "blind" doctor said about the patient. We found, however, that the patient almost always said the same thing about himself. Over time our Zung self-rating scale results (Zung 1970) correlate 0.95 with our Hamilton results.

DISCUSSION

Before trying to formulate our data it is useful to indicate areas of agreement and disagreement with previous authors.

In a general way we agree with Bunney *et al.* (1967) that, in untreated psychotic depression, excretion rates of VMA are high, along with those of other metabolites. We agree with Schildkraut, Gordon, and Durrell (1965) that NMN rises and VMA falls with treatment. We believe, however, that we have shown that these effects do not coincide with improvement but more or less systematically follow it. NMN changes in depression may have special significance since in normals imipramine produces opposite changes. We cannot agree with Maas, Fawcett, and Dekirmenjian (1968) that in depression MHPG tends to be low and to rise with recovery (Maas, personal communication). Furthermore, we rank-ordered our patients according to rate of improvement and could find no correlation between this parameter and either initial MHPG output or its change over time. Thus, we cannot confirm Maas *et al.* in their finding that good imipramine responders show low MHPG initially, with a rise during treatment (Maas, personal communication).

Concerning indoleamines, we agree with Rodnight (1961) and with Coppen *et al.* (1965) that TA is low initially and rises with recovery. We would add our datum that imipramine will produce this rise in normal women. A TA rise with recovery from depression is difficult to interpret because urinary TA is almost entirely a product of kidney decarboxylation (Sjoerdsma *et al.* 1959), and because Coppen (1967) has shown that in depression there is no whole-body failure of decarboxylation. Confirmed and reconfirmed biochemical findings in depression, however, are so rare that they should be cherished even when their interpretation is obscure. Our finding that 5-HIAA is elevated and increases with recovery is unexplained. We have found the increase to be produced by imipramine alone in normal women on a carefully controlled diet. A consensus seems to be emerging that in depression 5-HIAA in spinal fluid is diminished (Ashcroft *et al.* 1966; Dencker *et al.* 1966).

In formulating the present data we wish to emphasize that our findings pertain only to women. The few men we have studied have been excluded from the present report, but it is worth noting that their biochemical behavior seems quite distinct from that of women.

Moreover, we have indicated clear sex differences in response to imipramine and its enhancement by T3.

Our data, taken with other accumulating data, allow the following hypothesis: depressed women have a low level of aminergic receptor sensitivity. Considerable evidence pertains to catecholamines. Depressed women have a persistently low catechol-O-methyl transferase activity in red blood cells according to Cohn, Dunner, and Axelrod (in press), and this enzyme is probably part of the receptor complex. Depressed patients have a high level of catecholamines in plasma according to Wyatt *et al.* (1971), but they are normotensive. Depressed patients, mainly women, show less response to infused NE before, than after, recovery even when recovery follows placebo treatment, according to Prange, McCurdy, and Cochrane (1967). In the face of these conditions, we have found high initial 24-hour production of NMN and VMA. Catecholamines, we believe, only attempt to compensate for diminished receptor sensitivity. We first made this suggestion on the basis of our infusion studies (Prange, McCurdy, and Cochrane 1967), and Rosenblatt, Chanley, and Leighton (1969 a and b) have elaborated this position on the basis of their studies of excretion ratios of various catecholamine metabolites. Compensation in the periphery seems reasonably adequate judged by cardiovascular criteria. We believe it is less than adequate in brain. MHPG, which may be our best marker of catecholamine metabolism in brain, is only normal, a finding that must be compared to excesses of metabolites in the periphery.

A similar situation seems to obtain regarding indoleamines. Before treatment, the peripheral tissues of depressed women seem to produce nearly twice as much 5-HIAA as do the tissues of normal women. Again we view this as amine compensation for a decrement in receptor sensitivity. As in the case of catecholamines, compensation in the brain may be deficient. In suicidal depressed patients, levels of serotonin are slightly diminished (Bourne *et al.* 1968), and 5-HIAA in spinal fluid also tends to be reduced (Ashcroft *et al.* 1966; Dencker *et al.* 1966). In the brain, then, indoleamines seem not only to compensate inadequately but perhaps to contribute to a final diminution of synaptic transmission by their scarcity. We cannot explain the observed rise in 5-HIAA in our patients with continuing lapse of time and with improvement. The same effect was produced by imipramine-T3 in our normal subjects, and it may represent a pharmacological property of treatment not specifically related to depression.

Although we have spoken of receptor sensitivity, it is not necessarily the variable at issue. What we have observed is hyporesponse in the face of standard amounts of agonist (infusion study); or normal resting function (e.g., blood pressure) in the face of increased excretion of agonist metabolic products (present study).

From these findings and compatible ones concerning amines or their products in brain and spinal fluid, we have inferred a receptor failure in which the brain participates but which is compensated only in the periphery. The peripheral amine findings are similar to those produced by drugs known to produce receptor blockade (Dairman *et al.* 1968; Nybäck and Sedvall 1968). However, failure of the response systems, of which receptors are a part, could occur at other points, end organs, for example. Identification of the locus or loci of failure would be aided by knowing which ones are capable of exerting a feedback influence on amine synthesis. It is interesting to note that certain induced hormonal deficiencies in animals can produce increased amine synthesis with persistent hyporesponsiveness (Lipton *et al.* 1968).

That depression improves before chemical change is detected may mean that we have studied the wrong chemicals, though a wealth of evidence indicates that both catecholamines and indoleamines are involved in the same manner in the depression process. It is also possible that brain is responsive to chemical changes that must increase in magnitude before they can be detected in urine. We believe it is still more likely that the observed lag in chemical change occurs because such changes are the consequences of changes in amine distribution, produced by imipramine, and in receptor sensitivity, produced by thyroid hormones. In any case, the ability to accelerate recovery in such a manner as to separate mental and chemical change indicates the need to examine the role of aminergic receptors and their endocrine regulation.

ACKNOWLEDGMENTS

This work was supported by Public Health Service grants MH-15631 and MH-07520, Public Health Service career scientist award MH-22536 from the National Institute of Mental Health, and by a grant from Geigy Pharmaceuticals, Ardsley, N. Y.

The authors wish to thank Dr. Judson J. Van Wyk, professor of pediatrics (endocrinology), for his consultation; Drs. William J. Buffaloe, Robert L. Rollins, Jr., and Peter N. Witt for their cooperation and encouragement; and Mrs. Rachel A. Stikeleather, R.N., for immediate clinical supervision of the patients.

The imipramine used was supplied by Geigy Pharmaceuticals; the thyroid stimulating hormone by Armour Pharmaceutical Company; the Metrecal by Mead Johnson and Company.

REFERENCES

Ashcroft, G. W.; Crawford, T. B. B.; Eccleston, D.; Sharman, D. F.; MacDougall, E. J.; Stanton, J. B.; and Binns, J. K. 1966. 5-Hydroxyindole compounds in the cerebrospinal fluid of patients with psychiatric or neurological disease. *Lancet* 2:1049.

Bourne, H. R.; Bunney, W. E., Jr.; Colburn, R. W.; Davis, J. M.; Davis, J. N.; Shaw, D. M.; and Coppen, A. J. 1968. Noradrenaline, 5-hydroxytryptamine, and 5-hydroxyindoleacetic acid in hindbrains of suicidal patients. *Lancet* 2:805.

Bunney, W. E.; Davis, J. M.; Weil-Malherbe, H.; and Smith, E. R. B. 1967. Biochemical changes in psychotic depression: High norepinephrine levels in psychotic versus neurotic depression. *Arch. Gen. Psychiat.* 16:448.

Cohn, C. K.; Dunner, D. L.; and Axelrod, J. 1971. Reduced catechol-O-methyltransferase activity in red blood cells of women with primary affective disorder. *Science* 170:1323.

Coppen, A. 1967. The biochemistry of affective disorders. *Brit. J. Psychiat.* 113:1237.

Coppen, A.; Shaw, D. M.; Malleson, A.; Eccleston, E.; and Gundy, G. 1965. Tryptamine metabolism in depression. *Brit. J. Psychiat.* 111:993.

Dairman, W. R.; Gordon, R.; Spector, S.; Sjoerdsma, A.; and Udenfriend, S. 1968. Effect of alpha-blockers on catecholamine biosynthesis. *Fed. Proc.* 27:240.

Dencker, S. J.; Malm, U.; Roos, B. E.; and Werdinius, B. 1966. Acid monoamine metabolites of cerebrospinal fluid in mental depression and mania. *J. Neurochem.* 13:1545.

Earle, B. V. 1970. Thyroid hormone and tricyclic antidepressants in resistant depressions. *Amer. J. Psychiat.* 126:143.

Goetsch, E. 1918. Newer methods in the diagnosis of thyroid disorders: pathological and clinical. *New York J. Med.* 18:259.

Hamilton, M. 1960. A rating scale for depression. *J. Neurol. Neurosurg. Psychiat.* 23:56.

Lipton, M. A.; Prange, A. J., Jr.; Dairman, W.; and Udenfriend, S. 1968. Increased rate of norepinephrine biosynthesis in hypothyroid rats. *Fed. Proc. Abstracts* 27:399.

Long, C. (ed.) 1968. *Biochemist's Handbook.* Princeton, N. J.: D. Van Nostrand, p. 926.

Maas, J. W.; Fawcett, J.; and Dekirmenjian, H. 1968. 3-Methoxy-4-hydroxy phenylglycol (MHPG) excretion in depressive states. *Arch. Gen. Psychiat.* 19:129.

Maas, J. W. Personal communication.

McClane, T.; Wilson, I. C.; and Prange, A. J., Jr. The effects of imipramine and L-triiodothyronine on mental activity, thyroid state, and response to norepinephrine infusion in normal women. In preparation.

McClure, D. J.; and Cleghorn, R. A. 1968. Suppression studies in affective disorders. *Canad. Psychiat. Assoc. J.* 13:477.

Nybäck, H.; and Sedvall, G. 1968. Effect of chlorpromazine on accumulation and disappearance of catecholamines formed from tyrosine-C^{14} in brain. *J. Pharmacol. Exp. Ther.* 162:294.

Park, S.; Prange, A. J., Jr.; and Happy, J. The effects of altered thyroid state in phenothiazine response distribution and metabolism in the rat. In preparation.

Prange, A. J., Jr.; and Lipton, M. A. 1962. Enhancement of imipramine mortality in hyperthyroid mice. *Nature* 196:588.

Prange, A. J., Jr.; Lipton, M. A.; and Love, G. N. 1963. Diminution of imipramine mortality in hypothyroid mice. *Nature* 197:1212.

Prange, A. J., Jr.; Lipton, M. A.; and Love, G. N. 1964. The effect of altered thyroid status on desmethylimipramine mortality in mice. *Nature* 204:1204.

Prange, A. J., Jr.; McCurdy, R. L.; and Cochrane, C. M. 1967. The systolic blood pressure response of depressed patients to infused norepinephrine. *J. Psychiat. Res.* 5:1.

Prange, A. J., Jr.; Wilson, I. C.; Knox, A. E.; McClane, T. K.; and Lipton, M. A. 1970. Enhancement of imipramine by thyroid stimulating hormone: clinical and theoretical implications. *Amer. J. Psychiat.* 127:191.

Prange, A. J., Jr.; Wilson, I. C.; and Lipton, M. A. In preparation.

Prange, A. J., Jr.; Wilson, I. C.; Rabon, A. M.; and Lipton, M. A. 1968. Enhancement of imipramine by triiodothyronine in unselected depressed patients. *Excerpta Medica International Congress Series*. No. 180, p. 532.

Prange, A. J., Jr.; Wilson, I. C.; Rabon, A. M.; and Lipton, M. A. 1969. Enhancement of imipramine antidepressant activity by thyroid hormone. *Amer. J. Psychiat.* 126:457.

Rodnight, R. 1961. Body fluid indoles in mental illness. *Int. Rev. Neurobiol.* 3:251.

Rosenblatt, S.; Chanley, J. D.; and Leighton, W. P. 1969a. The investigation of adrenergic metabolism with $7H^3$-norepinephrine in psychiatric disorders--I. Temporal change in the distribution of urinary tritiated metabolites and the effects of drugs. *J. Psychiat. Res.* 6:307.

Rosenblatt, S.; Chanley, J. D.; and Leighton, W. P. 1969b. The investigation of adrenergic metabolism with $7H^3$-norepinephrine in psychiatric disorders--II. Temporal changes in the distribution of urinary tritiated metabolites in affective disorders. *J. Psychiat. Res.* 6:321.

Schildkraut, J. J.; Gordon, E. K.; and Durrell, J. 1965. Catecholamine metabolism in affective disorders: I. Normetanephrine and VMA excretion in depressed patients treated with imipramine. *J. Psychiat. Res.* 3:213.

Sjoerdsma, A.; Oates, J. A.; Zaltman, P.; and Udenfriend, S. 1959. Identification and assay of urinary tryptamine: application as an index of monoamine oxidase inhibition in man. *J. Pharmacol Exp. Ther.* 126:217.

Spencer, P. S. J.; and West, G. B. 1961. Sensitivity of the hyperthyroid and hypothyroid mouse to histamine and 5-hydroxytryptamine. *Brit. J. Pharmacol.* 17:137.

Taniguchi, K.; Kakimoto, Y.; and Armstrong, M. D. 1964. Quantitative determination of metanephrine and normetanephrine in urine. *J. Lab. Clin. Med.* 64.

Toth, S.; and Csaba, B. 1966. The effect of thyroid gland on 5-hydroxytryptamine (5-HT) level of brain stem and blood in rabbits. *Experientia* 22:755.

Udenfriend, S.; Titus, E.; and Weissbach, H. 1955. The identification of 5-hydroxy-3-indoleacetic acid in normal urine and a method for its assay. *J. Biol. Chem.* 216:499.

Wheatley, D. A comparative trial of amitryptyline with two dose levels of L-triiodothyronine in depressed outpatients. In preparation.

Wilk, S.; Gitlow, S. E.; Clarke, D. D.; and Paley, D. H. 1967. Determination of urinary 3-methoxy-4-hydroxyphenylethylene glycol by gas-liquid chromatography and electron capture detection. *Clin. Chim. Acta.* 16:403.

Wilk, S.; Gitlow, S. E.; Mendlowitz, M.; Franklin, M. J.; Carr, H. E.; and Clarke, D. D. 1965. A quantitative assay for vanillylmandelic acid (VMA) by gas-liquid chromatography. *Anal. Biochem.* 13:544.

Williams, E. D. 1968. 5-Hydroxyindoles and the thyroid. *Advances Pharmacol.* 6:(suppl.)151.

Wilson, I. C.; Prange, A. J., Jr.; McClane, T. K.; Rabon, A. M.; and Lipton, M. A. 1970. Thyroid-hormone enhancement of imipramine in nonretarded depressions. *New Eng. J. Med.* 282:1063.

Wyatt R. J.; Portnoy, B.; Kupfer, D. J.; Snyder, F.; and Engleman, K. 1971. Resting plasma catecholamine concentrations in patients with depression and anxiety. *Arch. Gen. Psychiat.* 24:65.

Zung, W. W. K. 1970. A self-rating depression scale. *Arch. Gen. Psychiat.* 12:63.

EFFECTS OF TRICYCLIC ANTIDEPRESSANTS ON NOREPINEPHRINE METABOLISM:

BASIC AND CLINICAL STUDIES

>
> Joseph J. Schildkraut, Paul R. Draskoczy,
> Elliot S. Gershon, Peter Reich, and Edwin L. Grab
>
> Massachusetts Mental Health Center and
> Harvard Medical School
> Boston, Massachusetts

The tricyclic antidepressants have been well established as clinically effective treatments for certain types of depressions, and these drugs have provided important tools for investigating those neurochemical changes that may be associated with alterations in affective state in man (Schildkraut 1970). Some years ago, in clinical studies of depressed patients, we observed a decrease in the urinary excretion of 3-methoxy-4-hydroxymandelic acid (VMA), the major deaminated O-methylated metabolite of norepinephrine during treatment with imipramine (a tricyclic antidepressant) as well as with phenelzine (a monoamine oxidase inhibitor) (Table 1) (Schildkraut et al. 1964; Schildkraut, Gordon, and Durell 1965). In these studies with imipramine, we showed that the decrease in VMA excretion was a pharmacological effect of the drug per se and not a secondary concomitant of the alteration in clinical state (Table 2) (Schildkraut, Gordon, and Durell 1965). On the basis of these findings, which have been confirmed by other investigators (Haskovec and Rysanek 1967; Maas, Fawcett, and Dekirmenjian 1968b and personal communication), we suggested that tricyclic antidepressants like monoamine oxidase inhibitors may decrease the deamination of norepinephrine. Subsequently, Glowinski, Axelrod, and Iversen (1966) showed that desmethylimipramine decreased the deamination of intraventricularly administered tritiated norepinephrine in rat brain, and we found a similar decrease in the deamination of intracisternally administered tritiated norepinephrine and a concurrent increase in levels of tritiated normetanephrine in rat brain after administration of various other tricyclic antidepressants (Table 3) (Schildkraut et al. 1967; Schildkraut, Dodge, and Logue 1969).

Amitriptyline, as well as imipramine, was initially reported to inhibit the uptake of norepinephrine in rat brain (Glowinski and Axel-

TABLE 1

Summary of Changes in VMA Excretion in Depressed Patients
During Treatment with Placebo, Phenelzine, or Imipramine

Treatment Group	Number of Patients	Pretreatment Mean VMA ± SEM	Treatment Mean VMA ± SEM	p*
Placebo	5	4.54 ± 0.40	3.97 ± 0.81	N.S.
Phenelzine	6	3.54 ± 0.81	1.09 ± 0.23	<0.05
Imipramine	6	5.12 ± 0.92	2.36 ± 0.36	<0.05

In this study of VMA excretion in depressed patients, the initial "pretreatment" placebo period was followed by an "active" treatment period during which phenelzine, imipramine, or placebo was administered. Mean urinary VMA excretion during each of the "active" treatments was compared with the corresponding pretreatment values. Levels of VMA excretion are reported in mg/24 hours.

*p = probability level for difference between pretreatment and treatment values.

Data from Schildkraut, Klerman, Hammond, and Friend 1964. Reprinted with permission of authors and J. Psychiat. Res. 2:257.

rod 1964), but in subsequent studies in our laboratory and elsewhere the uptake of norepinephrine in rat brain did not appear to be inhibited by amitriptyline (Table 3) (Schildkraut, Dodge, and Logue 1969; Stille 1968). (Uptake of norepinephrine into the presynaptic noradrenergic neuron is thought to be the major mechanism for removing norepinephrine from the synaptic cleft--i.e., terminating the activity of norepinephrine at receptors [Figure 1].) In contrast, a number of investigators have reported that serotonin uptake is inhibited by amitriptyline (Carlsson et al. 1969a; Himwich and Alpers 1970). Moreover, in one study, amitriptyline did not alter the turnover or synthesis of norepinephrine in rat brain, whereas the turnover and synthesis of serotonin were decreased by this drug (Schubert, Nybäck, and Sedvall 1970). Thus, some investigators have suggested, on the basis of these findings, that the clinical antidepressant actions of amitriptyline may be due to its effects on the uptake, turnover, and metabolism of serotonin rather than of norepinephrine (Carlsson et al. 1969b).

With respect to the possible biochemical mechanism of action of tricyclic antidepressants, it is, therefore, of considerable interest to know whether amitriptyline alters norepinephrine metabolism

TABLE 2

VMA Excretion in Depressed Patients Treated with Imipramine

Patient	Pretreatment Placebo Period		Imipramine Data Period		Posttreatment Placebo Period
	VMA Excretion Mean ± SD	p*	VMA Excretion Mean ± SD	p†	VMA Excretion Mean ± SD
N.B.	3.8 ± 0.4	0.10	2.7 ± 0.1	0.0005	4.5 ± 0.1
E.J.	1.7 ± 0.7	0.18	1.1 ± 0.2	0.06	3.0 ± 1.6
F.J.	7.0 ± 2.7	0.13	4.2 ± 2.5	0.10	6.8 ± 1.5
J.Q.	4.1 ± 0.3	0.01	3.1 ± 0.5	0.005	4.3 ± 0.6
N.J.	4.5 ± 0.8	0.05	3.1 ± 0.6	--	--

In this study of VMA excretion in depressed patients, the initial pretreatment placebo period was followed by a period of treatment with imipramine; a posttreatment placebo period followed the withdrawal of imipramine. Mean urinary VMA excretion in each patient was compared during the three periods. Levels of VMA excretion are reported in mg/24 hr.

*probability (one-tailed) - difference between pretreatment placebo and imipramine data periods.
†probability (one-tailed) - difference between posttreatment placebo and imipramine data periods.
(One-tailed t-tests were used since the directions of change were predicted on the basis of previous findings.)

Data from Schildkraut, Gordon, and Durell 1965. Reprinted with permission of authors and J. Psychiat. Res. 3:213.

in man. In our preliminary studies of the effects of amitriptyline on the metabolism of norepinephrine in depressed patients, we have found that amitriptyline decreases both the urinary excretion of VMA--the metabolite that may provide the best index of norepinephrine synthesis and metabolism in peripheral tissues, and the urinary excretion of 3-methoxy-4-hydroxyphenylglycol (MHPG)--the metabolite that may provide the best available index of norepinephrine synthesis and metabolism in brain (Schildkraut et al. in press).

TABLE 3

Effects of Tricyclic Antidepressants on the Uptake and Metabolism of ^{3}H-Norepinephrine in Rat Brain

Drugs	^{3}H-NE a	^{3}H-NMN b	^{3}H-DCM c	Total ^{3}H-DOM d	Free ^{3}H-DOM e
	Percent Control Mean ± SEM				
Desmethylimipramine	71 ± 2*	196 ± 7*	52 ± 2*	102 ± 3	100 ± 6
Protriptyline	67 ± 5*	174 ± 11*	45 ± 4*	92 ± 5	98 ± 5
Imipramine	81 ± 5†	176 ± 8*	50 ± 3*	94 ± 7	100 ± 12
Nortriptyline	80 ± 3*	151 ± 6*	48 ± 2*	93 ± 3	102 ± 9
Amitriptyline	100 ± 2	123 ± 4*	74 ± 3*	95 ± 2	94 ± 5

A tricyclic antidepressant (25 mg/kg) or isotonic saline was administered 90 minutes before the intracisternal injection of ^{3}H-norepinephrine, and animals were sacrificed 6 minutes after the intracisternal injection. In this series of experiments, the total number of animals administered each drug was: desmethylimipramine = 27; protriptyline = 6; imipramine = 6; nortriptyline = 15; amitriptyline = 29. Results for each drug were combined and are expressed as a percentage of the matched control mean (100%) ± standard error of the mean.

a – ^{3}H-NE = tritiated norepinephrine
b – ^{3}H-NMN = tritiated normetanephrine
c – ^{3}H-DCM = tritiated deaminated catechol metabolites, i.e., 3,4-dihydroxyphenylglycol and 3,4-dihydroxymandelic acid
d – Total ^{3}H-DOM = total tritiated deaminated O-methylated metabolites, i.e., 3-methoxy-4-hydroxymandelic acid (VMA), 3-methoxy-4-hydroxyphenylglycol (MHPG), and the sulfate conjugate of MHPG
e – Free ^{3}H-DOM = free tritiated deaminated O-methylated metabolites, i.e., VMA and MHPG

*p < 0.001; †p < 0.01

Reproduced from Schildkraut, Dodge, and Logue 1969. Reprinted with permission of authors and J. Psychiat. Res. 7:29.

NORADRENERGIC NEURON AND RECEPTOR

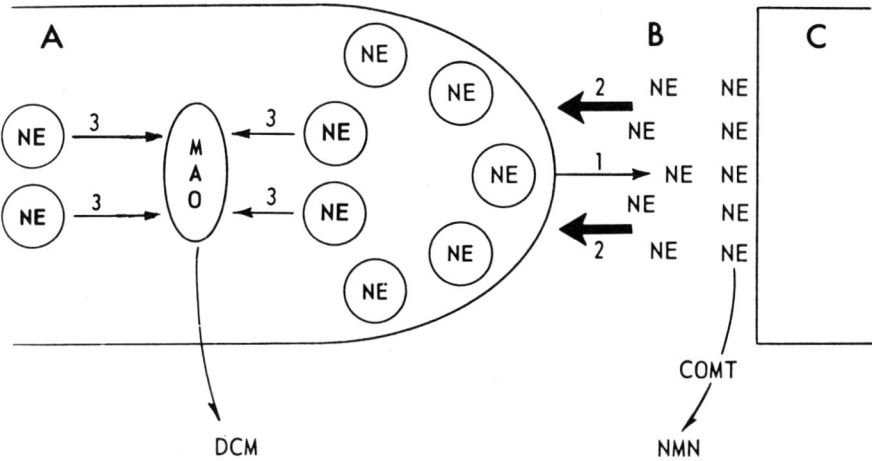

Figure 1. Schematic representation of a noradrenergic nerve ending (A), synaptic cleft (B), and receptor (C). NE = norepinephrine, NMN = normetanephrine, DCM = deaminated catechol metabolites, COMT = catechol-O-methyl transferase, MAO = monoamine oxidase (within a mitochondrion); 1 = discharge of norepinephrine into synaptic cleft, 2 = reuptake of norepinephrine from synaptic cleft, 3 = intracellular release of norepinephrine from storage granules into cytoplasm and onto mitochrondrial monoamine oxidase.

Table 4 shows that VMA excretion was lower during treatment with amitriptyline in the three patients studied. In two of these, VMA excretion was decreased by approximately 50 percent, and these differences were statistically significant ($p < 0.05$), whether the data were computed on the basis of VMA excretion per 24 hours or VMA excretion per gram of creatinine. In the third patient, a similar trend was observed but the decrease in VMA excretion was smaller. It is of some interest to note that the two patients with large decreases in VMA excretion showed rapid and dramatic clinical responses to treatment with amitriptyline; complete remissions of the depressions occurred within several weeks in these two patients. In contrast, the third patient with a smaller decrease in VMA excretion did not show a marked clinical response during the first month of treatment with amitriptyline; complete clinical remission, which could not necessarily be ascribed to the pharmacological effects of the drug, was gradually attained only after a period of many months.

TABLE 4

VMA Excretion in Depressed Patients
Before and During Amitriptyline Administration

Patient	Before Drug	During Drug	Difference	Δ%	p
B.O.	Weeks=4 4010 ± 810 (6750 ± 960) N=8	Weeks=2 1810 ± 180 (3690 ± 410) N=6	2200 (3060)	55% (45%)	<0.05 (<0.05)
B.L.	Weeks=3 3940 ± 550 (5540 ± 510) N=5	Weeks=4 1800 ± 250 (3240 ± 250) N=4	2140 (2300)	54% (42%)	<0.05 (<0.01)
E.S.	Weeks=6 3420 ± 520 (2660 ± 50) N=4	Weeks=29 2530 ± 190 (2280 ± 260) N=8	890 (380)	26% (14%)	<0.10 (---)

In this study of norepinephrine metabolism in depressed patients, which is reported in Tables 4 through 10, the initial pretreatment (Before Drug) period was followed by a period of treatment (During Drug) with amitriptyline, 150 to 225 mg per day. The data are expressed as the means ± standard errors of the means in micrograms per 24 hours. (The values in micrograms per gram of creatinine are indicated below in parentheses.) "Weeks" are the number of weeks in the period, "N" is the number of urine samples assayed during the period. The "difference" is the mean value before drug minus the mean value during drug. $\Delta\% = \frac{\text{difference}}{\text{mean value before drug}} \times 100$.

p = probability level for difference between "Before Drug" and "During Drug" values.

The design and methods of this study are described in specific detail in Schildkraut, Draskoczy, Gershon, Reich, and Grab: Catecholamine metabolism in affective disorders IV. Preliminary studies of norepinephrine metabolism in depressed patients treated with amitriptyline. J. Psychiat. Res. in press. Reprinted with permission of authors and J. Psychiat. Res.

The present findings suggest, therefore, that the magnitude of the decrease of VMA excretion produced by amitriptyline may in some way be related to the pharmacological effectiveness of this drug as a clinical antidepressant in any given patient. This relationship could be a trivial one since, for example, both the decrease in VMA excretion and the clinical effectiveness of the drug would be expected to vary as a function of drug dosage (or tissue concentration) without these two variables necessarily bearing a causal relationship to each other. However, the possibility of a nontrivial relationship and even a causal connection between this biochemical effect of the drug (i.e., the decrease in VMA excretion) and its clin-

TABLE 5

MHPG Excretion in Depressed Patients
Before and During Amitriptyline Administration

Patient	Before Drug	During Drug	Difference	Δ%	p
B.O.	Weeks=4 1210 ± 130 (2240 ± 200) N=7	Weeks=2 500 ± 90 (970 ± 70) N=6	710 (1270)	59% (57%)	<0.005 (<0.001)
B.L.	Weeks=3 2070 ± 220 (3190 ± 230) N=7	Weeks=4 1490 ± 140 (2710 ± 220) N=4	580 (480)	28% (15%)	<0.10 (--)
E.S.	Weeks=6 670 ± 150 (530 ± 70) N=4	Weeks=29 530 ± 30 (470 ± 30) N=8	140 (60)	21% (11%)	(--) (--)

See legend to Table 4.

ical antidepressant effects should not be excluded. For example, the magnitude of the decrease in VMA excretion may reflect the extent of the decrease in deamination of norepinephrine produced by amitriptyline (see below) and this, conceivably, could be one of the factors determining its clinical effectiveness as an antidepressant. Further studies in a larger number of patients are now in progress to test this hypothesis.

3-Methoxy-4-hydroxyphenylglycol (MHPG) was identified in cat brain (Mannarino, Kirshner, and Nashold 1963), and we found that the sulfate conjugate of MHPG was the principal metabolite of norepinephrine and normetanephrine in rat brain (Schanberg et al. 1968b). In dogs, most norepinephrine coming from brain is excreted in the urine as MHPG (Maas and Landis 1968). Although technical difficulties have prevented comparable studies of these routes of metabolism in human brain, we have identified MHPG and its sulfate conjugate in the cerebrospinal fluid of man (Schanberg et al. 1968a). The urinary excretion of MHPG in human subjects, therefore, may provide the best available index of norepinephrine synthesis and metabolism in the brain, although urinary MHPG may also derive in part from norepinephrine coming from peripheral sympathetic nerves. Maas and his collaborators have reported that MHPG excretion was decreased in a heterogeneous group of depressed patients (Maas, Fawcett, and Dekirmenjian 1968a), and we found that MHPG levels were decreased during depression and increased during mania in a small group of manic-depressive patients studied longitudinally (Greenspan et al. 1970).

Table 5 shows that urinary levels of MHPG were lower during treatment with amitriptyline than prior to treatment with this drug. The differences, however, were statistically significant in only one of the three patients studied. Similarly, in studies of the effects of imipramine on MHPG excretion, Maas and his associates have observed decreases in MHPG excretion during treatment with imipramine that were less pronounced and less consistent than the decreases in VMA excretion (Maas, Fawcett, and Dekirmenjian 1968b and personal communications). It may be of some interest to note that the patient (B.O.) who had the very marked decrease in MHPG excretion during treatment with amitriptyline, developed a manic episode severe enough to necessitate withdrawal of amitriptyline and further treatment with chlorpromazine.

Whereas levels of VMA prior to drug treatment were similar in these three patients (Table 4), marked differences were observed in MHPG levels. Urinary excretion of MHPG prior to treatment was considerably lower in the patient (E.S.) in whom we made the diagnosis of manic-depressive depression, than in the patients (B.O. or B.L.) in whom we diagnosed involutional depressions (Table 5). (Clinical diagnoses were made in accordance with criteria described elsewhere [Schildkraut 1970].) It may be relevant that the patient (E.S.) with the very low levels of MHPG did not show a clear-cut clinical response to treatment with amitriptyline, whereas the other two patients with higher pretreatment levels of MHPG showed marked and rapid clinical responses after treatment with this drug.

Maas and his associates have reported that depressed patients with low levels of MHPG excretion respond better to treatment with imipramine than do patients with higher levels of MHPG (Maas, Fawcett, and Dekirmenjian 1968b and personal communications); in line with this observation, patient E.S. gave a history of having responded well to imipramine during a previous depressive episode. In contrast, the two patients in the present study with higher levels of MHPG excretion responded rapidly to amitriptyline. These very preliminary findings, which suggest that patients with higher levels of MHPG may respond well to amitriptyline, if borne out in our ongoing studies, may provide a rational basis for choosing between amitriptyline and imipramine in the treatment of patients with endogenous depressions.

In our studies of imipramine in depressed patients, no consistent changes in normetanephrine excretion were observed when values obtained before and during drug treatment were compared (Schildkraut, Gordon, and Durell 1965; Schildkraut et al. 1966). Gradual increases in normetanephrine excretion were observed, however, in relation to the improvement in clinical state; and patients with retarded depressions were found to have lower levels of normetanephrine excretion during the period of depression than after clinical improvement (Schildkraut, Gordon, and Durell 1965; Schildkraut et al. 1966). Similarly, Table 6 shows that a consistent direction of change was not observed when levels of normetanephrine were compared before and during treatment with amitriptyline; however, low levels of normetanephrine were observed in the manic-depressive patient (E.S.) during the initial period of study when this patient was most depressed, and a gradual rise in normetanephrine excretion, which was highly correlated with the gradual decrease in depression rating scores, was observed during the six-month period of gradual clinical improvement.

In our previous studies, normetanephrine levels were not lower, and in some instances were even higher, during the period of depression in patients with agitated or involutional depressions (Schildkraut et al. 1966; Greenspan et al. 1970), and similar findings were observed in the two patients (B.O. and B.L.) with involutional depressions in the present study (Table 6). It has been suggested previously that factors tending to increase and factors tending to decrease urinary normetanephrine may be operative simultaneously in such patients (Schildkraut, Davis, and Klerman 1968). Agitation, anxiety, psychic turmoil, overt psychosis, and motor activity have been found to be associated with an increase in urinary norepinephrine and normetanephrine as well as epinephrine and metanephrine, presumably as a result of increased peripheral sympathetic and adrenal medullary activity (Schildkraut, Gordon, and Durell 1965; Karki 1956; Sachar et al. 1963; Nelson, Masuda, and Holmes 1966;

TABLE 6

Normetanephrine Excretion in Depressed Patients
Before and During Amitriptyline Administration

Patient	Before Drug	During Drug	Difference	Δ%	p
B.O.	Weeks=4 340 ± 90 (580 ± 120) N=8	Weeks=2 290 ± 40 (580 ± 80) N=6	50 (0)	15% (0%)	-- (--)
B.L.	Weeks=3 220 ± 29 (330 ± 20) N=6	Weeks=4 220 ± 12 (410 ± 43) ·N=4	0 (-80)	0% (-24%)	-- (<0.10)
E.S.	Weeks=6 110 ± 30 (90 ± 20) N=4	Weeks=29 250 ± 40 (210 ± 20) N=9	-140 (-120)	-127% (-133%)	0.05 (<0.05)

See legend to Table 4.

Bunney et al. 1967). In some patients with agitated or involutional depressions, the increase in peripheral sympathetic activity associated with the agitation or psychic turmoil may, therefore, mask any measurable decrease in noradrenergic activity that may be associated with the depression per se (Greenspan et al. 1970).

It has also been suggested that some depressed patients may have a relative (that is, functional), but not an absolute, deficiency of norepinephrine as a result of a decrease in the sensitivity of noradrenergic receptors (Schildkraut 1965). The finding of Prange and his associates (Prange, McCurdy, and Cochrane 1967) that the infusion of norepinephrine produces a smaller elevation in blood pressure in some depressed patients during depression than after recovery

TABLE 7

Norepinephrine Excretion in Depressed Patients
Before and During Amitriptyline Administration

Patient	Before Drug	During Drug	Difference	Δ%	p
B.O.	Weeks=4 28 ± 6 (50 ± 8) N=8	Weeks=2 20 ± 2 (40 ± 3) N=6	8 (10)	29% (20%)	(--) (--)
B.L.	Weeks=3 16 ± 2 (24 ± 2) N=6	Weeks=4 12 ± 1 (22 ± 2) N=4	4 (2)	25% (8%)	<0.20 (--)
E.S.	Weeks=6 5 ± 1 (4 ± 1) N=4	Weeks=29 17 ± 4 (13 ± 3) N=9	-12 (-9)	-240% (-225%)	<0.10 (<0.10)

See legend to Table 4.

is compatible with this hypothesis. Moreover, after administration of various phenothiazines, which are thought to block noradrenergic receptors, we have observed an increase in normetanephrine excretion and possibly also in MHPG excretion (Schildkraut, Gordon, and Durell 1965; Schildkraut, unpublished data). It is, thus, possible that some depressed patients with relatively high normetanephrine excretion may have a homeostatic increase in the output of norepinephrine from presynaptic neurons that partially compensates for a decrease in the sensitivity of postsynaptic noradrenergic receptors. This possibility has also been discussed by Prange et al. in this symposium.

Table 7 shows that a consistent direction of change in norepinephrine excretion was not observed when values obtained before and during treatment with amitriptyline were compared. Only in patient E.S. did the change in norepinephrine excretion approach statistical significance, and in this patient the gradual increase in norepinephrine excretion seemed to be correlated with the gradual decrease in depression rating scores.

A number of factors could contribute to the decreases in VMA and MHPG excretion that we have observed during treatment with amitriptyline. Such decreases would be expected to occur with a decrease in norepinephrine synthesis, as well as with a decrease in the deamination of norepinephrine or normetanephrine, or a decrease in the O-methylation of norepinephrine or its deaminated catechol metabolites (Figure 2).

A decrease in norepinephrine biosynthesis does seem to occur during treatment with amitriptyline, since the sum of norepinephrine and the various metabolites we have measured was, in each instance, lower during treatment with amitriptyline than prior to treatment with this drug (Table 8). There is no evidence to suggest that there may have been a compensatory increase in some other metabolite that we did not measure, although this possibility cannot be definitely ruled out. It is unlikely that the deaminated catechol metabolites, the only normally occurring metabolites we did not measure, would be increased by amitriptyline, since studies in animals suggest that these metabolites are decreased by this drug (Schildkraut, Dodge, and Logue 1969). Moreover, we are not aware of any data suggesting that amitriptyline leads to the formation of other (i.e., abnormal) metabolites of norepinephrine.

Similar changes have previously been observed with imipramine (Schildkraut, Gordon, and Durell 1965), and two possible mechanisms, which are not mutually exclusive, have been suggested to account for the decreased synthesis of norepinephrine (Schildkraut, Winokur, and Applegate 1970; Schildkraut et al. 1971). A decrease in the deamination of norepinephrine, which may be presumed to occur on the basis of our studies in animals (Schildkraut, Dodge, and Logue 1969), could cause an increase in free intraneuronal norepinephrine after administration of amitriptyline or other tricyclic antidepressants. This would be expected to decrease norepinephrine synthesis since, in other systems, free intraneuronal catecholamines have been found to inhibit tyrosine hydroxylase, the rate-limiting enzyme in the biosynthesis of norepinephrine (Weiner 1970). It has also been suggested that the rate of discharge of presynaptic noradrenergic neurons may be controlled, in part, by a negative feedback from the postsynaptic neurons. By increasing levels of norepinephrine at postsynaptic receptors, tricyclic antidepressants may, thus, cause a decrease in the rate of discharge of presynaptic neurons which, under steady state conditions, would lead to a decrease in the turnover

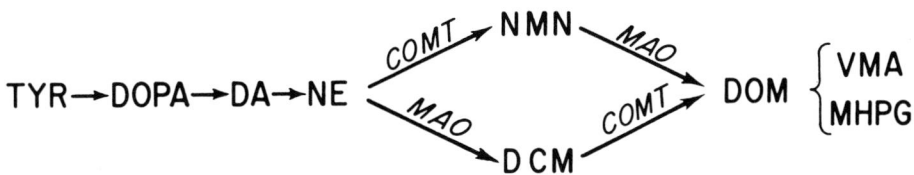

Figure 2. Synthesis and metabolism of norepinephrine. TYR = tyrosine, DOPA = dihydroxyphenylalanine, DA = dopamine, NE = norpinephrine, NMN = normetanephrine, DCM = deaminated catechol metabolites, DOM = deaminated O-methylated metabolites, VMA = 3-methoxy-4-hydroxymandelic acid, MHPG = 3-methoxy-4-hydroxyphenylglycol, COMT = catechol O-methyl transferase, MAO = monoamine oxidase.

TABLE 8

NE+NMN+MHPG+VMA Excretion in Depressed Patients
Before and During Treatment with Amitriptyline

Patient	Before Drug	During Drug	Difference	Δ%	p
B.O.	Weeks=4 4790 ± 600 (8670 ± 770) N=7	Weeks=2 2610 ± 280 (5280 ± 470) N=6	2180 (3390)	46% (39%)	<0.05 (<0.005)
B.L.	Weeks=3 6330 ± 790 (8890 ± 520) N=5	Weeks=4 3530 ± 370 (6380 ± 420) N=4	2800 (2510)	44% (28%)	<0.05 (<0.01)
E.S.	Weeks=6 4200 ± 640 (3280 ± 100) N=4	Weeks=29 3320 ± 210 (2970 ± 270) N=8	880 (310)	21% (9%)	<0.20 (--)

See legend to Table 4.

TABLE 9

NMN:VMA Ratio* in Depressed Patients
Before and During Amitriptyline Administration

Patient	Before Drug*	During Drug*	Difference*	Δ%	p
B.O.	Weeks=4 8.2 ± 0.8 N=8	Weeks=2 15.8 ± 1.3 N=6	-7.6	-93%	<0.001
B.L.	Weeks=3 6.2 ± 0.2 N=5	Weeks=4 12.9 ± 1.3 N=4	-6.7	-109%	<0.001
E.S.	Weeks=6 3.3 ± 0.8 N=4	Weeks=29 10.1 ± 1.7 N=8	-6.8	-206%	<0.05

"Weeks," "N," "Difference," and "Δ%" are defined in legend to Table 4.
*Ratios have been multiplied by 100.

and synthesis of norepinephrine (Schildkraut, Winokur, and Applegate 1970; Schildkraut et al. 1971). (This second mechanism may be of more importance with imipramine and other tricyclic antidepressants than with amitriptyline, since the uptake of norepinephrine into the presynaptic neuron, which is thought to be the major mechanism for terminating the activity of extraneuronal norepinephrine, may not be inhibited by amitriptyline [Table 3] [Schildkraut, Dodge, and Logue 1969].)

In order to provide further information concerning changes in metabolism which could contribute to the decreases in VMA and MHPG excretion, the ratios, NMN:VMA and NMN:MHPG, were examined before and during treatment with amitriptyline. The NMN:VMA and NMN:MHPG ratios were higher in all patients during treatment with amitriptyline than they were prior to treatment with this drug (Tables 9 and 10). The consistent increases of these ratios during treatment with amitriptyline suggest that the decreases in VMA and MHPG do not occur simply as a result of decreased norepinephrine biosynthesis, but that changes in metabolism also contribute to these findings.

TABLE 10

NMN:MHPG Ratio* in Depressed Patients
Before and During Amitriptyline Administration

Patient	Before Drug*	During Drug*	Difference*	Δ%	p
B.O.	Weeks=4 21 ± 2 N=7	Weeks=2 62 ± 11 N=6	-41	-195%	<0.005
B.L.	Weeks=3 11 ± 1 N=6	Weeks=4 16 ± 2 N=4	-5	-45%	<0.10
E.S.	Weeks=6 17 ± 5 N=4	Weeks=29 47 ± 8 N=8	-30	-176%	<0.05

"Weeks," "N," "Difference," and "Δ%" are defined in legend to Table 4.

*Ratios have been multiplied by 100.

A decrease in the deamination of norepinephrine during treatment with amitriptyline provides the most likely explanation of these findings. This could contribute to the decrease in MHPG and VMA and lead to the increases in the NMN:VMA and NMN:MHPG ratios (Figure 2). Since amitriptyline does not seem to decrease the deamination of tritiated normetanephrine and its conversion to deaminated O-methylated compounds in animal brain (Table 11), it is unlikely that a decrease in the conversion of normetanephrine to VMA or MHPG contributed to the changes we have observed. The elevated NMN:VMA and NMN:MHPG ratios in the present study, and the increases in tritiated normetanephrine (formed from intracisternally administered tritiated norepinephrine) in animal brain after treatment with amitriptyline (Schildkraut, Dodge, and Logue 1969) do not favor the possibility that amitriptyline decreases the O-methylation of norepinephrine. A decrease in the O-methylation of deaminated catechol metabolites could conceivably contribute to the findings we have observed, but we are not aware of any studies in animals or man to suggest that amitriptyline does, in fact, decrease the O-methylation of deaminated catechols.

TABLE 11

Effects of Amitriptyline on the Metabolism
of ^{3}H-Normetanephrine in Rat Brain

	Control	Amitriptyline
	(Percent Control ± SEM)	
6 minutes after ^{3}H-normetanephrine		
^{3}H-NMN	100 ± 6	104 ± 4
Total ^{3}H-DOM	100 ± 6	103 ± 6
Free ^{3}H-DOM	100 ± 6	94 ± 6
45 minutes after ^{3}H-normetanephrine		
^{3}H-NMN	100 ± 4	115 ± 6
Total ^{3}H-DOM	100 ± 6	103 ± 7
Free ^{3}H-DOM	100 ± 6	108 ± 6

Amitriptyline (25 mg/kg) or isotonic saline was administered i.p. 90 minutes before the intracisternal injection of ^{3}H-normetanephrine and animals were sacrificed 6 or 45 minutes after the intracisternal injection. Results are expressed as a percentage of the control means (100%) ± standard errors of the means. Abbreviations are defined in legend to Table 3.

CONCLUSIONS

The effects of the tricyclic antidepressants, as well as other drugs or electroconvulsive shock, on the turnover and metabolism of the biogenic amines, norepinephrine, dopamine, and serotonin, in the brain of the experimental animal, correlate fairly well with the clinical effects of these treatments on affective states in man (Schildkraut 1970). Despite some discrepancies, most findings seem compatible with the hypothesis that drugs that are antidepressants or euphoriants may increase one or another of the biogenic amines at receptor sites in brain, whereas drugs that cause depressions or are effective in the treatment of manias may decrease the activity of

TABLE 12

Summary of Effects of Psychoactive Drugs and Electroconvulsive Shock on Norepinephrine Metabolism and Mood

Drug or Treatment	Effects on Mood (Man)	Effects on Norepinephrine Metabolism in Brain (Animals)	Presumed Effect on Norepinephrine at Receptors
Monoamine Oxidase Inhibitors	Antidepressant	Inhibits deamination; increases NE; increases NMN; decreases DCM	Increase
----		----	
Tranylcypromine		May discharge NE and inhibit cellular uptake of NE	
Tricyclic Antidepressants	Antidepressant	Inhibits cellular uptake of NE; increases NMN; decreases DCM	Increase
----		----	
Amitriptyline		May not inhibit cellular uptake of NE; but increases NMN; decreases DCM	
Cocaine	Stimulant	Inhibits cellular uptake of NE; increases NMN; decreases DCM	Increase
Amphetamine	Stimulant	Inhibits cellular uptake of NE; discharges NE; increases NMN; decreases DCM	Increase
Electroconvulsive Shock	Counteracts Depression	Increases neuronal discharge of NE; increases NMN	Increase
Reserpine	Causes Depression	Depletes NE (with intracellular deamination); decreases synthesis of NE	Decrease
Lithium Salts	Counteracts Mania	Increases DCM; decreases NMN; high dose increases turnover of NE	Decrease

NE = norepinephrine; NMN = normetanephrine; DCM = deaminated catechol metabolites

Reprinted with permission from Schildkraut, J. J. 1970. *Neuropsychopharmacology and the Affective Disorders*, Boston: Little, Brown and Co., p. 36.

monoamines at receptors. Norepinephrine is the monoamine that has been studied most extensively, and the findings from these studies provide the most coherent body of data (Table 12). On the basis of these studies, as well as correlative studies of biogenic amine metabolism in patients with affective disorders, it has been suggested that functional deficiencies of norepinephrine or serotonin at critical receptor sites in brain may occur in, at least, some types of depressions, whereas elations may be associated with an excess of one or another of the monoamines (Schildkraut 1965 and 1970; Bunney and Davis 1965; Schildkraut and Kety 1967).

The decreases in MHPG and VMA excretion observed during treatment with amitriptyline suggest that amitriptyline decreases the synthesis of norepinephrine in the brain as well as in the peripheral sympathetic nervous system. The concurrent increases in the NMN:MHPG and NMN:VMA ratios during treatment with amitriptyline suggest that this decrease in norepinephrine synthesis is accompanied by and, in part, may even be caused by a decrease in the deamination of norepinephrine. As a result of this decrease in deamination (presumed to occur within the presynaptic neuron), a larger fraction of synthesized norepinephrine may be available for extraneuronal release onto receptors. These findings are consistent with the effects of imipramine on norepinephrine metabolism in depressed patients (Schildkraut et al. 1964; Schildkraut, Gordon, and Durell 1965), and with the effects of acute and chronic administration of tricyclic antidepressants on norepinephrine metabolism in animal brain (Schildkraut, Dodge, and Logue 1969; Schildkraut, Winokur, and Applegate 1970; Schildkraut et al. 1971).

In their studies of the effect of imipramine on VMA or MHPG excretion in depressed patients, Maas and his associates found that the decrease in VMA excretion was greater and more consistent than the decrease in MHPG excretion (Maas, Fawcett, and Dekirmenjian 1968b and personal communications). Similarly, during treatment with amitriptyline, the decrease in VMA excretion was more pronounced than the decrease in MHPG excretion. Studies in animals have shown that normetanephrine does not readily penetrate the brain-blood barrier, and that most normetanephrine is deaminated (i.e., converted to the sulfate conjugate of MHPG) before leaving the brain (Schanberg et al. 1968b). Thus, the deamination of normetanephrine in the brain, which does not seem to be altered appreciably by tricyclic antidepressants, may account for a substantial fraction of MHPG, the principal metabolite of norepinephrine coming from the brain. Normetanephrine which is formed in the periphery, however, may be excreted in the urine without undergoing deamination. Thus, the deamination of normetanephrine may account for a relatively smaller fraction of VMA, the principal metabolite of norepinephrine coming from peripheral tissues.

In contrast to imipramine, which has been reported to be most effective in depressed patients excreting the lowest levels of MHPG (Maas, Fawcett, and Dekirmenjian 1968b and personal communication), our preliminary findings tentatively suggest that amitriptyline may be more effective in depressed patients with relatively higher levels of MHPG. Since amitriptyline, unlike imipramine, may not inhibit the uptake of norepinephrine into presynaptic neurons, the antidepressant effects of amitriptyline may depend principally on the alterations in norepinephrine metabolism produced by this drug. An adequate rate of synthesis of norepinephrine in the brain (as reflected by the relatively higher levels of MHPG), therefore, may be necessary for amitriptyline to exert its clinical antidepressant effects. These very preliminary findings, if borne out in our ongoing studies, may provide a rational basis for choosing between amitriptyline and imipramine in the treatment of patients with endogenous depressions.

Our findings in no way exclude the possibility that alterations in the metabolism of other biogenic amines (e.g., serotonin) may play a role in the clinical antidepressant effects of the tricyclic antidepressants. They do, however, provide clear evidence that the clinical administration of amitriptyline, as well as of imipramine, produces changes in the metabolism of norepinephrine in depressed patients, and they suggest that these changes may be involved in the biochemical mechanism of action by which these and other tricyclic antidepressants produce their clinical antidepressant effects.

ACKNOWLEDGMENTS

The authors thank Karen Bozogan, research nurse; Dr. Peter Wohlauer, research psychiatrist; Dr. Martin Kelly and Dr. Stuart Hauser, clinical psychiatrists; Barbara Keeler, research assistant; and Pallas Sun Lo, chemist, for their collaborative assistance. This work was supported in part by USPHS grant MH 15,413 from the National Institute of Mental Health and by a grant from Merck Sharp and Dohme.

REFERENCES

Bunney, W. E., Jr., and Davis, J. M. 1965. Norepinephrine in depressive reactions. *Arch. Gen. Psychiat.* 13:483.

Bunney, W. E., Jr.; Davis, J. M.; Weil-Malherbe, H.; and Smith, E.R.B. 1967. Biochemical changes in psychotic depression. *Arch. Gen. Psychiat.* 16:448.

Carlsson, A.; Corrodi, H.; Fuxe, K.; and Hökfelt, T. 1969a. Effect of antidepressant drugs on the depletion of intraneuronal brain 5-

hydroxytryptamine stores caused by 4-methyl-alpha-ethyl-meta-tyramine. *Europ. J. Pharmacol.* 5:357.

Carlsson, A.; Corrodi, H.; Fuxe, K.; and Hökfelt, T. 1969b. Effects of some antidepressant drugs on the depletion of intraneuronal brain catecholamine stores caused by 4-alpha-dimethyl-meta-tyramine. *Europ. J. Pharmacol.* 5:367.

Glowinski, J., and Axelrod, J. 1964. Inhibition of uptake of tritiated noradrenaline in intact rat brain by imipramine and related compounds. *Nature* 204:1318.

Glowinski, J.; Axelrod, J.; and Iversen, L. L. 1966. Regional studies of catecholamines in rat brain IV. Effects of drugs on the disposition and metabolism of H^3-norepinephrine and H^3-dopamine. *J. Pharmacol. Exp. Ther.* 153:30.

Greenspan, K.; Schildkraut, J. J.; Gordon, E. K.; Baer, L.; Aronoff, M. S.; and Durell, J. 1970. Catecholamine metabolism in affective disorders III. MHPG and other catecholamine metabolites in patients treated with lithium carbonate. *J. Psychiat. Res.* 7:171.

Haskovec, L., and Rysanek, K. 1967. Excretion of 3-methoxy-4-hydroxy-mandelic acid and 5-hydroxyindoleacetic acid in depressed patients treated with imipramine. *J. Psychiat. Res.* 5:213.

Himwich, H. E., and Alpers, H. S. 1970. Psychopharmacology. *Ann. Rev. Pharmacol.* 10:313.

Karki, N. T. 1956. The urinary excretion of noradrenaline and adrenaline in different age groups, its diurnal variation and the effect of muscular work on it. *Acta Physiol. Scand.* 39: suppl. 132.

Maas, J. W.; Fawcett, J.; and Dekirmenjian, H. 1968a. 3-Methoxy-4-hydroxyphenyl glycol (MHPG) excretion in depressed states: A pilot study. *Arch. Gen. Psychiat.* 19:129.

Maas, J. W.; Fawcett, J.; and Dekirmenjian, H. 1968b. Catecholamine metabolism and the depressive states. Presented at the annual meeting of American Psychiatric Association, Boston.

Maas, J. W.; Fawcett, J.; and Dekirmenjian, H. Personal communication.

Maas, J. W., and Landis, D. H. 1968. In vivo studies of the metabolism of norepinephrine in the central nervous system. *J. Pharmacol. Exp. Ther.* 163:147.

Mannarino, E.; Kirshner, N.; and Nashold, B. S., Jr. 1963. The metabolism of (C-14) noradrenaline by cat brain in vivo. *J. Neurochem.* 10:373.

Nelson, G. N.; Masuda, M.; and Holmes, T. H. 1966. Correlations of behavior and catecholamine metabolite excretion. *Psychosom. Med.* 28:216.

Prange, A. J., Jr.; McCurdy, L. R.; and Cochrane, C. M. 1967. The systolic blood pressure response of depressed patients to infused norepinephrine. *J. Psychiat. Res.* 5:1.

Prange, A. J., Jr.; Wilson, I. C.; Knox, A. E.; McClane, T. K.; Breese, G. R.; Martin, B. R.; Alltop, L. B.; and Lipton, M. A. 1971. Thyroid-imipramine interaction: Clinical results and basic mechanism. This volume.

Sachar, E. J.; Mason, J. W.; Kolmer, H. A.; and Artiss, K. L. 1963. Psychoendocrine aspects of acute schizophrenic reactions. *Psychosom. Med.* 25:510.

Schanberg, S. M.; Breese, G. R.; Schildkraut, J. J.; Gordon, E. K.; and Kopin, I. J. 1968a. 3-Methoxy-4-hydroxyphenylglycol sulfate in brain and cerebrospinal fluid. *Biochem. Pharmacol.* 17:2006.

Schanberg, S. M.; Schildkraut, J. J.; Breese, G. R.; and Kopin, I. J. 1968b. Metabolism of normetanephrine-H^3 in rat brain--Identification of conjugated 3-methoxy-4-hydroxyphenylglycol as the major metabolite. *Biochem. Pharmacol.* 17:247.

Schildkraut, J. J. 1965. The catecholamine hypothesis of affective disorders: A review of supporting evidence. *Amer. J. Psychiat.* 122:509.

Schildkraut, J. J. 1970. *Neuropsychopharmacology and the Affective Disorders.* Boston: Little, Brown.

Schildkraut, J. J.; Davis, J. M.; and Klerman, G. L. 1968. Biochemistry of depressions. In *Psychopharmacology. A Review of Progress.* D. H. Efron et al. (eds.). Washington, D. C.: U. S. Govt. Printing Office, p. 625.

Schildkraut, J. J.; Dodge, G. A.; and Logue, M. A. 1969. Effects of tricyclic antidepressants on the uptake and metabolism of intracisternally administered norepinephrine-H^3 in rat brain. *J. Psychiat. Res.* 7:29.

Schildkraut, J. J.; Draskoczy, P. R.; Gershon, E.; Reich, P.; and Grab, E. L. Catecholamine metabolism in affective disorders IV: Preliminary studies of norepinephrine metabolism in depressed patients treated with amitriptyline. *J. Psychiat. Res.* in press.

Schildkraut, J. J.; Gordon, E. K.; and Durell, J. 1965. Catecholamine metabolism in affective disorders I: Normetanephrine and VMA excretion in depressed patients treated with imipramine. *J. Psychiat. Res.* 3:213.

Schildkraut, J. J.; Green, R.; Gordon, E. K.; and Durell, J. 1966. Normetanephrine excretion and affective state in depressed patients treated with imipramine. *Amer. J. Psychiat.* 123:690.

Schildkraut, J. J.; and Kety, S. S. 1967. Biogenic amines and emotion. *Science* 156:21.

Schildkraut, J. J.; Klerman, G. L.; Hammond, R.; and Friend, D. G. 1964. Excretion of 3-methoxy-4-hydroxymandelic acid (VMA) in depressed patients treated with antidepressant drugs. *J. Psychiat. Res.* 2:257.

Schildkraut, J. J.; Schanberg, S. M.; Breese, G. R.; and Kopin, I. J. 1967. Norepinephrine metabolism and drugs used in the affective disorders: A possible mechanism of action. *Amer. J. Psychiat.* 124:600.

Schildkraut, J. J.; Winokur, A.; and Applegate, W. 1970. Norepinephrine turnover and metabolism in rat brain after longterm administration of imipramine. *Science* 168:867.

Schildkraut, J. J.; Winokur, A.; Draskoczy, P. R.; and Hensle, J. H. 1971. Changes in norepinephrine turnover in rat brain during chronic administration of imipramine and protriptyline: A possible explanation for the delay in onset of clinical antidepressant effects. *Amer. J. Psychiat.* 127:1032.

Schubert, J.; Nybäck, H.; and Sedvall, G. 1970. Effect of antidepressant drugs on accumulation and disappearance of monoamines formed in vivo from labeled precursors in mouse brain. *J. Pharm. Pharmacol.* 22:136.

Stille, G. 1968. Pharmacological investigation of antidepressant compounds. *Pharmakopsychiatrie Neuropsychopharmakologie* 1:92.

Weiner, N. 1970. Regulation of norepinephrine biosynthesis. *Ann. Rev. Pharmacol.* 10:273.

BRAIN AMINES AND AFFECTIVE DISORDERS

      Overview: Seymour Kety
                      Harvard Medical School, Boston, Massachusetts

      Panelists: Joseph J. Schildkraut, chairman; William E.
                     Bunney, Jr., Alec Coppen, G. Curzon, Paul
                     R. Draskoczy, Morris A. Lipton, James W.
                     Maas, and Arthur J. Prange, Jr.

    SEYMOUR KETY: The discussion yesterday concerned itself with possible biochemical mechanisms in schizophrenia, and today the discussion has turned to the affective disorders. Among the differences between these two types of conditions one of the most interesting is that the affective disorders are composed of manifestations or symptoms that are much more familiar to all of us than are the manifestations of schizophrenia. It is difficult to identify with the symptoms of schizophrenic patients because, except in the dream state, the normal individual is not aware of bizarre thinking, hallucinations, and delusions in his own mental state. In the case of the affective disorders, all of these manifestations are part of our everyday life. It is not the abnormality of the individual manifestations that permits us to classify these as psychiatric disorders, but the fact that in some individuals these symptoms last too long or are inappropriately exaggerated under the circumstances associated with them. There is a sort of polarity in most of the affective symptoms, with the normal state lying somewhere in the middle, and the affective illnesses representing extremes of intensity, duration, or adaptiveness.

    The symptoms of the depressions may tell us something of value in our effort to define the possible biochemical mechanisms involved. Sadness may be treated as part of an axis of elation, happiness, sadness, grief. Hopelessness would lie at one extreme of a "coping" axis and, at the other, excessive confidence, aggression, or ambition. Retarded thought and activity would have, at its other extreme, the volatile thought processes one sees in a manic individual, and his heightened movements and activities.

There have been many theories to account for the affective disorders, but the theories implicating the biogenic amines seem to be most compelling, to make the most sense, and to be compatible with much of the knowledge that has recently been acquired about the affective disorders, the biogenic amines, and the drugs that act upon them.

The biogenic amine theories are about thirteen years old this year. I believe it is possible to trace them to the observation in 1957 in Brodie's laboratory by Shore and his associates that reserpine, the antihypertensive agent that was known to produce tranquilization and even depression in some of the patients who received it, caused a marked increase in the indoleamine metabolites in the urine. This was soon shown to be associated with a marked depletion of serotonin in the brain. The finding that reserpine depleted serotonin was quickly followed by another serendipitous finding: iproniazid, the antituberculosis agent, also caused excitement and was found to be a potent inhibitor of monoamine oxidase. It was then learned that iproniazid could elevate brain serotonin levels in animals, further strengthening belief in the likelihood that serotonin was involved in the behavioral action of that drug. These observations generated much confidence on the part of some that serotonin would eventually provide the explanation for changes in mood in man. Everything seemed to be reasonable and simple. Then some spoilsports showed that reserpine and iproniazid affect noradrenaline in much the same manner as they affect serotonin. Thus two contenders had now entered the race and the field has been more interesting, more exciting, and considerably more confusing as a result.

The proponents of these positions have produced and brought together much evidence that one or the other is crucially involved in affective disorder, evidence which it is very difficult, indeed, to ignore. Nor is it necessary to reject either one of them for it is quite possible that both may be correct.

The story is told that England and France had decided to undertake the building of a tunnel under the English Channel. Among the many bids that were received from construction companies, with estimates ranging in the billions of pounds, was one from an unknown outfit willing to undertake the task for an absurdly small sum. Further questioning elicited the information that these were two brothers who proposed to start digging on opposite sides of the channel until they met in the middle. When asked by the commission what would happen if they failed to meet, they replied, "Lucky you, you'll have two tunnels!"

We seem to be in the fortunate position today of having two tunnels. But neither has yet made it to the other side and, although each seems capable of accounting for much of what is known about the affective disorders and the ways in which drugs act upon them, somehow neither one of these theories completely fulfills all of the requirements.

Let me review the evidence that Coppen has presented and that I find rather compelling, concerning the possible role of indoleamines in the affective disorders. His evidence starts with such patients and attempts to get as close as possible to their neurochemistry in the living state. He does not quite get there, but by examining the cerebrospinal fluid of living patients and the brains of dead patients, he comes close to this aim. In previous studies on cerebrospinal fluid, three had shown a decrease in 5-hydroxyindoleacetic acid in depression, and two had failed to find a significant change. In their very systematic investigation, Coppen and his associates found a clearly significant decrease in the cerebrospinal fluid levels of 5-hydroxyindoleacetic acid in depression. Interestingly enough, this metabolite was depressed to the same level during remission, and, even more unexpectedly, was also significantly decreased during mania. The fact that this decrease occurs in mania, in depression, and in remission rules out many of the nondisease variables that confound biochemical research in mental illness (Kety 1959). It is difficult to entertain alternative hypotheses that diet, activity, or the action of drugs could explain this same finding in three quite different clinical states which would be expected to have no systematic dietary similarities, which would cover the entire range of activity, and which would be treated with no drugs or drugs with quite opposite effects.

I find it difficult to disregard the postmortem findings entirely. It is true, as Coppen has pointed out, that there are many problems in interpreting postmortem analysis of the brain for labile constituents, but unless some systematic difference occurred in the dietary or drug history, or in the postmortem handling of the brains, it should be more difficult, rather than easier, to find a significant difference between the suicide and control populations. In these studies, there was a significant decrease in 5-hydroxyindoleacetic acid in the brains of individuals after suicide.

When we turn from clinical observations to studies at a more fundamental level to support a hypothesis of the dependence of mood on serotonin, one finds the information rather sparse and far less compelling. Replacement of serotonin does not reverse the depressant effects of reserpine in animals and the actions of para-chlorophenylalanine, which depletes the brain more or less specifically of serotonin, are not suggestive of depression (Tenen 1967). Another approach is by producing lesions in the midline raphe. As Jouvet (1969) has demonstrated, these cause a marked depletion of brain serotonin and, in fact, of most of the serotoninergic system in the brain. These animals, however, do not exhibit many signs of depression, but they do show a change in sleep patterns. Animals without serotonin in the brain show decreased amounts or absence of slow-wave sleep. Another interesting finding is that animals without serotonin, or with low serotonin, have a low threshold to pain. As far as I know, these are the only significant behavioral changes produced by para-chlorophenylalanine. Of course, in man, when para-chlorophenylalanine was given in rather large doses in treatment for carcinoid lesions by Sjoerdsma and his group (not in doses large enough to deplete the brain of serotonin), there were changes in behavior and thought processes, but it would be difficult to call these changes depression (Kety 1967). The changes were more involved with anxiety, hallucinations, and with bizarre thinking, rather than with any clearcut manifestations of depression. Serotonin, if it is involved in behavior, seems to be important in producing sleep and a higher pain threshold. Perhaps serotonin has more to do with the sensitivity of the nervous system or its interaction with the environment than it does with affective state.

When we enter the catecholamine tunnel on the side of basic research and animal studies, we find the tunnel handsomely appointed, but as we move toward the clinical side it is quite incomplete. No one has yet demonstrated a change in brain catecholamines in depressed or manic patients; no one has even demonstrated a consistent change in the cerebrospinal fluid catecholamines or their metabolites in affective disorders. Our best evidence depends upon studies of the urine. Schildkraut has reviewed studies he and his colleagues have done, starting perhaps six or eight years ago, in which there was good correlation between improvement in depression and a specific metabolite--normetanephrine in the urine. These findings were confirmed by Bunney and by Prange, although Prange raised a question as to which came first. In any case, Schildkraut is the first to admit that these studies of the urine reflect the peripheral autonomic system largely, and while they are compatible with changes in the brain, they do not necessarily indicate their occurrence. As a matter of fact, with improvement in depression there is likely to be an increase in activity in the peripheral adrenergic system, and it is not at all surprising that the metabolites reflecting an increase in peripheral adrenergic activity are increased in such patients. That is an oversimplification, I know, and one can fractionate the patient populations and obtain more satisfying evidence but it is still far from compelling. The possibility that methoxyhydroxyphenylglycol (MHPG) may be more specifically related to the brain is, of course, a good one. In all the urinary studies, I suppose the use of MHPG is at present the one most likely to be reflected in changes in the brain. But here, again, Maas usually points out the difficulties in inferring too much from MHPG which also has extracerebral sources. Although it is interesting that this metabolite is decreased fairly significantly and consistently in the urine of depressed patients, I find it disappointing that MHPG did not increase with the use of drugs that improve depression. Although one can explain why this could happen and still be associated with an increase of norepinephrine at receptors, somehow that evidence is not as convincing as an increase or decrease in MHPG or another catecholamine metabolite in the cerebrospinal fluid of manic or depressed patients would be.

But here we are at the narrowest and darkest part of the catecholamine tunnel. As we go back toward the other end, it becomes wider, well lit, and beautifully tiled. The fundamental information on which the catecholamine hypothesis is based seems to be continually increasing in extent and significance. What is the evidence? In animals it concerns various types of affective behavioral states. DOPA has been shown to counteract reserpine depression much more promptly and completely than 5-hydroxytryptamine was ever shown to do. Conversely, the fairly specific catecholamine depleter, alpha-methyl-para-tyrosine, has now been used in a number of studies in animals and in man. Although the results are not the striking depression one sees with reserpine, the results are still quite compatible with an important role of catecholamines in affective states (Rech, Borys, and Moore 1966). That agent given to primates engaged in social interaction produces many of the symptoms one would imagine depressed primates to have (Redmond et al. 1971). Other studies suggest the same phenomenon. When alpha-methyltyrosine has been given in man, it has produced a mild depression in some and depressive symptoms in others.

Rage is becoming more clearly associated with catecholamines, largely as the result of work by Reis, Fuxe, and Gunne (1965, 1969). They showed in their earlier work that sham rage, produced in cats by two different techniques, caused a significant depletion of norepinephrine in the brain. Their more recent work, bolstered by histofluorescence and drug studies, suggests that drugs specifically acting upon catecholamine receptors in the brain are capable of blocking sham rage, and those potentiating adrenergic activity are capable of exaggerating it. A number of studies of fear, anxiety, stress, and pain indicate that these affective states are accompanied by an increased turnover of norepinephrine in the brain. Some interesting work by Weiss and associates at Rockefeller University (Weiss, Stone, and Harrell 1970) on coping behavior suggests that, norepinephrine is involved in coping with an unpleasant situation. There is a substantial amount of evidence that catecholamines are involved in appetitive or rewarding processes. Stein has been pursuing the interrelationship between catecholamines and self-stimulatory behavior. I find his most recent work especially compelling. He had previously found that a number of drugs affecting catecholamines of the brain also affect self-stimulating behavior. Drugs that deplete catecholamines block self-stimulating behavior, while drugs that potentiate, increase, or favor the release of catecholamines, such as amphetamine, increase self-stimulatory behavior (Stein 1964). But, of course, such studies suffer from a problem common to pharmacologic studies: one gives a drug for a particular purpose and tends to forget that no drug does only one thing. What happens may not be the result of the action for which the drug was used, but some unexpected side effect. Wise and Stein (1969) have now come fairly close to demonstrating the role of particular adrenergic receptors in such appetitive behavior. They had found that they could prevent self-stimulating behavior in rats by injections of disulfiram which blocks the dopamine-β-hydroxylase step in the conversion of dopamine to norepinephrine. This gave them a model with which they may test the ability of one or another putative transmitter to restore this behavior. They tested a number of agents --serotonin, dopamine, D-epinephrine, and L-epinephrine--and only norepinephrine was capable of restoring self-stimulating behavior. Even more compelling is the work of Slangen and Miller (1969) on highly specific adrenergic receptors in the hypothalamus that are involved in feeding, another form of appetitive behavior. They found a spot in the posterior hypothalamic and perifornical area that, when stimulated electrically, causes eating in a satiated animal. They could also stimulate the area with micro-pipets and test a wide variety of putative transmitters. Only norepinephrine appeared to be capable of inducing this behavior. Epinephrine and serotonin did not induce it; dopamine did, but only weakly and after a lag period, suggesting to them that dopamine was being converted to norepinephrine before it acted. They went further, testing the ability of particular alpha- or beta-adrenergic blockers to prevent or potentiate this behavior. They found this effect highly consistent with the involvement of alpha-noradrenergic receptors. At least, the phenomena they observed were entirely consistent with what would have been found in a peripheral adrenergic synapse of the alpha type. Here, again, one can hardly avoid concluding that, at least in the pathways involved in this kind of eating behavior, adrenergic systems seem to be crucially involved.

Finally, we have the effects of the catecholamines on arousal, activity, and attention. I find most interesting the report by Segal and Mandell (1970), who infused norepinephrine into the ventricles of rats in controlled dosage and found that very small doses of norepinephrine produced an increase in exploratory behavior, an increase in what seems to be attention and locomotor activity. With larger doses of norepinephrine, the more traditional effects of sedation occurred which had been described by Mandell earlier.

I would like to suggest on the basis of the evidence I have reviewed that the symptoms of the affective disorders may be related to changes in brain catecholamines, but that the existence of the affective disorder may be related to an insufficiency of indoleamines. In other words, I would like to break down the wall between the two tunnels and use them both. The finding of a low 5-HIAA in the cerebrospinal fluid of both manic and depressed patients which persists during remission suggests that this may be a constitutional factor--an inadequate production or action of serotonin, which may have the peculiar property of stabilizing and damping the central synapses that have to do with affective states. I would like to think of the level of serotonin as regulating the volatility, lability, or instability of such synapses, and of maintaining a reasonable homeostasis in the system. When there is a serotonin deficiency, there need not be depression or mania but simply a predisposition toward either. There is an enhanced likelihood that depression or mania will occur and if it does occur, it is mediated by undamped activity of the adrenergic system in the brain. If this is in the direction of increased adrenergic output or activity, then one may see the symptoms of mania or hypomania. If the changes happen to be a marked decrease of adrenergic activity in the brain, then the symptoms would be those of depression. These mood swings do not necessarily occur purely on the basis of spontaneous changes in the adrenergic synapses. Genetic and endocrinological factors and those associated with aging may operate. We can also imagine experience, psychological, and cognitive factors playing a role in producing these changes in mood, but through undamped or uncompensated adrenergic activity.

Curzon referred to Sir Aubrey Lewis's statement that the more one examines the antecedents of endogenous depression in an individual, the more one is convinced that the depression is a reactive one. Thus most endogenous depressions may be in response to environmental circumstances. The thing that makes them a mental illness and different from a normal response to similar phenomena is the exaggerated quality of the response, and the fact that, in a normal individual, that kind of situational change would hardly have produced the magnitude of the symptoms and the duration of an endogenous depression.

This hypothesis--that the central synapses mediating mood are catecholaminergic but modulated by serotonin--has no direct evidence to support it. I have been bold enough to suggest it because it is heuristic and because it parsimoniously accounts for many apparently contradictory observations. It would explain--in fact, it is based upon--the 5-hydroxyindoleacetic acid reduction in cerebrospinal fluid that Coppen observed in patients with both mania and depression persisting during remission. It would also be compatible with his unexpected observation that methysergide, a serotonin blocker, apparently worsens mania instead of alleviating it. If too much serotonin were responsible for mania, as had been suggested, then serotonin inhibitors should improve the condition. The hypothesis may also account for the effectiveness of tryptophan in patients with affective disorders. It is also compatible with the indirect evidence that decreased catecholamine activity occurs in the central nervous system in depression while mania is associated with an increase. It is also compatible with the effectiveness of α-MT in mania and with the pharmacological studies suggesting that most of the agents that affect depression also affect brain catecholamines (and quite possibly indoleamines as well) in a way that would be compatible with their decrease in depression (Glowinski and Axelrod 1966). It would be interesting to try a combined treatment for depression with tryptophan and DOPA. Bunney has come close to that with consecutive use of these two agents, but with rather disappointing results. I wonder what would happen if one tried a combination of drugs or precursors that elevated both the indoleamines and catecholamines in patients with affective disorder or increased indoleamines but decreased catecholamines in patients with mania. Would the combinations be more beneficial than altering only one amine? Such trials, if they could be carried out safely, would constitute fairly crucial tests of the hypothesis.

REFERENCES

Glowinski, J., and Axelrod, J. 1966. *Pharmacol. Rev.* 18:775.
Jouvet, M. 1969. *Science* 163:32.
Kety, S. S. 1959. *Science* 129:1528, 1590.
Kety, S. S. 1967. *New Eng. J. Med.* 277:1146.
Rech, R. H.; Borys, H. K.; and Moore, K. E. 1966. *J. Pharm. Exp. Ther.* 153:412.
Redmond, D. E.; Maas, J. W.; Kling, A.; and Dekirmenjian, H. 1971. *Psychosomatic Med.* (in press).
Reis, D. J., and Fuxe, K. 1969. *Proc. Nat. Acad. Sci.* 64:108.
Reis, D. J., and Gunne, L. M. 1965. *Science* 149:450.
Segal, D. S., and Mandell, A. J. 1970. *Proc. Nat. Acad. Sci.* 66:289.
Slangen, J. L., and Miller, N. E. 1969. *Physiol. Behav.* 4:543.
Stein, L. 1964. *Fed. Proc.* 23:836.
Tenen, S. S. 1967. *Psychopharmacologia* 10:204.
Weiss, J. A.; Stone, E. A.; and Harrell, N. 1970. *J. Comp. Physiol. Psychol.* 72:153.
Wise, C. D., and Stein, L. 1969. *Science* 163:299.

DISCUSSION:

BRAIN AMINES AND AFFECTIVE DISORDERS

ARNOLD J. MANDELL: I would like to hear more about the helpfulness or relevance of terms like alpha- and beta-adrenergic receptors when talking about the brain.

SEYMOUR KETY: I am the one who introduced these horrible words. I think they have the same potential usefulness in the brain as in the periphery and about as much meaning. After all, no one has ever seen an alpha or a beta receptor, and they probably don't have "alpha" or "beta" printed on them. They are phenomenological constructs--simply economical ways of putting together the actions of drugs. One could hope to do that for the brain just as readily as for the periphery, with some help in systematizing many diverse observations but not necessarily contributing any new information.

IRWIN J. KOPIN: Dividing receptors into alpha and beta has been useful. Many years ago, Ahlquist found that sympathomimetic amines could be rank-ordered with regard to their effectiveness in causing a particular type of response--such as pilomotor erection, cardiac acceleration, etc. He found that Isuprel was much more active than epinephrine, and epinephrine was more active than norepinephrine in producing cardiac acceleration. The blood pressure response to Isuprel, however, was slight. It did not cause a constriction of the arterial muscles, while epinephrine caused a greater response, and norepinephrine an even greater one. He reasoned that there are differences in the nature of the receptor, and divided receptors into two major categories. This was not widely accepted until a group of drugs was found to inhibit all of what he had called alpha responses. Subsequently, we found another group of drugs that inhibited all of the actions he had called beta responses. There are some things that do not fit into this whole pattern, but I think it is useful in terms of differentiating responses, because a receptor is a particular area or membrane that is sensitive to another substance. The receptors probably form a mosaic on the membrane surface of neurons. If one applies a transmitter to one area, one may facilitate the depolarization and impulse formation by the neuron. Activation of another, adjacent, receptor might tend to inhibit this cell from firing. With different kinds of receptors, there may be different mechanisms for facilitating or inhibiting. Catecholamine interaction with adenyl cyclase to form cyclic AMP is generally thought of in relation to beta receptors, but the identity has not been established. The concept of different receptors for a single transmitter is useful in thinking of how drugs or transmitters may modulate functions of neurons. Furthermore, neurotransmitters may have long-term, as well as very short, discrete effects. With cumulative experience the cell might change its metabolism over minute- or hour-, rather than millisecond, intervals. I think it would be worthwhile to examine the types of responses a cell can give. The types of molecular interactions causing these responses would also be included in the abbreviated concept, receptor. It is probably an unfortunate word, as Dr. Kety has indicated. No one has ever seen a receptor. What we have come to mean by it is some molecular configuration responsive to the appearance of a particular type of molecule. When this interaction occurs, a sequence of events leading to some change in the effector cell occurs. It is convenient for pharmacologists to talk about "receptors," as long as we define what we mean.

MANDELL: Suppose you wanted to look at receptors in the brain and you chose phenoxybenzamine, because it is the classic peripheral specific receptor blocker, injected it into the ventricle, and waited for some period of time for it to be distributed. Would you then be safe to get the protein it was bound to and call it an alpha-receptor protein?

KOPIN: The fact that a substance binds to a particular protein does not mean that protein is a receptor. Certainly, other proteins, perhaps involved in uptake or storage, may bind the amine. If phenoxybenzamine blocks this binding, this may be interpreted as supporting the view that the protein is involved in the receptor (or uptake) mechanism. If phenoxybenzamine did not block, however, the protein would not be an alpha receptor. I think negative evidence is much more important than positive; this holds for almost anything in science. We can identify a compound, or attempt to identify it by looking at its Rf in chromatography. It is compared with a known standard in forty different solvent systems and the two may have the same Rf in all forty systems. But if we find the forty-first solvent system in which the Rf is different, we can then say the compounds are different. This type of negative finding gives a lot more information.

JOSEPH J. SCHILDKRAUT: A notion that has often been disregarded, but which we might entertain with some justification, is that one or another of the biogenic amines in certain regions of the brain may be subserving a neurohormonal, rather than a neurotransmitter, function. One may ask whether there are regions of the brain in which one or another of the biogenic amines may, in fact, be modulating neuronal function in a hormonal sense, rather than being specific transmitters. It is only a bare speculation right now, but there is a possibility that some of our thinking about the role of biogenic amines in affective disorders--which has been relying largely on a neuronal model--might demand in addition, or instead, a more hormonal concept: namely, that neuronal activity may be altered by the concentration of biogenic amines in surrounding regions of the brain (but not necessarily the whole brain), and that the concentration of a specific neurotransmitter within a single synaptic cleft may not be the sole determinant of neuronal activity.

KOPIN: Two things support that idea. First, the distribution of the terminals of norepinephrine-containing cells in the brain. Many of these terminals are not, in fact, adjacent to the effector cell. The varicosities are distributed in a generalized fashion throughout the tissue of the brain in the cortex. Second, the arrangement of norepinephrine-containing cells and serotonin-containing cells are remarkably adapted to such a purpose. The arrangement of the cells of the brain is a great complex of wiring and cells in complicated patterns. But the norepinephrine cells are nearly always located in a very strategic place in the hind brain and so is the serotonin in the raphe nuclei. The axons from these go all over the brain; a stimulus in a very localized place can lead to a widespread release of amines all over the brain. Norepinephrine and serotonin are thus concerned with various phenomena and, by manipulating the background activity of neurons, recall, attention, memory, etc. may be facilitated.

MORRIS A. LIPTON: Another area which pertains to the question of the specificity and function of the various aminergic neurons derives from the recent work on Parkinsonism with DOPA. If dopaminergic neurons are exclusively required for the maintenance of appropriate muscle tone and movement, and if, as is apparently the case, these neurons are destroyed in Parkinsonism, it is difficult to see how treatment with DOPA could be effective, because dead neurons could hardly be expected to perform metabolic conversions. On the other hand, if under conditions of high DOPA administration the norepinephrine- or serotonin-containing neurons could decarboxylate the DOPA and thereby maintain a high humoral milieu of dopamine, one might still get restoration of the extrapyramidal system and functioning. I am trying to say, in agreement with Dr. Schildkraut and Dr. Kopin, that we still have much to learn about the specificity and interaction of the various aminergic systems.

The same considerations hold for depression. Here again it seems clear enough that we are not dealing with exclusive disturbances of catecholamines or indolealkylamines, but rather with the interaction between them. Clearly, as Dr. Kety indicated, we are learning a good deal about the specific functions of the catecholamines and the indoleamines in various forms of appetitive behavior and perhaps even in sleep. But clinical depression is a more complex and subtle phenomenon.

We can often get more stimulation from data which do not fit our hypotheses than from the data which do. And in the area of the affective disorders we have much data which do not conveniently fit. Dr. Coppen has informed us that hydroxyindoleacetic acid levels are high in the cerebrospinal fluid of manics and low in that of depressives, and he adds the intriguing finding that these levels are independent of the patients' clinical status. Recent work from Dr. Axelrod's laboratory (*Science* 170:1323, 1970) reveals that women who have unipolar depression have low COMT levels in their red cells, and that the level stays low even when clinical remission has occurred. We still do not know whether these findings are the product of a genetic diathesis or whether they are related to aging or alterations in endocrine state.

The changes in urinary catecholamine metabolites which occur during the treatment of depression are also puzzling. VMA levels are low during depression. They rise while the patient is improving, but I am not persuaded that they continue to stay high when the patient is well. This is tedious work to perform and so data are not as complete as one would like, but I am not yet convinced that the urinary VMA levels are different when the patient is ill from those when he is clinically well.

There are also the puzzling data derived from human clinical pharmacology. Alpha-methyl-tyrosine administered to patients with pheochromocytoma in doses which (from animal data) should lower central catecholamines markedly, and which certainly lower peripheral catecholamines in these patients, produces singularly mild effects on the mood. Parachlorophenylalanine, an inhibitor of serotonin synthesis, administered in large doses to patients with carcinoid syndrome also has relatively little effect on mood. L-DOPA, administered in the huge doses required in Parkinsonism should, by bypassing the rate-limiting step in catecholamine biosynthesis, lead to substantial increases in norepinephrine as well as dopamine, and yet the consequences on mood are mild and infrequent. The carboline of which Dr. Ho spoke should also produce major changes in serotonin but does not produce major changes in mood. So there is the strange paradox that the endogenous mood disorders are associated with small changes in the biogenic amines, while much larger changes in these amines induced with pharmacological agents do not result in striking mood disorders. Dr. Schildkraut's recent findings about the differences between acute and chronic imipramine administration in animals also fit the existing hypotheses with difficulty. All of these data are explainable in one way or another, but they require ad hoc explanations which must be added on to our original hypotheses. We are constantly violating the law of parsimony, but I suppose that is the present state of the art.

I am much intrigued by Dr. Kety's suggestion, which may integrate much of our disparate data, that serotonin may be involved with general reactivity of the portions of the nervous system involved with mood, whereas the catecholamines have more to do with specific symptoms. This suggestion is in accord with the data from comparative biology which suggest that serotonin may have evolved earlier as a transmitter or modulator than did the catecholamines. The suggestion is testable in the laboratory, and will require the simultaneous measurement of serotonin and catecholamine metabolism in the same patient.

As a psychiatrist I must always invoke the environmental components, which are usually psychological, in our considerations of the affective disorders. During this entire symposium, we have talked mainly about 20 percent of our clinical depressions, the so-called endogenous ones. Other types of depression, the neurotic and reactive types, are much more common. Do the biological changes that occur in the endogenous depressions also occur in these? Is there some common path that might integrate all of the mood disorders? Is it possible, for example, that one might have a genetic diathesis in the form of a less efficient aminergic system that somehow requires a more consistent environmental input in order to maintain optimum mood? Finally, we must not ignore data from other disciplines that would indicate that we must find a way to bring cognitive factors into consideration. It seems quite possible that a common basic physiological state may exist for more than one emotion, and that the specificity of the emotion is more determined by the ideas attached to the state than by the state itself.

SCHILDKRAUT: This slide (Table A) is in partial response to Dr. Kety's and Dr. Lipton's questions apropos the finding that, in patients treated with amitriptyline, 3-methoxy-4-hydroxyphenylglycol (MHPG) was decreased during treatment, even at the time of clinical improvement. We suggested earlier that this decrease might have occurred because amitriptyline decreases the synthesis and deamination of norepinephrine, thereby decreasing MHPG. Some years ago, Jack Durell, Ken Greenspan, and I, at the National Institute of

TABLE A

MHPG Excretion in Patients Treated with Lithium Carbonate

Patients	MHPG Excretion (μg/24 hr)		Difference*	p**
	Pretreatment Period	Treatment Period		
Hypomanic Patients				
A.C.	2,750±290 (4)	2,210± 80 (3)	+540	<.20
O.E.	2,810±230 (5)	2,170±200 (5)	+640	<.10
Normothymic Patients				
H.B.	2,470±280 (3)	2,240±290 (4)	+230	--
G.S.	2,720±140 (5)	2,730±370 (5)	- 10	--
Agitated Depressed Patients				
W.J.	1,330±210 (5)	1,580±270 (5)	-250	--
C.S.	1,520± 50 (5)	1,940±220 (5)	-420	<.20
C.O.	1,590±110 (5)	2,130±170 (4)	-540	<.05

MHPG excretion was studied in patients who were initially hypomanic, normothymic, or depressed (agitated). All patients received placebo during the pretreatment period and lithium carbonate during the treatment period. During the treatment period, all patients were clinically normothymic. The number of 24-hour urine specimens analyzed is given in parentheses. The values for MHPG excretion are expressed in μg/24 hr and reported as the means ± SEM.

*Difference = pretreatment mean minus treatment mean
**p = level of statistical significance of the difference between the pretreatment and treatment means and is indicated only for p < 0.20.

Data from Greenspan, Schildkraut, Gordon, Baer, Aronoff, and Durell 1970. Reprinted with permission from *J. Psychiat. Res.* 7:171.

Mental Health, did the study of manic depressive disorders that is partially summarized in this table. We had a small group of hypomanic patients, a small group of normothymic patients, and a small group of patients with depressions, all of them initially studied before treatment and after clinical improvement. Lithium was administered in this study. I am not asserting that lithium was the clinically effective agent because the study was conducted in a highly intensive therapeutic milieu. Our first and most striking observation, which confirms Dr. Maas's findings, was that MHPG excretion seemed to be lower in the depressed patients when they were depressed than in the normothymic or the hypomanic groups. Moreover, when the depressed patients improved, there was a tendency for MHPG to increase. When the hypomanic patients (who initially showed a slight MHPG elevation) improved there was a tendency for the MHPG to decrease. The normothymic patients showed no apparent change in MHPG. So, in this case, in which we gave a drug that presumably does not decrease norepinephrine deamination and MHPG formation, we saw some coupling of the change in clinical state with the direction of change of MHPG.

I would like to go one step further because this table is misleading in a way. From the data on the normothymic patients, one might conclude that lithium does not affect MHPG excretion, since the levels before treatment and after several weeks of lithium were not very different. But we have recently observed, in an extensive day-by-day study of one manic-depressive patient over about six months, that the changes in MHPG excretion during the first several weeks of lithium treatment may be quite striking. Lithium carbonate was started at a low dose, 300 mg daily, then gradually increased to 1200 mg by the end of the first week. We saw virtually no change in MHPG during the first four days. On the fifth day, with the first measurable level of serum lithium, we began to see an increase in MHPG which spiked quite dramatically during the course of a week and then decreased to baseline levels or lower. After several months of treatment with lithium, the patient's MHPG levels were significantly lower than they were prior to, or during, the initial phase of treatment. One of the initial effects of lithium administration, therefore, may be an increase in MHPG excretion, which may be analogous to the increase in MHPG produced by reserpine as reported by Sandler and Youdim (*Nature* 217:771, 1968). VMA excretion, which we studied concurrently in this patient, was altered by lithium, but did not show changes as dramatic as the changes in MHPG.

As we know, lithium is an extremely effective agent for treating mania. Lithium has a rather rapid action in that it acts in five to ten days, roughly corresponding to this peaking of MHPG, which may be a reserpine-like effect. The prophylactic action of lithium in preventing recurrences of manic-depressive episodes, however, seems to take much longer. These data suggest the possibility that, with chronic administration over several months, lithium may cause enduring changes in the rate of synthesis and metabolism of catecholamines that might possibly account for the prophylactic effects reported in some long-term clinical studies. In this context, one may recall that Schou (*J. Psychiat. Res.* 6:67, 1968) has stated that a patient may have to be maintained on lithium for several months to a year before prophylactic effects occur. In the patient I have described, there seemed to be a gradual trend toward lower MHPG, lower normetanephrine and lower VMA, after several months of treatment with lithium. The really outstanding and dramatic finding, however, was the marked peak in MHPG during the initial phase of treatment, when the first measurable lithium blood levels occurred.

LIPTON: Both the rise and the fall of MHPG during the lithium treatment are equally impressive. There seems to be an alteration in the aminergic state that is rapid initially and then slower. We don't know whether it is at the affector level, the receptor level, the synthetic level, or the membrane level, but there is something about a change in state of the activity of the system that somehow permits the amine levels to return to what they were before the patient became ill.

SCHILDKRAUT: It is relevant to point out that this was a woman who was fired a number of times from responsible positions because of manic episodes. These occurred with such increasing frequency that she finally consented to treatment with lithium. During the past year's treatment, she has been quite well and she is back at her job. Her supervisor reports she is better than she has been in many, many years. Her psychological reactivity has certainly been changed by this treatment.

JAMES W. MAAS: Dr. Coppen, how long after the patients were treated did you get these measures of 5-hydroxyindoleacetic acid in cerebral spinal fluid? Was it two months or fourteen months, or were they randomly distributed?

COPPEN: Randomly distributed. When one thinks about the epidemiology of the affective disorders, one is very struck by one's ignorance and one ought to keep in mind that we are dealing with a disorder that occurs in middle age. It is almost certainly recurrent. If untreated, it is self-limiting; the average period of untreated affective disorder is about six months, and the period between attacks decreases with age and previous attacks. At the moment, we really have no hypothesis why someone goes into an attack. We may have some feeling about the mechanism of a recurrence; when the patient becomes ill, there may be changes in the amines, but it is very difficult to suggest an analogy in the rest of medicine for this sort of recurrent periodic behavior. I have been very intrigued by the European studies of Angst (Angst and Weiss 1967, Excerpta Medica Foundation I.C.S. 129, p. 703) and others on the natural history of the affective disorders, which I think we tend to forget. It is a recurrent self-limiting condition, a very curious thing, and difficult to bring into our integrated scheme of this afternoon. Dr. Curzon suggested that sort of an endocrinological stimulus may provoke these changes. Unfortunately, I don't believe cortisol is the cause. We have just obtained some data on cerebrospinal fluid cortisol levels in patients suffering from affective disorders. After the patients are settled in a research ward, they show very little evidence of plasma cortisol changes. My hunch is that we ought to be looking more at endocrinological factors to get the sort of changes for which you provided a model; there must be something triggering these attacks. Sometimes it may be environmental stress, but I am not convinced that this occurs on every occasion. Can anyone think of a similar illness that has this curious recurrent behavior?

MANDELL: You might say that the so-called periodic diseases are somewhat similar. There is a whole group of exotic periodic diseases, from periodic peritonitis, hepatitis, to acute intermittent porphyria, which may have some metabolic triggers. The porphyria model is a very seductive one but it has a latent metabolic disturbance that can be brought into fruition with a barbiturate load. It has manifestations in psychiatric disease, with metabolic signs and spontaneous remission.

ARTHUR J. PRANGE: Periodic catatonia, of course, is a mental disorder, and here we know that endocrine factors, particularly thyroid factors, are bound up with what is seen clinically (Gjessing 1938, *J. Ment. Sci.* 84:608).

I agree with Dr. Curzon and Dr. Coppen that endocrine changes may contribute to the precipitation of affective attacks. I also think they may contribute to recovery. Unfortunately for purposes of untangling the web, interplay between hormones is probably at least as complex as interplay between amines.

Sometimes treatment effects may help clarify matters. Dr. Schildkraut has just shown us the remarkable biphasic effects of lithium in MHPG excretion. In his patient it would also be useful to know the effects of the lithium treatment on thyroid state. It is now known that lithium in man can produce a marked and often prolonged drop not only in bound thyroxine but also in free thyroxine (Cooper and Simpson 1969, *Curr. Ther. Res.* 11:603), the metabolically significant fraction. I think it is quite possible that such an endocrine shift could activate the recovery process or at least contribute to its activation.

LIPTON: It seems to be emerging that the biological systems controlling mood are very complex and that one can, perhaps, intervene in the system of interlocking circles. Dr. Prange's data, for example, on the clinical change preceding the catecholamine change indicate that, if you take the tryptamine data, they would coincide with the clinical change. So maybe it is tryptamine that alters catecholamines, which then alter something else. Alternatively, it may be that the receptor is initially altered by the thyroid. Changes in receptor sensitivity may initiate a series of changes that will follow consequently. I believe we will have to do careful sequential studies before we can get a real picture of the pathobiology of the mood disorders and of the changes that accompany getting ill or getting well.

SCHILDKRAUT: To a certain extent, the work of the past ten years may have delineated some of the cast of characters, but it has not really told us how they interact in the play. Perhaps for the next ten or 200 years, we will be trying to figure out how the characters talk to one another.

YUTAKA KOBAYASHI: Do you think it will ever be possible to classify the various mental illnesses according to a biochemical or pharmacological profile? Some of the data given this morning are relevant to this. Dr. Schildkraut suggested that, with one type of MHPG level, you might select one sort of treatment whereas, with a lower MHPG level, another type of treatment would be indicated. If this is so, it would be interesting in terms of treatment, but it would also have some real consequences for understanding some of the processes involved.

A situation I was faced with some years ago, when I first got into this area, occurred in a study on histamine metabolism in schizophrenics (Kobayashi and Freeman 1961, *J. Neuropsychiat.* 3:112). When it was all over, it turned out that there was a great deal of confusion or disagreement whether or not we were actually dealing with schizophrenics. I am wondering whether there is any better way to decide this besides by interview. There must be some biochemical measurement on which you can hang your hat.

SCHILDKRAUT: By analogy, I would say that we really are at the level of talking about the fevers and the pneumonias when discussing the clinical signs and symptoms of affective disorders. I think all of us hope that some day we shall have the equivalent of bacteriological cultures in this field. Even if we are lucky enough to develop certain biochemical discriminators, my expectation, at least within the future I can foresee, is that the clinical psychiatric syndromes and clinical psychiatric interview techniques will continue to provide the basis for clinical diagnosis, even if supplemented by biochemical or pharmacological criteria.

KOBAYASHI: Is there one biochemical criterion on which you can all agree that is consistent with depression?

MAAS: I do not think it is clearly a one-to-one sort of thing. I would guess the answer to your question would be, no.

PRANGE: I can't think of one either. My hunch is that resting values may never be of much help either in identifying depression or in devising a biochemical classification of depression. If the syndrome has several contributing causes, if they are interrelated, and if a function can contribute to cause on one occasion and partially compensate for some other contributary cause on another occasion, then there is not much hope of looking at resting values and finding something that is more than frequently present. For example, I think we have shown that frank hypothyroidism is usually, if not always, accompanied by depression (Whybrow, Prange, and Treadway 1969, *Arch. Gen. Psychiat.* 20:48), that depressed patients as a whole tend to have rather low normal thyroid function (Prange *et al.* 1969, *Amer. J. Psychiat.* 126:457) but that some depressed patients show thyroid activation when most severely sick (Whybrow *et al.*, *Arch. Gen. Psychiat.* in press). Thus, in a given depressed patient, you may find thyroid state to be low normal, or elevated. I think this means that thyroid state is involved in the depression process, but not specifically, and certainly not exclusively.

There might be a chance, however, of establishing some kind of biochemical classification based upon challenging techniques, something akin to what is useful in the diagnosis of diabetes, say, with challenging doses of glucose. There might be kinds of depression one could differentiate on the basis of response to infused norepinephrine, say, or on the basis of blood level after infused doses of tryptophan. With this kind of challenging technique one might find subclasses, but I would be doubtful of diagnosis based on unchallenged resting values.

LIPTON: Let me remind you that, in clinical medicine, there are relatively few biochemical indices. In pneumonia, for example, there are really no biochemical indices. One uses x-ray or percussion indices, as well as hematological and other clinical findings, but there are no specific biochemical findings. So I don't necessarily see biochemical indices as the Holy Grail. If there is one, it will be under challenging circumstances, as Dr. Prange said, but physiological indices may well arrive--through electroencephalograms, for example, or perhaps through relatively simple clinical data. If someone today showed me a patient and said, "This is his blood pressure response to infused norepinephrine," and if I felt it to be distinctly low, I would be inclined to begin, at least, by saying, "Either he is hypothyroid, or he has Addison's disease, or he is depressed." That would be a kind of index. I would not want to make the diagnosis exclusively on that, but it would be at least a biological index.

GERALD KLERMAN: In answer to the biochemist's query about a classification scheme: A story is told about the man who had twin sons about the age of nine whom he classified, one as the optimist, the other as the pessimist. On their birthday, they both wanted a pony. The father, being in a somewhat sadistic mood, decided to test the boys. He dumped a large pile of manure in their playroom, and when the twins saw the manure, one son burst into tears and went crying to his mother. That was the pessimist. The optimist got a shovel and started digging. When the father asked him why he was digging, he said, "Well, with all this manure, there's got to be a pony somewhere." I would say that, with all these data, there has to be an amine somewhere.

A specific question, though, about the data concerning MHPG: why don't people on lithium get depressed? In other words, one of the challenges of lithium was to reconcile it with the catecholamine model in terms of too much or too little MHPG. Why don't patients get depressed on lithium?

SCHILDKRAUT: In contrast to the tenor of the question, I think that one does see patients who become depressed on lithium. I know of this from anecdotal reports, and I have seen several such patients myself; but it does not seem to occur consistently. It is likely that lithium does not totally deplete catecholamines, as does reserpine. Indeed, even with reserpine, one only finds depression in a small number of patients. Moreover, I should emphasize that chronic administration of lithium did not reduce MHPG to grossly subnormal levels. Lithium simply caused a transient increase in MHPG excretion that was followed by a slight decrease. The prior state of a system, when the drug is applied, may be relevant also; that is, if you administer a drug to a patient with a very rapid turnover rate of norepinephrine--i.e., a very high level of noradrenergic activity--the effect of lithium may well bring this down to normal. But we also know from our studies in animals that lithium can increase norepinephrine turnover; so lithium may, in fact, have opposing actions. If the noradrenergic system is functioning at a very high level, lithium may bring it back down, but it may also be able to bring the system back up if it is functioning at too low a level. At a biochemical level it may, in fact, be the kind of normalizer that it has been suggested to be at a clinical level.

MAAS: It is important to think of manic-depressive illness as a process. In terms of the catecholamine hypothesis, we say that there should be a lowering of norepinephrine or a slowing of the rate of synthesis, and it seems to me one ought to be able to induce in animals a process that will culminate in a decrease in norepinephrine synthesis in brain. Furthermore, one ought to be able to induce the process with the use of nonphysiologic agents. Most of our present methods increase the rate of synthesis, except alpha-methyltyrosine, which is an artificial type of intervention. If we had an animal model in which we could produce a slowing of the rate of synthesis of norepinephrine in brain by physiologically possible methods, it would be interesting to see how that animal behaved.

LIPTON: Apropos Dr. Klerman's question, I have never seen a reserpine depression, so I know only what I read. The figures of about 20 percent of reserpine-treated patients becoming depressed has always puzzled me, but in rereading some of the earlier literature, one of the things that impressed me again was the prolonged duration of reserpine depression. I know that the pharmacological action of reserpine lasts for weeks, but the depression in some patients continues for many months. Again we face the puzzling question of what has been done--how have we altered the state of the organism? After several months without reserpine, I would guess that the patient is biologically normal, at least catecholamine-wise. But psychologically speaking, he is certainly not back to normal. Again we come back to this peculiar business of altering states which are very difficult to verbalize. But we still do not fully understand the elimination of mania with chronic lithium, or the prolonged reserpine depression long after the drug is discontinued.

COPPEN: I also looked up some of the old reserpine literature, and I mentioned it this morning. The reserpine was used in treating manic patients who were maintained on it for months (Watts 1958, *J. Neurol. Neurosurg. Psychiat.* 21:297). The patients very seldom got depressed. The dosages were much higher than those used in the treatment for hypertension, so here is a very complex proposition.

SCHILDKRAUT: There is an odd finding that hypertensive patients are more susceptible than other patients to depression with reserpine treatment. One might argue that most of the patients who have been treated with reserpine were treated for hypertension. But some years ago, Bernstein and Kaufman (*J. Mt. Sinai Hosp. N.Y.* 27:525, 1960) did a controlled study of the effects of reserpine in a dermatology clinic and a hypertension clinic. A syndrome resembling depression and characterized by diminished psychomotor activity occurred much more frequently in the hypertensive than the dermatology patients. If one can jump from one species to another, Yamori, Lovenberg, and Sjoerdsma (*Science* 170:544, 1970) have reported that, in spontaneously hypertensive rats, there seems to be a lowering of endogenous norepinephrine in various brain regions. It is just barely possible (as Dr. Lipton has said on occasions) that there may be people who are operating with marginal norepinephrine reserves, e.g., hypertensives and perhaps others as well, who, when challenged with reserpine, will become much more prone to depression than those people who may have more adequate norepinephrine reserves. This may, in part, account for the greater incidence of reserpine-induced depressions in hypertensive patients.

WILLIAM E. BUNNEY, JR.: I would like to make some comments about reserpine. There were a few large studies of the use of reserpine in both moderate and severe depressions, and very few of these reported that the patients' condition worsened. Reserpine treatment seemed to help the neurotic depressions. The psychotic depressions were essentially unchanged. Another interesting finding was that a number of the patients reported to have become depressed on reserpine had previous histories of depression--again suggesting some kind of sensitization or defect.

MAAS: This is what I mean by thinking about process. One should remember that when a person falls ill changes occur in the psychosocial context which may affect the way the person behaves and feels, even though the "illness" factor may change. In our primates, for example, we gave alpha-methyl-para-tyrosine to an ape who was number two in a hierarchy of five. She developed some behaviors which were akin to those seen with human depressions and she dropped in rank to number three, becoming submissive to a smaller animal over whom she had been dominant for a year. Except for rank, all behaviors returned to normal after we stopped the drug, that is, she remained number three in the hierarchy. She had been off the enzyme inhibitor long enough so there could be little doubt as to biological normality, but something happened during the treatment period to both her and the group as a whole which prevented her from regaining her original dominance position. The final behavior of the animal was a function of a transient biochemical change which resulted in an enduring behavioral change which in part was probably due to the change in the psychosocial milieu.

LIPTON: If one were able to probe the feelings of your ape, I suspect that one might call her characterologically depressed because she has gone from number two to number four and that might predispose her to future depression.

MAAS: Right. My point is that sometimes these things become self-fulfilling prophesies for the person or animal.

SCHILDKRAUT: There is a clinical belief that depression itself tends to make people depressed. Conversely, mania tends to precipitate further mania, and there is the tendency to escalation. In the clinical treatment for mania, one contains the patient's behavior and decreases the environmental input. The fact that reserpine depression may last beyond the presence of the drug may be related to the notion that there may be positive feedback loops in depression, feeding into decreased noradrenergic activity leading to further depression or, conversely, in mania, feeding into heightened noradrenergic activity leading to further mania. As a clinical application of this, in treating a depressed patient with a tricyclic drug, once I am assured that the patient is no longer a suicidal risk and shows the first glimmerings of clinical improvement, I will intervene in a way that will promote activity and aggressiveness (in a sense of outgoing behavior, not necessarily hostility), on the assumption that once the pump has been primed by imipramine and improvement starts, one can accelerate and enhance it by interpersonal maneuvers (Schildkraut 1970, *Neuropsychopharmacology and the Affective Disorders*. Boston: Little, Brown, p. 49). Similarly, after reserpine, one may have a kind of vicious circle that keeps feeding itself, so that even after the drug effect is gone, you have a system that has been damped out and remains damped out because there is no impetus to bring it back up.

G. CURZON: It may be relevant to the question of the depressant effect of reserpine that in a study of a group of migrainous patients (Curzon *et al.* 1969, *J. Neurol. Neurosurg. Psychiat.* 32:555) we found a marked negative correlation between age and the increase of urinary 5-HIAA or VMA after reserpine. Thus, it may be that age also plays a part in determining mood changes due to reserpine.

LIPTON: But this would not hold for the hypertensive patients who are probably in this age group, too.

CURZON: I would like to comment also on another topic. We wondered about the feasibility of determining brain amines and metabolites after prolonged frozen storage and therefore we studied the data published by Dr. Coppen's and Dr. Bunney's groups (Bourne *et al.* 1968, *Lancet* 2:805) in which they determined 5-HIAA and 5-HT in the brains of coronary controls and depressed suicides at various times after death. We found that if both groups are taken together, there is a highly significant regression line relating to 5-HIAA storage: 5-HIAA in ng/gm brain = 415 + 5.91 × days stored. As the mean time between death and determination for the coronary controls was greater than the mean time between death and determination for the depressives, this relationship might explain why the depressive 5-HIAA's were lower than the mean of the control group. There was no significant relationship between the concentrations of 5-HT and 5-HIAA and no significant relationship between 5-HT and time after death.

COPPEN: We examined the correlation between storage time and concentration of 5-HIAA in our postmortem material and found no significant correlation in the material as a whole or in any of the subgroups except that of coronary controls in which a positive correlation was found.

The only direct data on this matter that I know are from Dowson (*Lancet* 1:596, 1969) who found a decrease in serotonin and 5-HIAA in stored brains up to 25 days and then little change up to 75 days.

He does not rule out further changes with longer storage time, but I suspect that the apparent opposite correlation in the coronary controls is a chance finding. The statistical significance in 5-HIAA concentrations between controls and suicide brains is, at any rate, unaffected by this factor and, indeed, Dowson's work suggests that the difference between the control brains (average storage time 185 days) and the suicide brains (average storage time 160 days) was in fact diminished by the longer storage time of the control brains. As we have pointed out, work on postmortem material is fraught with difficulties and the fact that significant findings did emerge in spite of such a lot of background noise is encouraging.

GEORGE BREESE: Dr. Maas, could you elaborate on your study with apes--were they "depressed" or did they have any impairment of motor activity after drug treatment?

MAAS: In this work, incidentally, the senior author is Dr. Gene Redmond, a research resident in our group. It was presented at the Psychosomatic Society (Washington, D.C. 1970) and is now in press in *Psychosomatic Medicine*. We used ethological observations of social behavior in a group of five *Macaca speciosa* as described previously by Dr. Arthur Kling, who was a co-author. Specific social behaviors, such as grooming, threats, attacks, submissions, social-sexual presentations, and copulations were observed per unit of time and behaviors were divided further as to initiating and responding animal. Two animals that received the alpha-methyl-para-tyrosine initiated fewer social interactions and assumed postures and expressions somewhat like depressed patients. Otherwise they were apparently healthy. These changes in behavior seemed clearly related to the treatment with alpha-methyl-para-tyrosine and the animals rapidly improved when we stopped administering the drug. We have been using some other drugs that are relevant to this conference, and we will be publishing these data also.

BREESE: After the intracisternal administration of 6-hydroxydopamine to rats pretreated with pargyline, our laboratory (Breese and Traylor 1970, *J. Pharmacol. Exp. Ther.* 174:413) has found brain levels of norepinephrine and dopamine to be reduced 75 to 80 percent. This depletion is the result of a selective degeneration of catecholamine-containing fibers. Except for a slight decrease in body weight and a lack of groomed appearance, "centrally sympathectomized" rats are difficult to distinguish from control animals. Behaviorally we have determined that a single dose of 6-hydroxydopamine does not alter general activity nor does this treatment alter a scheduled behavioral task. However, we have found that 6-hydroxydopamine will block self-stimulation behavior. Since drugs such as chlorpromazine and α-methyl-tyrosine have been reported to reduce responses in these tests, the inability of 6-hydroxydopamine to produce similar results has been difficult to reconcile. Since such data have been used to support various interpretations of affective behavior, perhaps someone would like to comment on these findings.

SCHILDKRAUT: Our group has done some work on this in collaboration with Dr. Ernest Hartmann's group, and we are working up this material for publication now. We do not agree with all of the findings to date that 6-hydroxydopamine does not block certain aspects of amphetamine behavior. We found that certain behavioral responses to amphetamine were diminished in animals treated with 6-hydroxydopamine. The main point of the study, however, was to examine the effects of 6-hydroxydopamine on REM sleep. We have used a number of substances in rats to determine whether there is a relationship between norepinephrine levels, turnover or metabolism, and REM sleep. The findings Hartmann has accumulated in man and now, in collaboration with us, in animals, suggest that there might actually be an inverse relationship. We find that orally administered alpha-methyltyrosine caused the expected decrease in norepinephrine levels and a reciprocal increase in REM sleep. In the experiments we ran with 6-hydroxydopamine in which there was about a 60 to 70 percent depletion of brain norepinephrine, we found that these animals had an increase in REM sleep. So there are behavioral effects after 6-hydroxydopamine. But I would not want to stretch the analogy between this paradigm and the suggestions that there may be pressure for REM sleep in some depressions.

PAUL R. DRASKOCZY: Dr. Coppen mentioned that he has given monoamine oxidase inhibitors in conjunction with tryptophan. In patients who were given high doses of oral tryptophan, Hartmann found increased REM sleep time (unpublished data). I wonder whether this contributed to improving depression. It might be possible that the improvement was an artifact of the Hamilton rating scale that would show an improvement in depression if the patient reported better sleep.

COPPEN: I do not believe that the improvement in depression with tryptophan is simply a reflection of the improvement in sleep. In the last investigation we did with Dr. Prange, we looked to see whether there was any sort of differential improvement in tryptophan-treated patients compared to the imipramine-treated patients, for example. We did not find any.

CURZON: The regression line one gets by using coronary controls plus depressed suicides is almost identical to the regression line for coronary controls only. It is true that if the depressed patients alone are taken, there is no correlation with number of days of storage but the range of time of storage of this group was rather small, while that of the coronary control group was larger. Also, if one takes the nondepressed suicides, the 5-HIAA levels again fall around the same regression line while a miscellaneous control group shows a large scatter.

The sum of 5-HT and 5-HIAA goes up dramatically with number of days postmortem, because 5-HIAA values were very much higher than those of 5-HT, which vary little. The high 5-HIAA values made us suspect the validity of the determinations as it seemed rather striking that in determinations of 5-HT and 5-HIAA in animal brain it is almost invariably found that amounts of each are fairly comparable, while in human brain such a large excess of 5-HIAA over 5-HT was found.

PRANGE: One more thing about sleep and amino acids: while the effects of DOPA on sleep have been attributed to an increase in norepinephrine, other factors should be considered. Our laboratory (Breese and Prange 1971, *Europ. J. Pharmacol.* 13:259) has shown in the rat that, after the last of a series of chronic doses of DOPA, norepinephrine levels in heart start to fall within a few hours. By ten to twelve hours, there is as much as a 50 percent decrement. Butcher and Engel (*Brain Res.* 15:233, 1969) have reported a similar tendency in brain after administering DOPA with a decarboxylase inhibitor. It could be that DOPA is permitting less norepinephrine to be available rather than more. The mechanism would presumably be due to a feedback inhibition on tyrosine hydroxylase. Furthermore, we have found serotonin to be reduced after DOPA, suggesting that serotonergic fibers are also being influenced by this amino acid. In the face of all of these factors, dopamine levels are increasing to four to five times those of controls. It would seem that interpretation of effects of DOPA on sleep would be difficult at best.

SCHILDKRAUT: Some data that might throw the interpretation of all the DOPA treatment studies into further confusion were reported by O'Gorman *et al.* (*Clin. Chim. Acta* 29:111, 1970). They found that patients maintained on DOPA had markedly decreased excretion of various metabolites of norepinephrine, namely, normetanephrine and VMA. One explanation would be that this decrease is due to the competitive inhibition of catechol-O-methyltransferase, because both of these are methylated compounds. But they tend to rule this out because they did not find a compensatory elevation of norepinephrine. They concluded, therefore, that one of the effects of chronic administration of DOPA may be to decrease, rather than increase, the overall turnover of norepinephrine in man, and they postulate that this may be due to the formation of a false transmitter in noradrenergic neurons.

KETY: There is increasing evidence of the biochemical effects on the brain by a large dose of L-DOPA. These effects are much more complicated than we have imagined, and they do not simply involve an increase in the catecholamine substrates. In addition to possible formation of false transmitters, and in addition to the transmethylation effects of L-DOPA, there is also the fact that L-DOPA competitively inhibits the uptake of other amino acids by the brain. There is considerable evidence now that L-DOPA affects serotonin metabolism, possibly by affecting tryptophan uptake. How all of these things interrelate to explain the effects and the side effects of L-DOPA can well be the subject of another symposium.

BREESE: To our surprise, we have found the amount of labeled dopamine formed from radioactive DOPA to be lowered only slightly (20 to 25 percent) in 6-hydroxydopamine-treated rats, while the amount of labeled norepinephrine was found to be reduced by 90 percent. These data would suggest that the decarboxylation of DOPA can occur in other than dopaminergic fibers in brain (Breese and Traylor 1971, *Brit. J. Pharmacol.* in press).

MAAS: You can expect that, because the decarboxylase enzyme is soluble and ubiquitous, whereas the dopamine-beta-hydroxylase is not.

BREESE: This view fits the comments Dr. Kopin made earlier. Presumably in Parkinson's disease the dopaminergic neurons are destroyed, resulting in a loss of all synthesizing enzymes. Nevertheless, the benefits of DOPA in Parkinson's disease are well documented and are thought to result from the decarboxylation of DOPA. Can such views and data be compatible? The work with 6-hydroxydopamine would suggest that they can.

HETEROGENEOUS DISTRIBUTIONS OF SCHIZOPHRENIA

George Wilson McBee

Texas Research Institute of Mental Sciences
Houston, Texas

In reviewing the heterogeneous distributions of schizophrenia, the primary interest is in the area of epidemiology, particularly in the epidemiology of mental illness, with corollary interest in biostatistics and demography.

A substantial amount of the work in brain chemistry and mental disease is based on the assumption of inborn errors in metabolism predicated on genetic inheritance (Roman and Trice 1967). Therefore, selected studies in the area of genetics and a few on the effect of environment are to be reviewed. This review will be used to reach some conclusions, and to pursue the implications of those conclusions.

GENETICS

In the investigation of human genetics, most of the studies relating to the role of heredity in schizophrenia fall into three categories. First, there are the monozygotic and dizygotic twin studies. Both types of twins are compared with respect to concordance. Concordance is expressed as a rate of similar occurrence of any characteristic in both twins. Second, a number of genealogic studies have investigated the rate of occurrence of schizophrenia in terms of familial relationships. Third, a fairly recent entrant in the area of schizophrenia etiology is the adoptive or foster home study. Its basic design is to compare adopted individuals whose biological parents are schizophrenic with adopted individuals whose biological parents are not schizophrenic.

A number of twin studies concerning schizophrenia have been carried out by investigators in a number of different countries. Some

TABLE 1

Concordance Rates for Schizophrenia in Twins

Study	Monozygotic		Dizygotic	
	No.	Percentage	No.	Percentage
Tienari 1968	16	6-36	-	-
Kringlen 1968	55	25-38	90	7-10
Essen-Möller 1941	7	15-71	24	17
Luxenburger 1928	17	67	33	0
Rosanoff et al. 1934	41	67	101	10
Slater 1953	41	76	115	14
Kallmann 1946	174	86	296	15
Kallmann 1953	268	86	685	15

Sources: Kringlen, E. 1964. Schizophrenia in male monozygotic twins. In *Heredity and Environment in Functional Psychoses*. Oslo, Norway: Universitetsforlaget. Reprinted with permission.
Rosenthal, D., and Kety, S. S. 1968. *The Transmission of Schizophrenia*. New York: Pergamon Press. Reprinted with permission.

of the results are shown in Table 1. In most of the earlier studies the concordance rates for monozygotic twins are much higher than those for dizygotic twins. The values range from Kallmann's oft-quoted value of 86 percent to the 67 percent given by Kringlen (1964). More recent studies show a lower rate of concordance for monozygotic twins. A range of concordance is usually presented in later studies also, with the lower values based on a broad definition of schizophrenia. Clearly, a wide overall range of values has been reported. For monozygotic twins the percentage concordance ranges from 6 to 86 percent (Kringlen 1964). Dizygotic values range from 0 to 17 percent with clustering in the 10 to 15 percent bracket (Rosenthal and Kety

TABLE 2

Proportions of Relatives of Schizophrenics
Who Are Also Schizophrenics

Relative	Age-Corrected Proportion	Standard Error	Study
General population	0.008	0.0008	Fremming 1951
Children of first cousins	0.011	-	quoted by Slater 1953
Parents	0.093 0.041	0.008 0.011	Kallmann 1950 Slater 1953
Children of one or two schizophrenics	0.164	0.013	Kallmann 1938
Children of two schizophrenics	0.634 0.454 0.392	0.075 0.063 0.130	Kallmann 1938 Schulz 1940 Elsässer 1952
Full siblings	0.142 0.054	0.008 0.009	Kallmann 1950 Slater 1953
Half siblings	0.071	0.029	Kallmann 1950
Nephews and nieces	0.039	-	quoted by Kallmann 1946
First cousins	0.026	-	quoted by Kallmann 1946

Source: Gregory, I. 1960. Genetic factors in schizophrenia. Reprinted from Amer. J. Psychiat. 116:961. Copyright 1960, the American Psychiatric Association.

1968). While these results do not fit any single gene model with precision, the relatively higher percentage concordance for monozygotic twins lends support to the concept of a genetic factor in schizophrenia.

Table 2 is taken from Ian Gregory's work (Gregory 1960) and

TABLE 3

Schizophrenic Children Reared in Foster Homes

	Schizophrenic Biological Mother		Nonschizophrenic Biological Mother	
Schizophrenic	5	11%	0	0%
Nonschizophrenic	42	89%	50	100%
TOTAL	47	100%	50	100%

Source: Heston, L. L. 1966. Psychiatric disorders in foster home reared children. *Brit. J. Psychiat.* 112:819. Reprinted with permission.

Schizophrenic Children Reared in Adopted Homes

	Schizophrenic Parent		Nonschizophrenic Control	
Schizophrenic	3	8%	0	0%
Nonschizophrenic	36	92%	47	100%
TOTAL	39	100%	47	100%

Source: Rosenthal, D., and Kety, S. S. 1968. *The Transmission of Schizophrenia.* New York: Pergamon Press. Reprinted with permission.

shows the proportions of schizophrenics among the relations of schizophrenics. We can observe that, for the classes of relatives of whom independent studies exist, the estimates are variable. Most of the confidence intervals do not overlap. After fitting a series of gene-

TABLE 4

Migration

Rates per 100,000 for Schizophrenics among Norwegian Emigrants in Minnesota and Norwegians in Norway			Rates per 100,000 for Native-Born and Migrant Schizophrenics in Texas		
Sex	Norwegian Emigrants	Norwegians in Norway	Sex	Migrants	Native-Born
Male	24	15	Male	20	23
Female	30	13	Female	34	29
TOTAL	28	14	TOTAL	27	26

Source: Ödegaard, Ö. 1932. Emigration and insanity: a study of mental disease amont the Norwegian-born population of Minnesota. *Acta Psychiatrica et Neurologica*, Suppl. 4. Reprinted with permission.

Source: Jaco, E. G. 1960. *The Social Epidemiology of Mental Disorders*. New York: Russell Sage Foundation. Reprinted with permission.

tic models to the data in Table 2, Gregory concludes that no single gene theory fits all the data, even in a relational sense.

Table 3 shows the results of two studies of the outcome of rearing children, whose biological parents are schizophrenic, in foster homes. Both studies included appropriate control groups. Heston (1966) indicated that 11 percent of the children whose biological mothers were schizophrenic later developed schizophrenia, although the children were separated at a very early age. Similarly, Rosenthal and Kety (1968) found that 8 percent developed schizophrenia, as compared with none in the control group. Certainly, these findings are consistent with interpretations of the interaction of heredity and environment.

Considered as a whole, these data, particularly of twins, are quite variable. They do seem to point to a conclusion, however. While heredity seems to play a role in various forms of schizophrenia, the data in a general sense do not support the hypothesis that a single or major gene causes the observed difficulties. The observed data fit no Mendelian distribution of phenotype.

EFFECTS OF ENVIRONMENT

A number of environmental effects have been stressed as important in the etiology of schizophrenia. The following is a somewhat biased sample of these studies. Table 4 shows the results of two studies on the effect of migration. On the left, the results of the Ödegaard (1932) study show that Norwegian emigrants evidenced a higher rate of schizophrenia than those who stayed at home. This was true for both men and women.

Migration as an explicatory mechanism, however, is not borne out in Jaco's data (Jaco 1960). While women migrants show a slightly higher rate of schizophrenia than do native born women, the relationship is inverted for men. Further, the overall ratios are similar.

As noted by Mishler and Scotch (1965), a large number of studies points to an association between social status and incidence and prevalence measures of schizophrenia. Yet, Clausen and Kohn report no difference in their Hagerstown study.

Table 5 shows the results of Hollingshead and Redlich's study (1958) on the left, and Jaco's (1960) on the right. The Hollingshead and Redlich study evidences a consistent correlation between both the incidence and prevalence of schizophrenia and social class. Jaco's study simply does not show the same smooth gradient. The rates by occupational groups are quite varied while the rates by educational level are obviously curvilinear.

Table 6 shows the mean age of admission for the studies of Hollingshead and Redlich (1954) and Cooper (1961). Hollingshead and Redlich's data show a clear increase in mean age from high to low class, while, with a single exception, Cooper shows exactly the opposite.

Table 7 presents the results of studies of the social mobility of schizophrenics compared with the mobility of paired controls. Clausen and Kohn (1959) found no reliable differences between schizophrenics and their paired controls. In sharp contrast, Lystad (1957) found more downward mobility among schizophrenics with a corresponding lack of upward mobility for this group. Again, there is a dissonance in the results.

CONCLUSIONS

For each of these hypotheses it is fairly easy to show a set of divergent findings. A series of explanations suggest themselves:

1. Differences in method and general procedure.

TABLE 5

Social Class

Distribution of Schizophrenia Across Social Classes in New Haven, 1950 (rates/100,000)

Class	Incidence	Prevalence
I, II	6	111
III	8	168
IV	10	300
V	20	895

Source: Hollingshead, A. B., and Redlich, F. C. 1958. *Social Class and Mental Illness*, p. 236. New York: John Wiley and Sons. Reprinted with permission.

Relation of Occupation and Education to Rates of Schizophrenia in Texas, 1951-1952 (incidence/100,000)

Occupational Group	Rate
Professional, semi-professional	61
Managerial, official, proprietary	19
Clerical, sales	54
Service	64
Agriculture	51
Manual work	33
Unemployed	295

Educational Level	Rate
College	39
9-12 years	28
5-8 years	27
1-4 years	28
No education	45

Source: Jaco, E. G. 1960. *The Social Epidemiology of Mental Disorders*. New York: Russell Sage Foundation. Reprinted with permission.

---

2. Questions as to the reliability of the diagnosis of schizophrenia, and

3. to carry these questions a step further -- all of these studies are based on the assumption that schizophrenia is a homogeneous entity.

These data are consistent with the conclusion that schizophrenia as variously reported is not a homogeneous entity. Heterogeneous distributions have been observed on numerous occasions, and the most plausible assumption on the basis of current information is that schizophrenia is a group of disorders.

TABLE 6

Age by Social Class

Mean Age of Schizophrenics by Social Class at First Admission		Distribution of Age by Social Class at First Admission	
Class	Mean Age (years)	Class	Mean Age (years)
I, II	29	I, II	34.5
III	31	III	33.3
IV	32	IV	30.9
V	33	V	31.7

Source: Hollingshead, A. B., and Redlich, F. C. 1954. Schizophrenia and social structure. Reprinted from *Amer. J. Psychiat.* 110:695. Copyright 1954, the American Psychiatric Association.

Source: Cooper, B. 1961. Social class and prognosis in schizophrenia, Part 1. *Brit. J. Prev. Soc. Med.* 15:17. Reprinted with permission.

Thus, concerning schizophrenia, the question of nosology is a serious problem. Over the years, a number of nosological changes have been offered. The revisions proposed, however, have not met wide acceptance. Direct pursuit of nosology does not seem to yield immediate results.

In re-examining the studies, one finds that the only inferential statistics used are forms of chi-square analysis and unpaired t-tests. Such techniques as multivariate analysis of variance, discriminant function analysis, and canonical correlation procedures are conspicuous by their absence.

Biological, psychological, and sociological variables have been analyzed largely in an independent fashion. Yet, simultaneous consideration of these three forms of variables seems necessary to sorting out the heterogeneous groupings in schizophrenic patients. Advanced inferential statistical techniques have been designed largely for this purpose. Ideally, the outcome of applying these forms of analysis would be variations in patterns that would point to classification systems yielding more homogeneous groupings.

TABLE 7

Mobility

Intergenerational Mobility in Schizophrenics' Occupation Status as Compared to Parents			Comparison of Shifts in Class Levels of Schizophrenics and their Parents		
Occupation	Schizophrenic (%)	Paired Control (%)	Mobility	Schizophrenic (%)	Paired Control (%)
Higher than parents	34	30	Upward	13	20
Equal to parents	43	52	Absent	41	56
Lower than parents	23	18	Downward	46	24
TOTAL	100	100	TOTAL	100	100

(Based on 44 cases in each group.)

(Based on 94 cases in each group.)

Source: Clausen, J. A., and Kohn, M. L. 1959. Relation of schizophrenia to the social structures of a small city. In *Epidemiology of Mental Disorder*. B. Pasamanick, (ed.). Washington, D. C.: American Association for Advancement of Science, p. 69. Reprinted with permission.

Source: Lystad, M. H. 1957. Social mobility among selected groups of schizophrenic patients. *Amer. Sociol. Rev.* 22:288. Reprinted with permission from American Sociological Association.

The techniques often lead to assumptions about the data that are difficult to validate in practice. The more advanced of the techniques present serious problems in interpreting and communicating the results. The distributive forms of the test statistics are not widely known, particularly in canonical analysis. Results sometimes will not tell anything we do not already know. Obviously, these types of analyses are not a panacea.

These difficulties suggest that the techniques should be used to build models and probably not to test hypotheses at this time.

Such models could contribute much to the development of hypotheses that will be useful in the research dealing with the etiology of schizophrenia.

REFERENCES

Clausen, J. A., and Kohn, M. L. 1959. Relation of schizophrenia to the social structure of a small city. In *Epidemiology of Mental Disorder*. B. Pasamanick (ed.). Washington, D. C.: Amer. Assoc. Advanc. Sci. p. 69.

Cooper, B. 1961. Social class and prognosis in schizophrenia, Part 1. *Brit. J. Prev. Soc. Med.* 15:17.

Gregory, I. 1960. Genetic factors in schizophrenia. *Amer. J. Psychiat.* 116:961.

Heston, L. L. 1966. Psychiatric disorders in foster home reared children. *Brit. J. Psychiat.* 112:819.

Hollingshead, A. B., and Redlich, F. C. 1954. Schizophrenia and social structure. *Amer. J. Psychiat.* 110:695.

Hollingshead, A. B., and Redlich, F. C. 1958. *Social Class and Mental Illness*. New York: Wiley.

Jaco, E. G. 1960. *The Social Epidemiology of Mental Disorders*. New York: Russell Sage Foundation.

Kringlen, E. 1964. *Schizophrenia in Male Monozygotic Twins*. Oslo, Norway: The Norwegian Research Council for Science and the Humanities.

Lystad, M. H. 1957. Social mobility among selected groups of schizophrenia patients. *Amer. Sociol. Rev.* 22:288.

Mishler, E. G., and Scotch, N. A. 1965. Sociocultural factors in the epidemiology of schizophrenia. *Int. J. Psychiat.* 1:258.

Ödegaard, Ö. 1932. Emigration and insanity: a study of mental disease among the Norwegian-born population of Minnesota. *Acta Psychiat. Neurol.* Suppl. 4.

Roman, P. M., and Trice, H. M. 1967. *Schizophrenia and the Poor*. Ithaca, New York: Cayuga Press.

Rosenthal, D., and Kety, S. S. 1968. *The Transmission of Schizophrenia*. New York: Pergamon Press.

FREQUENCY OF GENETIC POLYMORPHISM:

IMPLICATIONS FOR MENTAL DISEASE

        Charles R. Shaw

        The University of Texas M. D. Anderson Hospital
        and Tumor Institute at Houston

        Houston, Texas

    The total number of genes occurring in the cells of higher animal organisms, such as man, is not accuratedly known. The figure most often quoted is 50,000, but this is no more than a slightly educated guess. The total amount of DNA contained in the nucleus would account for something like one hundred times that number of genes, but a large amount of the DNA, probably most of it, does not carry genetic information.

    The function of most genes, as far as is known, is to determine the specific structure of the various proteins; these proteins are mainly enzymes and the structural proteins making up the supporting materials of membranes, microtubules, etc. Other genes, perhaps a few, perhaps a great many, are involved in regulating the activity of those mentioned above; still others determine the structure of various ribonucleic acids that are a part of the machinery of protein assembly.

    A change in a gene (mutation) may have one or more of the following effects on the gene product:

        1. No change (synonymous mutation)
        2. Altered structure but normal activity
        3. Altered activity (more, less, none)
        4. Altered amount of protein (more, less, none)

    Mutants have been a major tool of the geneticist ever since the inception of the science with Mendel. Until recently, mutations were studied by analysis of their effects on the organism, called phenotypic effects. The phenotype is the outward manifestation of the gene. Thus, such phenotypic traits could be studied as eye color, shape of the wing, etc. In man, many of the phenotypic effects of most interest and considerable study have been those that produce disease. All such mutants obviously must affect activity or function of the gene products, since they produce phenotypic effects.

A major feature of any species is genetic variability. Within any species, such as *Homo sapiens*, there is a high degree of genetic homogeneity: all men look very much alike and are easily distinguishable from any other species. On the other hand, there is much obvious difference. Geneticists have long wondered and long been trying to find out whether most of the genes within a species are mostly alike or mostly different. Methods available until recently have not been very useful for answering the question, but the general supposition has been that most genes in man, or in any single species, are mostly alike. A subquestion of the general question has been, how many "deleterious" (hereditary disease-transmitting) genes does a population, and a single individual, carry? It has been estimated that each individual carries about a half-dozen deleterious genes, designated the "genetic load." When an individual mates with a person carrying one of the same defective genes (assuming the genes are recessive), one-fourth of the offspring will be homozygous and will have the disease. Alternatively, if the deleterious gene is dominant and has complete penetrance, every person carrying it will have the disease, and one-half of his offspring will also have it.

As to the amount of genetic variation in the individual and in the population that is not deleterious, transmitting the so-called neutral or partially neutral traits such as hair color, body size, etc., little useful information for accurate estimate has been available in the past.

METHODS AND RESULTS

Recently developed methods (Hunter and Markert 1957) have made such an estimate feasible. These methods are based on direct examination of the gene products, the proteins. They utilize the fact that very minor alterations in protein structure, that is, substitution of a single amino acid by a different one, are frequently detectable by gel electrophoresis (Shaw 1965). This class of mutants must retain at least some of the activity of the enzyme or they could not be detected on the gel. Rapid screening of a relatively large number of individuals and of different enzymes is now possible, using an aqueous extract of a tissue, such as erythrocytes. A small sample (about 10λ) is applied to the electrophoretic medium, usually a starch gel. Following electrophoresis by application of a direct current through the gel for periods of time ranging from one to

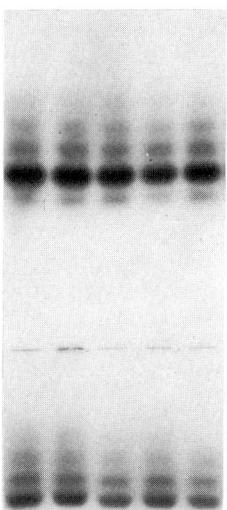

Figure 1. Photograph of a starch gel of kidney extracts of five deer mice, developed for the enzyme malate dehydrogenase. Anodal direction is toward top of gel. Sample slots are near center.

twenty-four hours, the position of a specific enzyme is determined by specific staining for that enzyme activity. An example of a stained gel, called a zymogram, is shown in Figure 1. The dark bands show the location of malate dehydrogenase (MDH) in extracts from the kidneys of five different mice. There are two different MDH's in this tissue; the upper form is present in the cytoplasm of the kidney cells, the lower form is from mitochondria (the multiple sub-bands are artifactual). Note that all occur at the same position, indicating that there is no genetic difference in these animals for the genes controlling this enzyme. Figure 2, on the other hand, shows clear differences in the supernatant form of the enzyme in these five animals.

Application of this method to a number of natural populations, including man, the deermouse *(Peromyscus)*, housemouse *(Mus)*, several species of fish, the horseshoe crab, and several others, all have led to the same general conclusion: about one-third of all the genes within a species show variation (Hubby and Lewontin 1966; Harris 1970; Selander et al. 1969 and 1970; Shaw 1970). Actually, the ratio is probably higher than this, for a number of reasons. First, the electrophoretic technique does not detect all of the amino acid substitutions, because about two-thirds of substitutions do not change the net charge on the molecule. Additionally, many of the studies were based on relatively small samples; if more individuals were

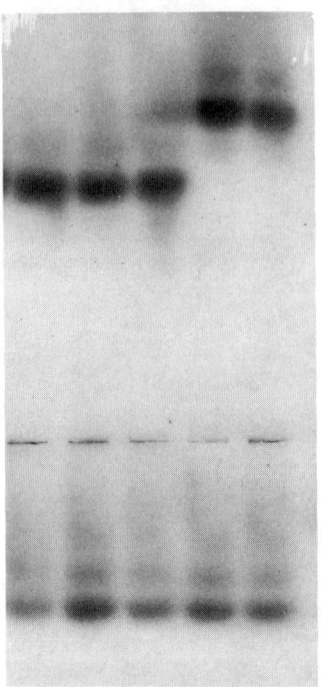

Figure 2. Same as Figure 1, but from five different animals, showing genetic variation of the anodal form of the enzyme.

examined, undoubtedly some additional fairly rare mutants would have been discovered. In fact, Ayala *et al.* (1970) recently studied a rather large sample of four *Drosophila* species and found variation in every protein examined!

DISCUSSION

There are several important inferences to be made from these findings. One is that genetic variation is far more common than was previously supposed. Another is that there must be a mechanism that causes "neutral" mutations to be incorporated into a population. The latter hypothesis is still a matter of some controversy, but it is gaining considerable support. It is in opposition to a major tenet of evolution theory, that is, that any mutation incorporated into a population at a significant level (arbitrarily, more than one percent) must have some selective advantage. Conversely, a mutation that is neutral or disadvantageous will be soon eliminated.

Recent advances in population genetics have provided mathematical models to explain the incorporation of neutral or nearly neutral mutations (Kimura 1968; King and Jukes 1970). Stated briefly, these models demonstrate that chance factors can account for at least some proportion of this phenomenon.

Implications of these findings have only begun to be appreciated. The high frequency of genetic polymorphism allows the acceptance of a theory of multigenic inheritance for a large number of diseases, including schizophrenia. In the past, the multigenic theory has come up against a numbers problem since, by earlier computations, the theoretically possible number of deleterious genes was several orders of magnitude lower than the number necessary to accommodate all of the diseases with all the genes that could be contributing to them. We are no longer in this quandary because we now have thousands of genes to "work with." Thus, the multigenic theory for the inheritance of schizophrenia seems more plausible. Actually, this theory has always fit the clinical picture better, although the single-gene theory continues to have its supporters. The multigenic theory also conforms better to the widely held position that schizophrenia probably is a heterogeneous group of disorders.

The findings fit well, too, with the position that many of the genetic variations are neutral or nearly neutral in their individual effects but that, in combination with certain of the other forms of other genes, they have the combined effect of producing the schizoid or schizophrenic state. Many workers, including myself, believe there is a continuum from a high level of reality testing at one end to severe schizophrenia at the other (Shaw and Lucas 1970). Included somewhere on the continuum of related functions is a variety of other capacities such as creative thinking, artistic feeling, abstraction, etc. Moreover, the success of any such complex population as man depends upon the infinite variety of behaviors and capabilities among its members. This implies, of necessity, that some members will receive from their parents particular combinations of genes producing extremes of behavior that are maladaptive, and that we call mental illness.

ACKNOWLEDGMENT

Supported in part by Grant GM 15597 from National Institutes of Health.

REFERENCES

Ayala, F. J.; Mourao, C. A.; Perez-Salas, S.; Richmond, R.; and Dobzhansky, T. 1970. Enzyme variability in the *Drosophila willistoni* group, 1. Genetic differentiation among sibling species. *Proc. Nat. Acad. Sci.* 67:225.

Harris, H. 1970. *The Principles of Human Biochemical Genetics*. New York: American Elsevier.

Hubby, J. L., and Lewontin, R. C. 1966. A molecular approach to the study of genic heterozygosity in natural populations 1. The number of alleles at different loci in *Drosophila pseudoobscura*. *Genetics* 54:577.

Hunter, R., and Markert, C. 1957. Histochemical demonstration of enzymes separated by zone electrophoresis in starch gel. *Science* 125:1294.

Kimura, M. 1968. Evolutionary rate at the molecular level. *Nature* 217:624.

King, J. L., and Jukes, T. H. 1969. Non-Darwinian evolution. *Science* 164:788.

Selander, R. K.; Hunt, W. G.; and Yang, S. Y. 1969. Protein polymorphism and genic heterozygosity in two European subspecies of the house mouse. *Evolution* 23:379.

Selander, R. K.; Yang, S. Y.; Lewontin, R. C.; and Johnson, W. E. 1970. Genetic variation in the horseshoe crab *(Limulus polyphemus)*, a phylogenetic "relic." *Evolution* 24:402.

Shaw, C. R. 1965. Electrophoretic variation in enzymes. *Science* 149:936.

Shaw, C. R. 1970. How many genes evolve? *Biochem. Genet.* 4:275.

Shaw, C. R., and Lucas, A. R. 1970. *The Psychiatric Disorders of Childhood*. 2nd Ed. New York: Appleton-Century-Crofts.

PURINE METABOLISM AND ABNORMAL BEHAVIOR IN CHILDREN

William L. Nyhan

University of California, San Diego

La Jolla, California

The study of the interrelationships of purine metabolism and behavior is, to some extent, in its infancy. It seems to us, however, that the study of human patients with heritable disorders of metabolism might, in fact, begin to give us some clues to a more molecular understanding of at least some forms of behavior. All forms of behavior are probably open ultimately for understanding on a molecular basis, but this is a more complicated problem for investigation.

We have been concerned for a number of years with the study of infants and children with inborn errors of metabolism. We are involved in clinical pediatrics, which has always seemed to us to be an appropriate place to study genetic disease, particularly disease of metabolism. A number of these diseases are detectable at birth and, furthermore, disease tends to occur in relatively pure form in childhood. This has been a rewarding field in which to look for new diseases and to find patients in whom one might get better understanding of already known diseases. It had, on the other hand, seemed likely that as pediatricians we would be protected from studying the most classic of the diseases of metabolism. Gout, which is the classic disorder of metabolism, has been known as a genetic disorder since antiquity. In fact, gout was recognized first by Hippocrates, who also recognized that this was a disease of the adult male; in the female it occurred rarely and then usually after the menopause. Obviously, there are no one hundred percent rules in human biology or medicine. As it turns out, a number of diseases of purine metabolism occur early in life, and I believe we can predict now with some confidence that further exploration will yield information on a number of others. The study of these disorders has focused attention, for the first time, on patterns of abnormal behavior and their biochemical correlates.

Figure 1 provides one conception of a relationship between purines and behavior. This ancient formulation considered the gout as the child of Bacchus and Aphrodite. We now know that this is not really the case. There are relationships between clinical attacks of gout and the ingestion of alcohol, but it is now clear that gout is an inherited disease. It is not as complicated as schizophrenia, but it is already apparent that gout may be caused by a number of genes, only a few of which have as yet been identified.

Table 1 presents another approach to the problem. This is a partial list of men who have been important to the development of Western civilization, who have also had gout. When one considers the frequency of the disease, which occurs in about two per thousand population, one comes away with the feeling that there is an association between gout and greatness, and, at least as measured by this kind of performance, that this is unlikely to have been fortuitous.

The argument was further developed on a theoretical basis by Orowan (1955), who pointed out that among the animals, only man and the higher apes had a significant concentration of uric acid in the blood. This is consistent with the fact that the other animals have a very active uricase in liver. Uric acid is rapidly destroyed by this highly specific enzyme. Another element in the story (Figure 2) is that uric acid, as a purine, has a chemical structure similar to compounds that are well known as central nervous system stimulants. These include caffeine, theophylline, and theobromine. In this sense, Orowan considered that the mutation responsible for the loss of hepatic uricase might have led to selective advantage.

Among the first tests of this hypothesis was the study of Stetten and Hearon (1959), who correlated the serum uric acid concentrations in a large series of Army inductees with their results on the Army General Classification Test. They found a low but statistically significant correlation. This has been followed by other studies of this type. Recent studies have tended to indicate that an elevated concentration of uric acid in the serum is related more to qualities of drive, ambition, and performance than to intelligence. They have focused on leadership qualities and behavior rather than on the more apparently inborn qualities one might classify as intelligence. It has been postulated that a tendency to gout is a tendency to the executive suite. A number of studies have indicated a relatively high level of performance, upward social mobility, or maintenance of high social status in populations in which uric acid concentrations tended to be high.

Table 2 illustrates a study of uric acid concentrations in university professors. It was carried out by Brooks and Mueller (1966) at the University of Michigan, on a sample of over 100 members of

Λυσιμελον Βάκχου, και λυσιμελους Αφροδίτης,
Γεννασαι θυγατηρ, λυσιμελης ποδαγρα.

Ut Venus enervat vires, sic copia vini,

Et tentat gressus, debilitatque pedes.

from Scudamore, C., 1823

Figure 1. A classic consideration of the gout. The conceptualization is expressed first in Greek and then in Latin.

TABLE 1

Partial List of Persons Important in the Development of Western Civilization Who Have Suffered from Gout

Alexander the Great	Thomas Gray
Isaac Newton	Johann Wolfgang von Goethe
Charles Darwin	James Russell Lowell
William Harvey	Alfred Tennyson
Benjamin Franklin	Edward Gibbon
Martin Luther	Henry Fielding
John Calvin	Horace Walpole
John Wesley	Samuel Johnson
Cardinal Wolsey	Lord Chesterfield
John Milton	Francis Bacon
Ben Johnson	Stendhal
William Congreve	Guy de Maupassant

Total incidence of gout: 2/1000 population.

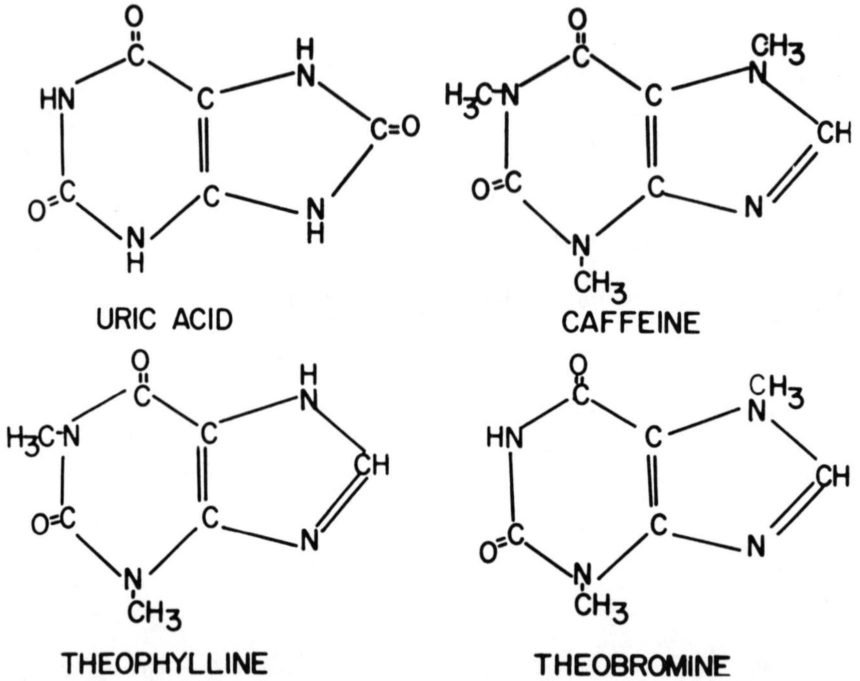

Figure 2. Structural formulas of uric acid and of some methylated purines known to have activity as central nervous system stimulants.

their faculty. They studied the correlation of uric acid concentrations (and a number of other chemical determinations which did not turn up any relationships) with a variety of other data obtained by a clinical psychologist in a two-hour semistructured interview. The mean serum uric acid value found in the total sample was 5.66, which is close to the normal mean but a little higher. It compares favorably with a series of executives who were found to have a 5.73 level. Within the series, it is of interest that full professors had the highest mean serum uric acid concentration. Their mean was 5.95, and that of the associate professors and assistant professors was 5.5. The differences were not large, but they are in the right direction. Listed in the table are correlation coefficients between serum urate values and either total behavior scores or scores for qualities of drive, achievement, and leadership. These have correlated positively, and correlations were statistically significant.

TABLE 2

Correlations of Uric Acid Concentration with Behavioral
Characteristics in University Professors

Behavioral Item	Pearsonian Correlation Coefficient
Drive	0.57
Achievement	0.54
Leadership	0.54
Pushing self	0.43
Emphasis on research	0.19
Total behavior score	0.66

Table derived from data reported by Brooks and Mueller (1966).

TABLE 3

Mean Concentrations of Uric Acid in Serum of High School
Students Ranked in Accordance with
Their Later Attendance at College

Group	mg/100 ml
CC	5.19
AC	5.88
NC	4.89

Group CC completed college and NC never entered, while group AC attempted college but was not able to complete the experience. Data reported by Kasl, Brooks, and Cobb (1966).

Table 3 presents a study by Kasl, Brooks, and Cobb (1966) of male high school students. This study provides additional evidence that the type of behavior that can be designated as achievement-oriented is related to the serum concentration of uric acid. This table presents mean serum uric acid values for three different groups. Group CC completed college; group AC attended college and then dropped out; and group NC never went to college. The highest value, 5.88, was found in the group that attended college (AC). The overall results are consistent with the concept that one could measure uric acid concentrations in high school students and determine whether or not they would go on to college. These levels of uric acid were obtained while the students were still in high school. Whether they went to college and what they accomplished there was determined by follow-up study. Interpretation of the results in terms of achievement orientation would suggest that the students in the AC group were less well prepared intellectually but had the drive that got them to college. Unfortunately, they were not able to stay there. This interpretation led to the prediction that, within the CC group, the people who went to college and stayed there, there might also be relationships to serum uric acid, and there are some data supporting this notion.

In Table 4, it can be seen that the length of time the individual remained in college was not related to past scholastic achievement but, rather, that longer attendance in college was related to the concentration of uric acid in the blood. Furthermore, in the CC group who stayed in college and graduated, the highest concentrations of uric acid were obtained from the blood of those whose grades were lowest. Thus, it seems that their drive got them through.

TABLE 4

Relationship Between Concentrations of Uric Acid and Grades in College for CC Group Only

Grades	mg/100 ml
Poor	6.16
Average	5.45
Good	5.03

Data reported by Kasl, Brooks, and Cobb (1966).

These rather general correlates of overall behavior are probably a low-power look at relationships of purine metabolism and behavior. When we have tried to study these at a higher magnification, we have had to look not at this end of the spectrum, but at the other, at patients who were not great scholars or intellectual achievers, but patients with mental retardation. Figure 3 illustrates a patient (S. M.) we have reported with Drs. James, Teberg, Sweetman, and Nelson in the *Journal of Pediatrics* (1969). This was not our first entry into the area of purines and behavior, but it seemed to be more closely relevant to the question of schizophrenia under consideration. At the time the photograph was taken, the patient was about three years of age. He seemed to be normal when he was examined at birth, except for a minor anomaly, a small degree of hypospadias. He was admitted to a hospital when he was four months old for cor-

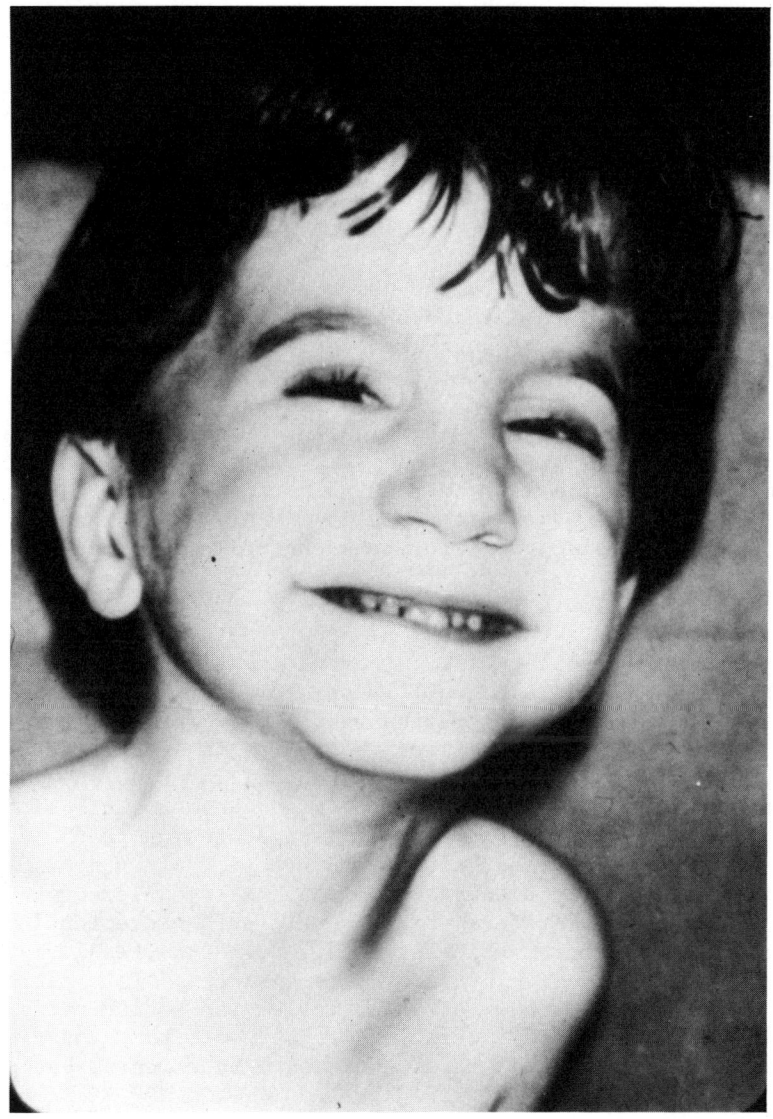

Figure 3. S. M. at three years of age. His characteristic, somewhat odd grin is illustrated, as are the dysplastic teeth.

rection of the hypospadias. He was given anesthesia and a certain amount of fasting, and repaired by surgical procedure. It was a relatively minor procedure from the urological point of view, but he became quite sick postoperatively. His temperature rose, and he had some trouble passing his urine. The small amount of urine passed was found to be full of crystals. The concentration of uric acid in his blood was high, a very unusual finding in a four-month-old baby. He grew up in a foster home. His foster mother noticed that he never shed tears when he cried, and that condition has remained. When his teeth erupted, they were very small and dysplastic. He began to walk and to develop in a motor sense, but he never began to talk. At five or six years of age, he still had no speech. A number of developmental tests indicated that he was not very retarded; his IQ or DQ has ranged from about 60 to 75. Speech retardation has been more profound. His "language" has been a kind of growling or humming, sounds we tend to associate with autistic children. Other factors in his behavior have suggested he was behaving in an autistic fashion. During the age of about two to five, he was oblivious of other people in his environment. He was living in a good foster home with the foster mother's three normal children, but he gave no evidence of relationship with them. The same was true of his relationships with examiners with whom he made no contact at all, although he saw the same people month after month. He had wide, inappropriate mood swings from giddy behavior to uncontrollable frustration.

This patient's growth in height and weight are illustrated in Figure 4. He followed a fairly normal growth pattern up to about three years of age, albeit at the bottom of the normal growth curve. His growth seems to be leveling off to some extent. A series of examinations of uric acid concentration gave a range of 9.5 to 11.6 mg/100 ml. Such high levels reflect the limits in solubility of uric acid in plasma, and they are distinctly unusual in children. A first assessment of whether or not the patient might have a metabolic abnormality was done by measuring the level of excretion in the urine. The total milligrams of urate excreted in a period of 24 hours is a more meaningful figure in a standard adult than in children who vary in age and size. We therefore express uric acid excretion in terms of milligrams per milligram of creatinine. Most individuals, even most adults with gout, have levels of less than one. This patient has had concentrations of two to three, reflecting a distinctly unusual level of excretion of uric acid. It suggests that the elevated concentration seen in the plasma is not caused by a renal, but a metabolic defect.

In almost a thousand determinations of uric acid in plasma reported by Seegmiller, Laster, and Howell (1963) in adult males, the mean level closely approximated 5 mg/100 ml. This provides a baseline for the interpretation of the behavioral studies discussed previously. A diagnosis of gout is supportable in patients with plasma uric acid over 6, and, because of variations in renal excretion, peo-

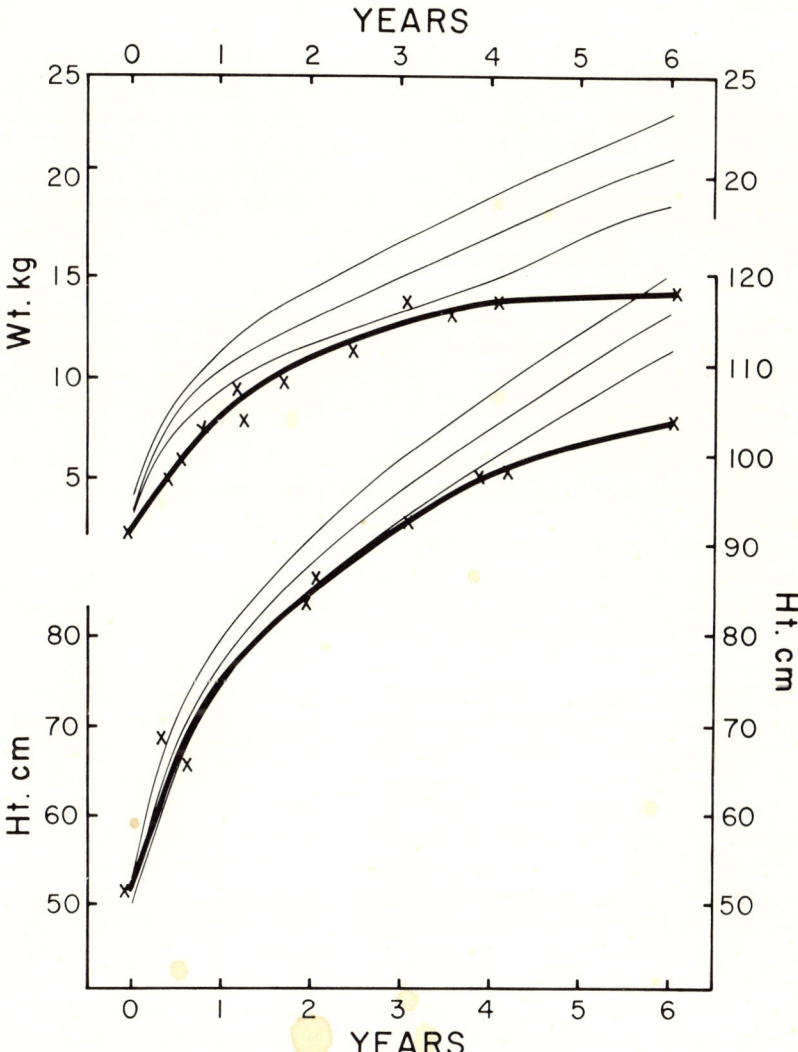
Figure 4. Growth and development of S. M.

ple with gout have concentrations ranging from 6 to well over 10 mg/100 ml. If the concentrations are much over 10, the patients probably have renal disease.

Urate excretion in man has been studied in carefully selected series of people who were eating no exogenous purine, and who were on such a diet for at least three days before the study. This kind of information then provides a look at the endogenous synthesis and breakdown of purines. Most adults excrete less than about 500 mg of urate in a 24-hour period, and, of course, so do most adults who have gout. It has also been known for some time that there is a smaller number of adults with gout, who were thought of as hyperexcretors because they excreted more than about 600 mg of uric acid in the urine in a 24-hour period. If we assess the milligram-per-kilogram excretion of the patient discussed above, it would be about 24, considerably higher than the levels observed in a normal or gouty adult. On the other hand, we have in the past studied some children with disordered purine metabolism who had an even more dramatic overexcretion of uric acid in the range of 40 to 50 milligrams per kilogram of body weight. Patients of this type will be discussed below.

Figure 5 illustrates some of the interrelations involved in the endogenous synthesis of purines. The pathway proceeds from such relatively simple precursors as glutamine, glycine, and formate, and the structure is slowly built up, always with the ribonucleotide attached, culminating in ring closure of this complicated molecule to form inosinic acid.

This information has been helpful in the study of purine synthesis in animals or man. The simple two-carbon amino acid, glycine, for instance, is incorporated whole into the four, five, and seven positions of uric acid. It is possible to start out with ^{14}C-labeled glycine which, injected into the patient, forms inosinic acid, and is then broken down to uric acid. We isolate this from the urine and measure its radioactivity. In the little boy we have presented, the curve obtained was distinctly different from the curve of normal individuals. It is easy to distinguish this kind of patient from a control population. The patient's curve indicates that uric acid is being made very rapidly from glycine, probably by a route different from that of the ordinary person. A normal individual shows no peak at all, probably reflecting the course of nucleic acid synthesis in which the glycine goes slowly into the nucleic acids and then slowly comes out with no change in rate. The abnormal pattern, in contrast, shows a rapid process that has been called a shunt pathway. Maximum specific activity occurs in the first twelve hours. These data represent the fastest conversions of glycine to uric acid we have seen. In previous studies of patients with overproduction of purine *de novo*, we have generally found the peak to occur between 24 and 48 hours.

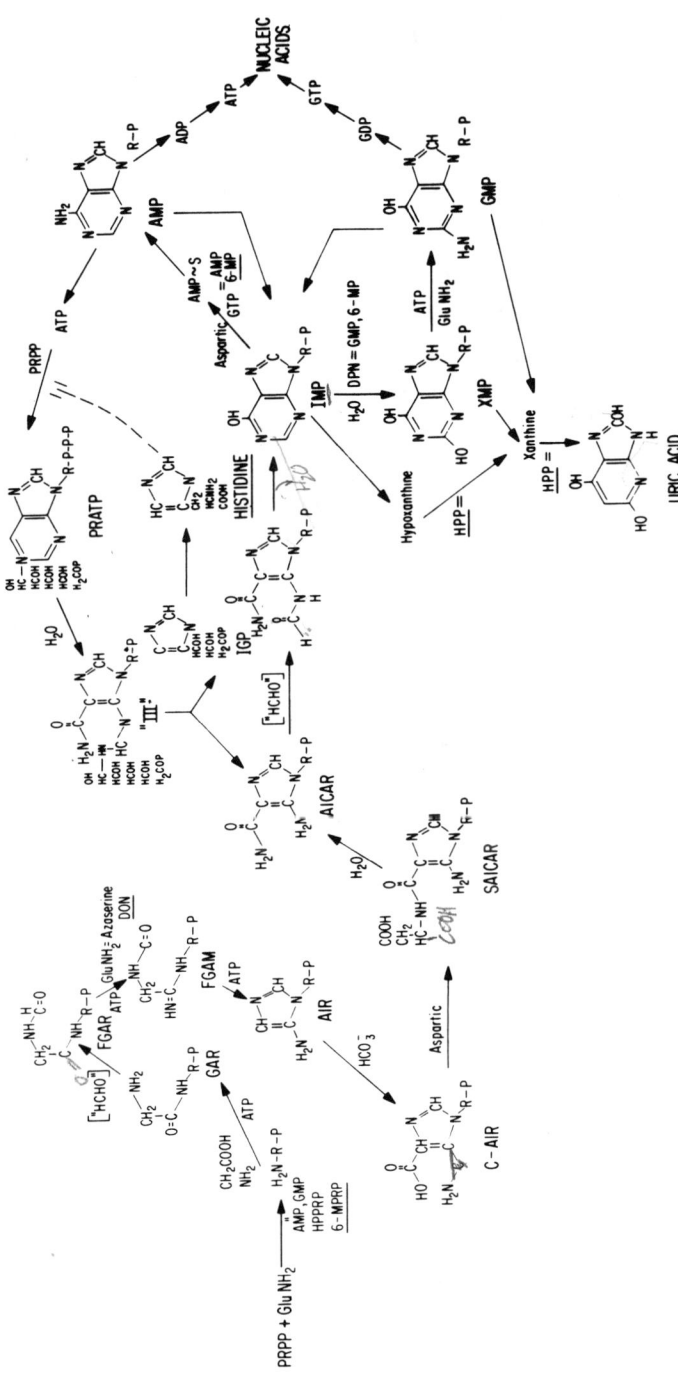

Figure 5. Pathways in *de novo* synthesis of purines.

A comparison of this type, in adults who did and did not have gout, would not discriminate between the two populations. Investigators studying gout in this fashion, therefore, have tended to evaluate the data in terms of the cumulative percentage of injected ^{14}C excreted as uric acid in the period studied. In seven days, a control child or adult would incorporate about one-tenth of one percent of the administered glycine into uric acid. This represents, then, a very small part of the overall metabolism of glycine, most of which is metabolized to CO_2 within 24 hours of injection. In the patient presented above, this analysis showed an enormous overproduction of inosinic acid, or overproduction of purine, which ultimately shows up in the breakdown product, uric acid. The difference between patient and control was of the order of seven times. In adults with overproduction gout, the level is usually about two times higher than control. This patient, therefore, had a very rapid rate of overproduction of purine.

In contrast, studies we did a few years ago on some children to be discussed next showed an even greater degree of overproduction of purine *de novo*. Four patients were studied, two of them related and two others unrelated. They had such massive overproduction that it accounted for about two percent of the total metabolism of glycine. This is a big drain in terms of glycine metabolism, and certainly an overproduction way out of the range one sees in any other disease.

These four patients were first presented in a report of studies carried out with Dr. Michael Lesch (Lesch and Nyhan 1964); they are the patients with whom we began our studies of behavior. Their syndrome has come to be known as the Lesch-Nyhan syndrome. Virtually all patients with this syndrome are markedly mentally retarded. They present a very different picture from the boy discussed above. These patients have a severe motor defect: they have never learned to walk; they cannot sit unassisted. Examination of muscles reveals a very marked increase in tone. Deep-tendon reflexes are increased. Overall, the neurological picture is that of spastic cerebral palsy. These children also have dramatic, writhing, rhythmic movements, both choreic and athetoid in character. All children with this abnormality have had choreoathetosis. Some other features of the disorder are relevant to behavior. It is possible to get a feeling for these patients by looking at their faces. They often have a nice smile and they seem to relate to people. They look brighter than one would expect of a patient with an IQ of around 50, as tested. This is classic for all children with this syndrome; those taking care of them have always felt that they were smarter than their tests showed, that they were somehow prevented by their neurological abnormality, spasticity, and athetosis from behaving as successfully as they could. I believe there is something in this as I study these children in the institutions for the retarded. Because of their motor defect, they are almost invariably placed in a ward in which all of the children are bedridden. Then we look at their faces, and these children look much brighter than any of the others on the ward. Then we begin to look at their behavior, and we see the way they relate to the staff. Usually on such a ward the patient with this disease is the favorite of the nurses, the aides, and everybody else. So they do relate to people. This is very different from the sort of thing we talked about in the first patient. One of these patients developed a relationship somehow with the mayor of Dade County in Florida, and he ultimately was given the key to the county. This, then, is one side of the personality.

Another more important aspect of behavior is illustrated in Figure 6, self-mutilation. One generally sees the patient in protective wrappings resembling mittens or boxing gloves. Wherever one sees patients with this disease--I have visited wards in England and in France and throughout the United States--one finds that the staff has learned this kind of tricks in managing them. As I see these patients with their athetoid movements, with mittens on their hands, and with their somewhat tragic, comic sense of humor, I am reminded of the principal character of the ballet, *Petrouschka*. Figure 6 shows the hands of a little boy (M. J.). The thumb of one hand illustrates his mutilative behavior; he has bitten his thumb and produced a certain amount of damage. He had a predilection for damaging that particular thumb and, on his other hand, he has damaged the little finger. The lesion can also be seen in Figure 7, the x-ray of that hand. The little finger had only two phalanges; he has produced an amputation of the tip.

This patient had lived at home and he was, as you might imagine, a terrible problem in management. The mother had not understood the relationship between restraint and behavior. She told me, when I first saw the child at two, that no one in the house had slept through the night since his teeth first developed. Every night he would go to bed and scream. This is a common history among these patients. We thought the reason he screamed all night was because he realized that if he was not protected from himself, he would chew himself to bits. We showed the mother how to restrain the child in sleep, and they all began sleeping through the night.

Figure 8 illustrates another patient with the same disease. This boy shows the clinical hallmark of this condition, mutilation of the lip. There is distinct loss of tissue, which in the individual case may represent the upper or lower. Some patients, but not many, mutilate both lips.

We have published an even more serious example of the same problem (Nyhan 1968). Destruction of tissue was so great that most physicians would think he had been born with a harelip and cleft palate, but this was not the case. He was born intact, and all of the mutilation around the mouth was self-induced. This biting, picking, and other mutilative activity is a very dramatic and bizarre example of

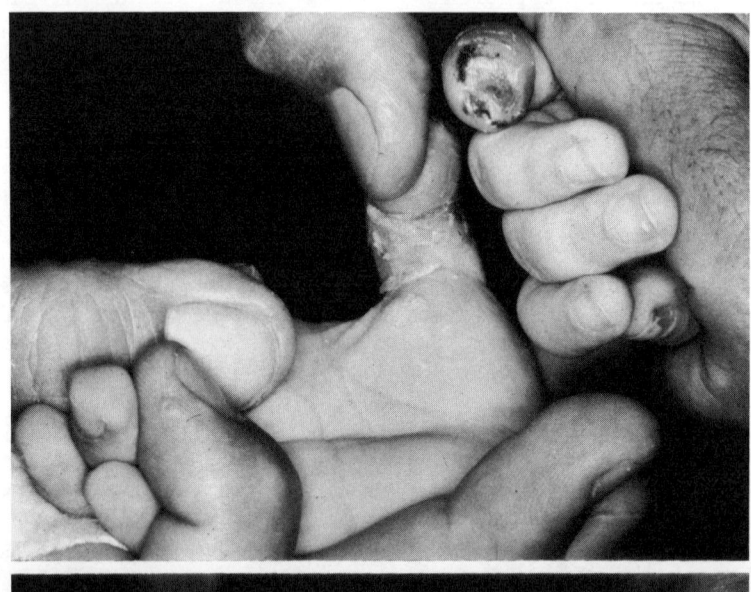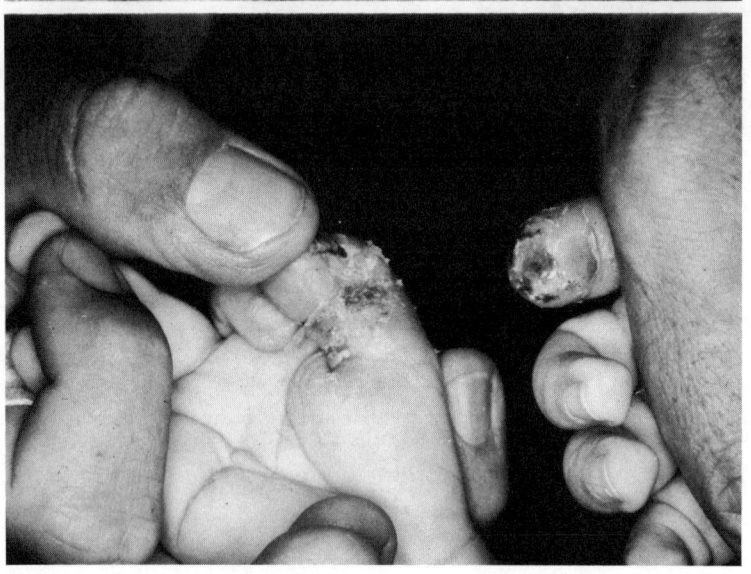

Figure 6. Hands of M. J., illustrating self-mutilation of right thumb and left fifth finger.

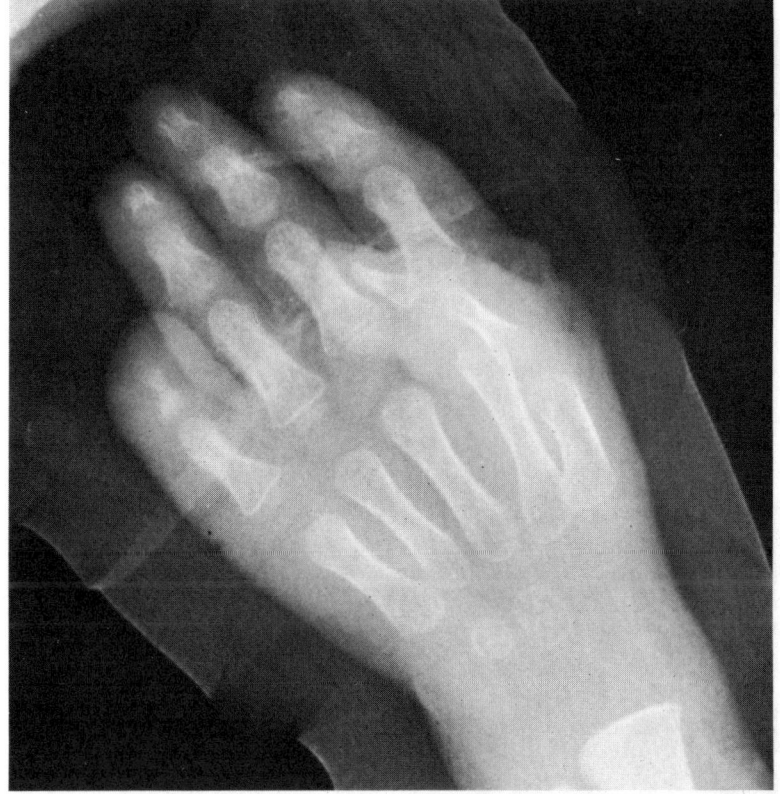

Figure 7. X-ray of the hand illustrating partial amputation of left fifth finger.

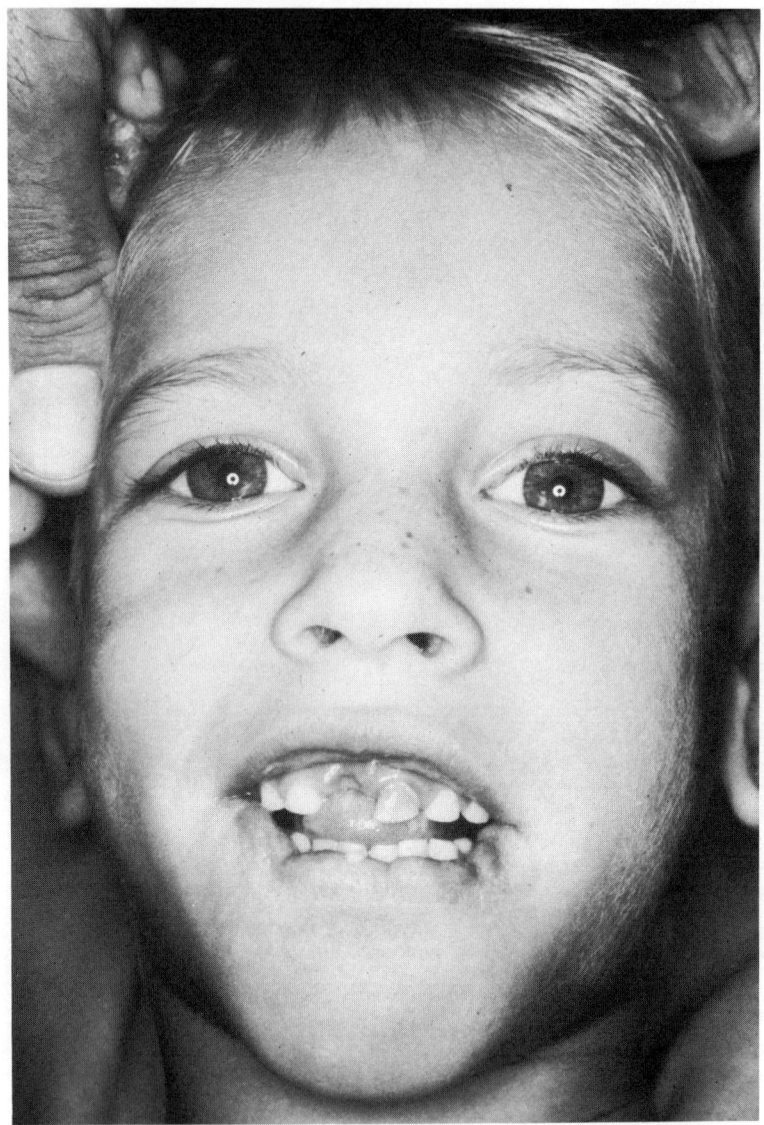

Figure 8. Face of M. J. Loss of tissue about the lip following biting is clinical hallmark of syndrome.

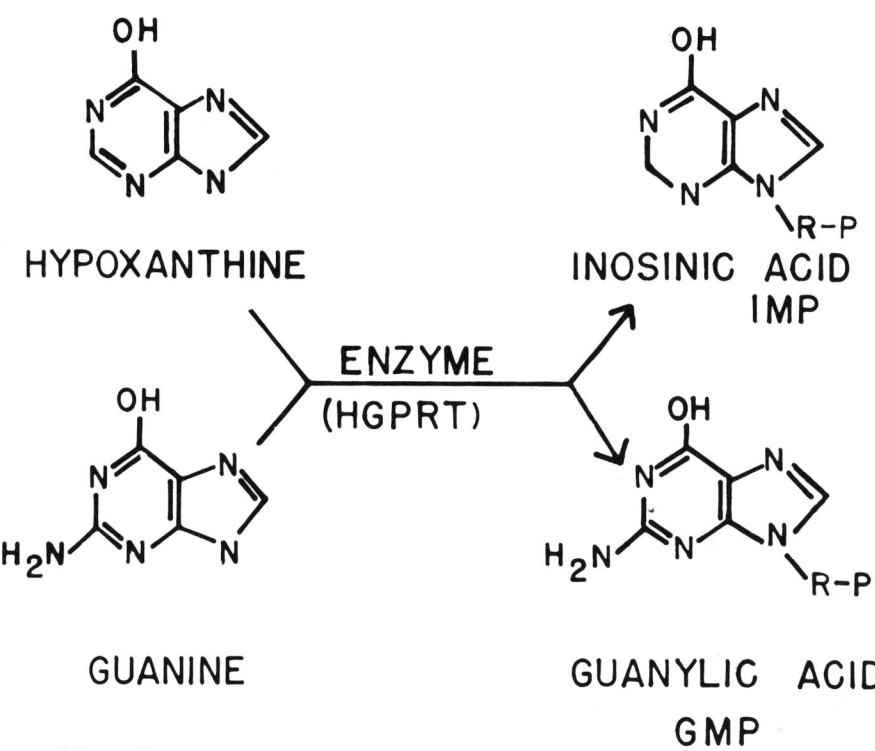

Figure 9. The hypoxanthine guanine phosphoribosyl transferase (HGPRT) reaction.

unusual behavior.

Current molecular understanding of this behavior must start with the reaction illustrated in Figure 9. The relationship of this enzyme, hypoxanthine guanine phosphoribosyl transferase (HGPRT), to the disease was first elucidated by Seegmiller, Rosenbloom, and Kelley (1967). Patients with the Lesch-Nyhan syndrome have a single gene defect in which the mutant gene, which is on the X chromosome, determines that this enzyme is almost completely inactive. HGPRT catalyzes the conversion of hypoxanthine and guanine in the presence of 5-phosphoribosyl-1-pyrophosphate (PRPP) to their respective ribonucleotides, inosinic acid and guanylic acid. It is a relatively nonspecific enzyme that makes these two and other purine nucleotides. It is relevant to the metabolism of nucleic acids.

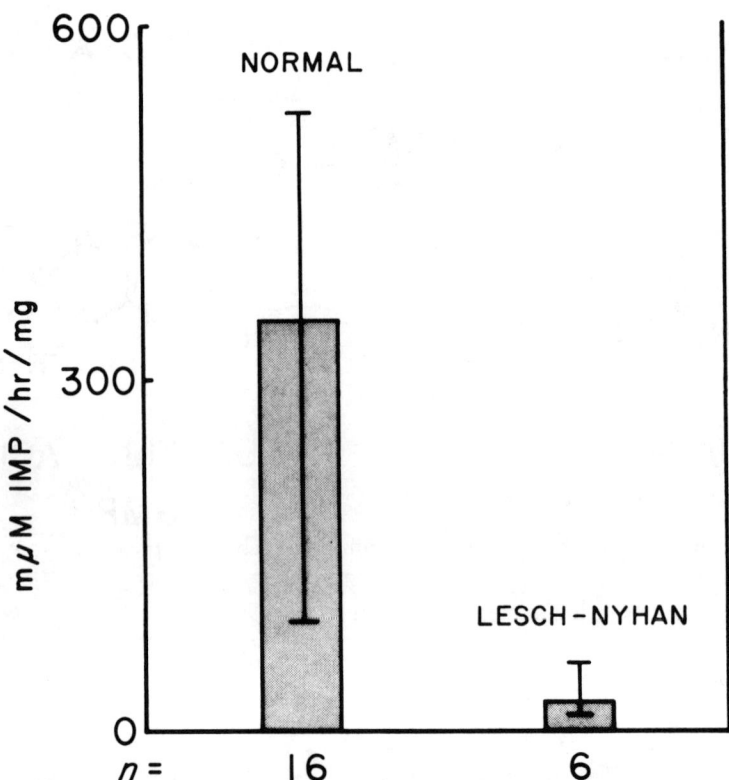

Figure 10. HGPRT activity in extracts of fibroblasts. Fibroblasts were studied from six patients and sixteen controls. Shaded bars represent means and bracketed line the ranges of values obtained.

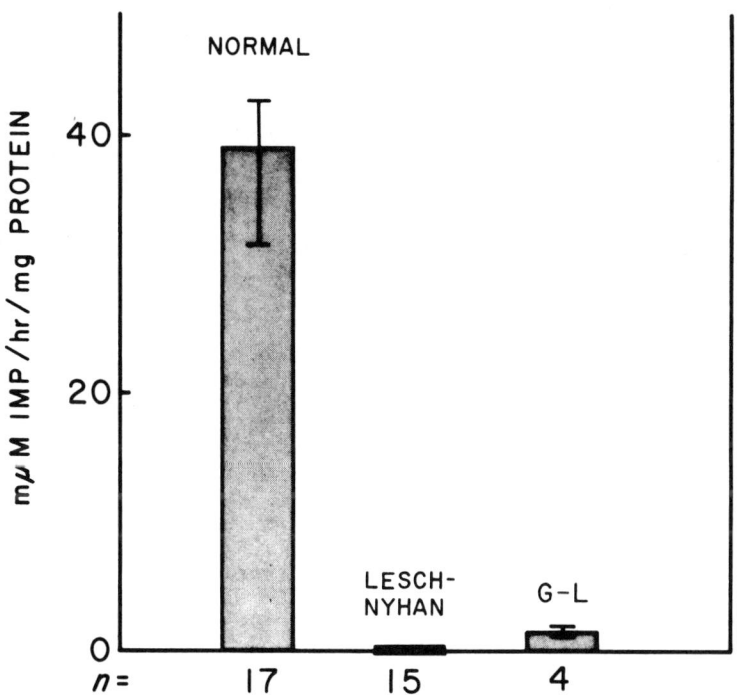

Figure 11. HGPRT activity in erythrocytes. The activity in the patients with the Lesch-Nyhan syndrome could not be distinguished from zero.

Our data on this enzyme were originally obtained by utilizing skin biopsy and cell culture. Fibroblasts from human skin are diploid cells, containing many of the enzymes one expects in all of the cells of the individual. They permit the study of enzymes in nucleated cells. Some of our data on HGPRT activity in human fibroblasts are illustrated in Figure 10. In this assay, we measured IMP, or inosinic acid, as indicated in Figure 9, but the fibroblast contains a nucleotidase that hydrolyzes inosinic acid very rapidly to inosine. We must, therefore, measure inosine as well, and we express the sum of inosinic acid and inosine. This yields a reproducible value in control individuals with modest variation about the mean. Patients with the disease, as illustrated, have virtually no activity of HGPRT. In fact, we have never found activity in IMP. We have wondered until very recently whether this enzyme might not be completely lacking. We now have data indicating that there is a small amount of activity that is significant.

We have also had experience with patients with partial deficiency of HGPRT. One such family has recently been reported (Kogut *et al*. 1970). In the involved individuals in this family, nothing was wrong with their behavior. Their IQs were normal. They did have high concentrations of uric acid in blood and urine, and some of them developed renal stone disease very early in life.

Figure 11 illustrates the activity of HGPRT in the erythrocyte. This assay is much easier to do than the fibroblast assay. It is now evident that the enzyme is present in the normal erythrocyte. HGPRT can be measured on the inosinic acid or the guanylic side, but there is no erythrocyte nucleotidase so one does not have to measure inosine. Adenine phosphoribosyl transferase (APRT), which makes the nucleotide of adenine, is a different enzyme. If we consider control individuals to have one hundred percent of normal activity, patients with the Lesch-Nyhan syndrome have levels of activity of HGPRT that cannot be distinguished from zero. In this assay, then, there is no activity at all. The adenine enzyme, however, is increased in activity. Data on the family reported by Kogut *et al*. (1970) indicate a defect in the HGPRT enzyme. It is genetically true. The levels obtained were the same in two siblings and in two of their cousins. All had about five percent of normal activity. They had an elevation of the adenine enzyme also. The little boy we discussed first, who had the semi-autistic behavior and the overproduction of hyperuricemia, has also been studied from the point of view of these enzymes. He had no abnormality in HGPRT. In terms of control of purine metabolism, he did have an elevation in the adenine enzyme. His molecular defect remains to be established.

REFERENCES

Brooks, G. W., and Mueller, E. 1966. Serum urate concentrations among university professors. *J.A.M.A.* 195:415.

Kasl, S. V.; Brooks, G. W.; and Cobb, S. 1966. Serum urate concentrations in male high-school students. *J.A.M.A.* 198:713.

Kogut, M. D.; Donnell, G. N.; Nyhan, W. L.; and Sweetman, L. 1970. Disorder of purine metabolism due to partial deficiency of hypoxanthine-guanine phosphoribosyltransferase. *Amer. J. Med.* 48:148.

Lesch, M., and Nyhan, W. L. 1964. A familial disorder of uric acid metabolism and central nervous system function. *Amer. J. Med.* 36:561.

Nyhan, W. L. 1968. Seminar on the Lesch-Nyhan syndrome. *Fed. Proc.* 27:1027.

Nyhan, W. L.; James, J. A.; Teberg, A. J.; Sweetman, L.; and Nelson, L. G. 1969. A new disorder of purine metabolism with behavioral manifestations. *J. Pediat.* 74:20.

Orowan, E. 1955. The origin of man. *Nature* 175:683.

Seegmiller, J. E.; Laster, L.; and Howell, R. R. 1963. Biochemistry of uric acid and its relation to gout. *New Eng. J. Med.* 268:712.

Seegmiller, J. E.; Rosenbloom, F. M.; and Kelley, W. N. 1967. Enzyme defect associated with a sex-linked human neurological disorder and excessive purine synthesis. *Science* 155:1682.

Stetten, D., Jr., and Hearon, J. Z. 1959. Intellectual level measured by Army classification battery and serum uric acid concentration. *Science* 129:1737.

CHEMOTHERAPY OF SCHIZOPHRENIA

Leo E. Hollister

Veterans Administration Hospital, Palo Alto,
and Stanford University School of Medicine

Stanford, California

Few illnesses compare with schizophrenia in the toll they take of the most useful years of an individual's life. Few illnesses have been so frustrating to explain or treat. Few illnesses create such sadness and guilt in those who cannot find ways to help their affected loved one. "Cures" are rare indeed; probably less than fifteen percent of individuals seriously affected who require any kind of prolonged hospitalization ever again function "normally." Schizophrenia and alcoholism are the two major problems in psychiatry; they deserve far more attention than they have been given.

No one with any regard for scientific evidence would argue that drugs are not effective for treating this disorder. The peculiar prejudices against drug therapy that existed in psychiatry fifteen years ago led to the most massive scientific overkill to establish their efficacy. In fact, as drugs are compared with other types of treatment, increasing evidence indicates that in the case of schizophrenics drugs contribute the most therapeutic benefits; there is little direct evidence that many traditional therapies add more. This is a most unfortunate situation, for good as antipsychotic drugs are, they are not yet good enough. We have too many patients who are better and too few who are well.

Although the disaster that is schizophrenia has been partially mitigated by drugs, our knowledge of the pathophysiological mechanisms of this disorder is still meager. The impetus provided by the success of drugs in treating this disorder resulted in many inquiries into the biological bases for it. Some of these have already been reviewed in this volume. Older notions that schizophrenia is a reaction to social-psychological influences, such as that it represents a disordered learning process initiated and sustained by conflicting messages from mother, have few remaining adherents. The present tendency is to regard schizophrenia as a genetically determined disorder with biological mechanisms whose phenotypic expression may be influenced in part by life experiences. As antischizophrenic drugs were discovered fortuitously, our continuing lack of knowledge of the pathogenesis of the disorder has limited development of more effective drugs. We have new chemicals, but old drugs.

CHEMICAL STRUCTURES

Seven chemical classes of drugs have the two unique pharmacological properties of neuroleptic or antipsychotic drugs: the ability to ameliorate schizophrenia and to evoke extrapyramidal syndromes. Chemical resemblances between the various subgroups of phenothiazines, or between this class and the thioxanthenes, are quite obvious, but less so when the other classes are considered (Figure 1). The structures of most antipsychotic drugs can be viewed as tertiary, or rarely secondary, amines derived from methylamine (-C-C-N-C). Phenothiazine antipsychotics have the following common S-shaped configuration, regardless of the subfamily to which they belong (R-N-C-C-C-N-C). Thioxanthenes are similar, as are the butyrophenones (R-C-C-C-C-N-C) (Janssen 1970). Presumably this S-shape is crucial to the fit of the molecule with its receptor, although an adequate model of the receptor for antipsychotic drugs has not yet been proposed. For practical purposes we are concerned with only three chemical classes: phenothiazines, thioxanthenes, and butyrophenones, the first two having strong chemical resemblances to each other. The members of these classes are listed in Table 1, which shows those drugs available at present in the United States.

The phenothiazine derivatives are the most important antipsychotics by virtue of both their long history and their great popularity. Partly because of chemical differences, but also because of variations in pharmacological actions and potency, it is well to distinguish between the three chemical subfamilies of phenothiazines as determined by their side chains. Compounds with an aliphatic dimethylaminopropyl side chain, such as chlorpromazine, are relatively low in potency and high in sedative effects. Substitution at the 2-position of the phenothiazine nucleus results in a more potent compound than no substitution (chlorpromazine > promazine), and some substituents, such as the trifluoromethyl group, confer more potency than a simple chlorine atom (triflupromazine > chlorpromazine). The nuclear substituents may increase potency by increasing fat solubility of the molecule.

The piperidine side-chain family is represented by thioridazine,

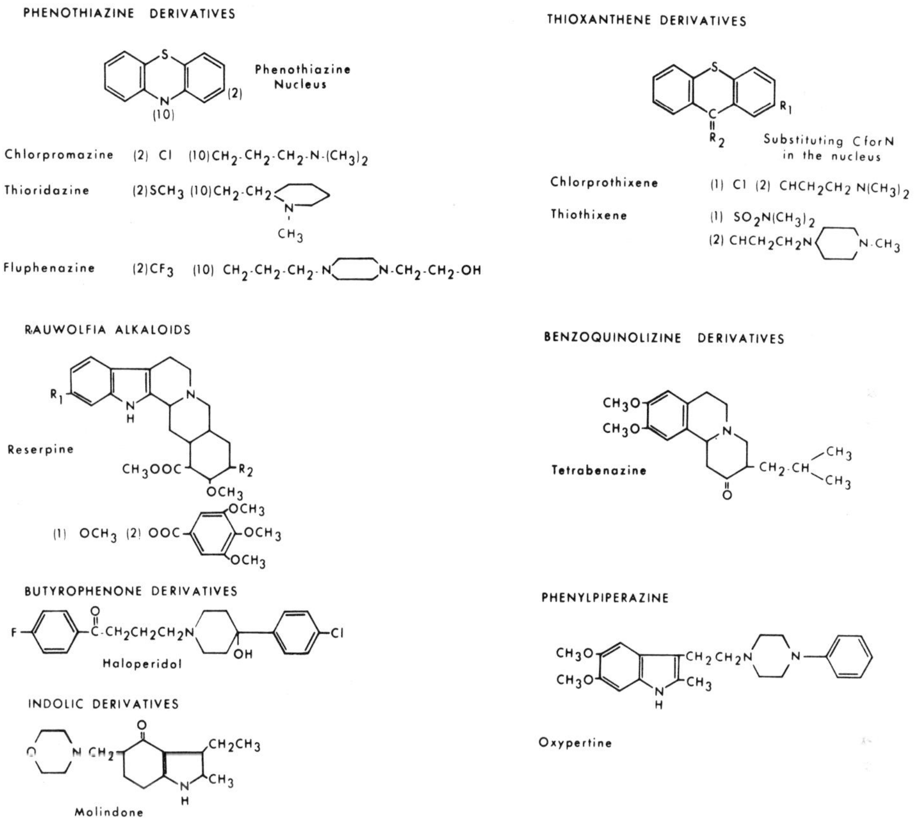

CHEMOTHERAPY OF SCHIZOPHRENIA

Figure 1. Structural representation of seven chemical classes of antipsychotic drugs.

which is no more potent than chlorpromazine but is most different from the other phenothiazines in pharmacological actions. Technically, piperacetazine is a piperidine derivative, but its structural geometry is closer to that of the piperazines, as are its pharmalogical properties. Three variants of the piperazine side chain, along with variations of the ring substituent, create a rather large class of piperazinylphenothiazines. These compounds are even more potent than their ring-substituted analogs in the aliphatic series. They tend to be less overtly sedative, at least in relation to antipsychotic effects, than the other two classes but are more prone to produce extrapyramidal reactions.

TABLE 1

Antipsychotic Drugs Available in the United States

	Estimated Equivalent Dose (mg)
Phenothiazines	
Aliphatic	
Chlorpromazine (Thorazine)	100
Triflupromazine (Vesprin)	25
Piperidine	
Thioridazine (Mellaril)	100
Piperacetazine (Quide)	10
Piperazine	
Acetophenazine (Tindal)	20
Butaperazine (Repoise)	10
Carphenazine (Proketazine)	25
Fluphenazine (Prolixin)	2
Perphenazine (Trilafon)	10
Prochlorperazine (Compazine)	15
Thiopropazate (Dartal)	10
Trifluoperazine (Stelazine)	5
Thioxanthenes	
Chlorprothixene (Taractan)	100
Thiothixene (Navane)	2
Butyrophenone	
Haloperidol (Haldol)	2

Nearly all antipsychotic drugs are highly surface-active, lipophilic and weakly basic. Such physicochemical properties would favor accumulation in brain and other tissues. They may also be subject to many routes of biotransformation, leading to as many as 164 postulated metabolites for chlorpromazine alone (Green and Forrest 1966). The relationship between specific metabolites and therapeutic or unwanted effects from these drugs is still uncertain.

TABLE 2

Pharmacologic Aspects of Antipsychotics

Postulated Bases of Antipsychotic Effects

    post-synaptic block of noradrenergic or dopaminergic receptors

    interaction with neuronal membrane to decrease excitability

    metabolic inhibition of oxidative phosphorylation, altering ionic pumps and decreasing neuronal excitability

Pharmacological Screening Tests

    reduce exploratory behavior without undue sedation

    induce a cataleptic state

    induce palpebral ptosis reversible through handling

    inhibit conditioned avoidance behavior

    inhibit intracranial self-stimulation in reward areas

    inhibit amphetamine- or apomorphine-induced stereotypic behaviors

    protect against epinephrine- or norepinephrine-induced mortality

PHARMACOLOGICAL PROPERTIES

The exact mechanism of the antipsychotic action has not been fully worked out. Some of the more prominent possibilities are shown in Table 2 (top). Evidence is mounting that all antipsychotics produce a postsynaptic dopamine receptor blockade, and that this action may be of primary importance. It is ascribed to stabilization of the membrane at the receptor site so that the neurotransmitter does not have access to it. Generally, this type of block is associated with an increased turnover rate of the blocked transmitter. From a neurophysiological point of view, phenothiazines stimulate the amygdaloid nucleus, a portion of the limbic system, depress the hypothalamus, and depress the reticular activating system. Thus these antipsychotics affect the three major integrating systems of the brain in a way that might be expected to diminish the emotional response to external or internal stimuli.

Some of the more predictive animal pharmacological screening tests for drugs with clinical antipsychotic activity are shown in Table 2 (bottom). It is still uncertain which of these activities may be most specifically related to antipsychotic activity, and one must bear in mind that for several years inhibition of apomorphine-induced vomiting in dogs was the test most highly correlated with antipsychotic activity simply because most known antipsychotic drugs were also antiemetics. Unfortunately, such screening batteries seem only able to allow the development of newer drugs that resemble those we already have.

The aliphatic phenothiazines are highly sedative, with strong adrenergic-blocking actions. Thus they are most useful in patients for whom some sedative effect is desirable. The piperidine derivative, thioridazine, is similar to the aliphatic derivatives in its sedative and adrenergic-blocking action. Like the aliphatics, thioridazine would be considered a "high-dose" phenothiazine. Unlike the other phenothiazines, thioridazine has little tendency to produce extrapyramidal effects and is devoid of antiemetic action. Its peripheral adrenergic-blocking action is the greatest of all these drugs.

The piperazine group of phenothiazines may be considered as low-dose drugs because of their greater potency. Although they are often claimed to have an "activating" action, this may be spurious. They are less overtly sedative in the usual therapeutic doses than the others, but the differences are not tremendous. They also tend to increase the motor activity of patients, but this is usually a purposeless, driven, and highly uncomfortable side effect termed akathisia.

The thioxanthenes also share many of the properties of the phenothiazines. One derivative, chlorprothixene, may be considered a high-dose drug while the other, thiothixene, is a low-dose drug. Haloperidol, the butyrophenone derivative, is also quite potent, with strong tendencies to evoke extrapyramidal syndromes and akathisia.

CLINICAL EFFICACY OF ANTIPSYCHOTICS

Reports of well-controlled studies from many sources indicate that most of these drugs effectively control symptoms of schizophrenia, allowing the rehabilitation of many patients who appeared doomed to a lifetime of hospitalization. The relationship of drug therapy to the practice of psychiatry, as well as the balance between therapeutic and side effects have been reviewed elsewhere (Hordern 1961; Kinross-Wright 1967).

With the exception of mepazine and promazine, both of which

are too weak in antipsychotic action to justify their hazards, the
phenothiazine derivatives have been repeatedly found to be equally
efficacious when the responses of groups of patients have been
compared (Casey *et al.* 1960 a and b; Kurland *et al.* 1961; Lasky
et al. 1962; Adelson and Epstein 1962; Michaux *et al.* 1964; NIMH-
PSC Collaborative Study Group 1964). The efficacy of these drugs
has been proved in every kind of schizophrenic patient, from those
suffering their initial schizophrenic symptoms to those who had
been exiled to hospitals for years. It is regrettable, in retro-
spect, that so much time, talent and money were expended to prove
what should have been obvious to any unbiased clinician who treated
several schizophrenics with these drugs: something new and different
and exciting was happening. Still, the effort has at least refined
the methodology for studying the effects of treatments for schizophrenia to such an extent that it is now beginning to be possible
to evaluate others in the same precise way that drugs have been
studied.

The impressive efficacy of antipsychotic drugs for an illness
that had seemed to respond only to the whims of fate clearly established drug therapy as the primary treatment of schizophrenics. In
fact, it became increasingly apparent from the many controlled studies that drug therapy was the only one whose ameliorative effects
could be definitely distinguished. After some initial restriction
of other "therapies" as possible confounding variables, it became
customary to evaluate drugs within the context of a full hospital
treatment program. Under such conditions, patients treated with
effective antipsychotics improved, while those who received ineffective drugs or placebos were little changed. This does not mean
that none of the latter patients improved, but rather that each
improved patient was offset by one who became worse, while the majority were unchanged. Not all patients treated with antipsychotic
drugs are helped. Many who are helped still leave much to be desired.

Another fact soon became apparent. The benefits from antipsychotics were not due simply to sedation. Rather, many prominent
symptoms of schizophrenia that had failed previously to respond to
sedatives were ameliorated. Disturbed thinking, paranoid symptoms,
delusions, emotional and social withdrawal, and personal neglect
improved as well as anxiety and agitation, symptoms that might be
expected to respond to conventional sedatives. Regardless of how
it was accomplished, the alleviation of such characteristic psychotic
symptoms by these drugs justified the epithet "antipsychotic."

THE QUESTION OF SPECIFIC INDICATIONS

Despite their overall efficacy, individual patients respond
differently to these drugs, doing poorly on some and better on

others. The more sedative phenothiazines, such as chlorpromazine or thioridazine, were thought initially to be preferable for patients with agitation; less sedative drugs, such as trifluoperazine and perphenazine, were considered best for patients with symptoms of withdrawal and retardation. But such a differential action was based more on armchair reasoning than on experimental evidence.

A few systematic approaches to the problem have been attempted with uncertain results. Schizophrenics were divided into three types: "paranoid," "core," and "depressed," using pattern probability models based on presenting signs and symptoms. All three schizophrenic subtypes responded equally to perphenazine, but paranoid patients responded more favorably to acetophenazine (Overall et al. 1963). A later study by the same group failed to replicate such a difference, indicating rather that paranoid patients in general tended to respond somewhat better than the other types (Hollister et al. 1967). Data from both a Veterans Administration study and a National Institute of Mental Health cooperative study indicated that regression equations could be derived that might be expected to predict the most suitable drug (either chlorpromazine or fluphenazine) for patients with a given initial profile of symptoms. When tested against actual results, the interactions were significant (Klett and Moseley 1965). A later attempt to replicate this approach was unsuccessful (Galbrecht and Klett 1968). The division of patients into the older categories of "hyperdynamic" and "hypodynamic," based on the degree of activity and socialization, failed to reveal any differential response between carphenazine, trifluoperazine, and chlorpromazine, despite the fact that the first two drugs were reputed to be better for the "hypodynamic" type (Platz, Klett, and Caffey 1967). Schizophrenic patients were divided into four types: "core," "paranoid," "bizarre," and "depressive," and the actions of three phenothiazines were compared in each group. Evidence suggested that chlorpromazine was the most efficacious for core, acetophenazine for bizarre and depressive, acetophenazine and chlorpromazine more effective than fluphenazine in paranoid, and fluphenazine most suitable for depressive patients (NIMH-PRB Collaborative Study Group 1967).

A later review of the entire subject of predicting responses to antipsychotic drugs by one of the participants of these studies concluded that the present evidence for a differential action of antipsychotic drugs was highly inconclusive (Goldberg 1968). This conclusion seems eminently reasonable, especially when one considers that the various schizophrenic groupings were based on retrospective analysis of group data; the proper choice of drug in advance for individual patients would be a vastly greater problem.

CHOICE OF ANTIPSYCHOTIC DRUG IN THE CLINIC

The wide array of antipsychotic drugs available for clinicians in the United States is shown in Table 1, which lists fifteen. From this bewildering array of drugs a choice of one must be made to be given an empirical trial in a given patient. This situation is analogous to the case of the numerous corticosteroids, antihistaminics, diuretics, and digitalis preparations that confront the clinician. The usual dictum has been to learn to use a few drugs well rather than all poorly. The differences between the proper and improper use of a drug will probably exceed any actual difference between drugs. One of the most rational ways to narrow the choice of antipsychotics would be to master one of each of the three types of phenothiazines, one of the two thioxanthenes, and a butyrophenone.

With five drugs chosen on this basis, one should be able to exploit the full range of pharmacological differences among the various antipsychotics. As one example of the array of drugs that could be obtained from such a choice, the following might be listed: triflupromazine, thioridazine, acetophenazine, thiothixene, and haloperidol. Obviously, many other combinations are possible, although thioridazine and haloperidol are the only available members of their particular classes.

SPECIAL CONSIDERATIONS IN CHOOSING FOR SPECIFIC PATIENTS

The patient's past experience is a fairly reliable guide. If he has done well previously on some drug, and especially if he has done less well on others, one would be foolhardy to change drugs or to reinstitute lapsed treatment with a different drug. To the objective response of the patient must also be added his subjective response. Unless a patient tolerates a drug well, he is not likely to maintain treatment faithfully. A patient who is made unbearably restless by a drug may much prefer no drug. On the other hand, some patients may prefer restlessness to impairment of their sexual capacity. The importance of various side effects to the patient should be a guide in choosing his specific treatment.

While high-dose drugs, such as chlorpromazine and thioridazine, are more sedative than low-dose drugs, sedation is not the most wanted effect. Antipsychotic drugs should be used to treat symptoms of schizophrenia. It may be better to rely on conventional sedatives, hypnotics, or antianxiety drugs to manage excited states, anxiety, or sleeplessness. Sedation alone should not dictate the choice of antipsychotic drug although, if the combination of effects is appropriate, so much the better.

Another problem with high-dose drugs is that if treatment is long continued (and for many patients, it may be for life), choosing these drugs commits one to a course that will eventually lead to the administration of kilograms of drug. We simply do not know whether it is preferable to give 20 mg daily of a foreign molecule rather than 200 mg. In view of the fact that harmful effects of drugs or chemicals in the environment are not appreciated for decades after their introduction, it seems prudent to reduce the total body burden as much as possible. Several years elapsed before it was recognized that lenticular deposits were a dose-related effect of chlorpromazine. Consequently, one might do well to consider only short-term rather than long-term use of the high-dose drugs, substituting whenever possible low-dose drugs for chronic treatment.

Many clinicians seem to prefer to choose two or more drugs in combination rather than seeking to use only one. In fact, in reviewing an order for a patient, one frequently finds the following conglomeration: two phenothiazines (one high-dose and one low-dose), a tricyclic antidepressant (the patient is withdrawn), an anti-parkinson drug (even if the patient has never shown any signs; this drug is completely superfluous in the presence of the anticholinergic tricyclic antidepressant), something for sleep, and something during the day to keep the patient awake. Such a choice of drugs is no choice at all and has many irrational aspects. Small wonder that some patients seem to improve after drugs are withdrawn! Ever since the early days of clinical psychopharmacology, when a combination of reserpine and chlorpromazine was touted as being better than either drug alone, it has been widely believed that two drugs are better than one. A fair number of systematic studies of drug combinations has now been completed, with no convincing evidence that any combination is superior for treating schizophrenics than a properly chosen single drug (Casey *et al.* 1961).

Some patients may tolerate antipsychotic drugs so poorly that no drug treatment should be given. As these patients tend to be less psychotic than most schizophrenics, with retention of insight and marked somatization, it may be that they represent a "schizophreniform" group rather than true schizophrenia. One should bear in mind that to take antipsychotic drugs, one must be crazy, either literally or figuratively. The ability to tolerate these drugs seems to be directly correlated with the severity of the psychosis.

SPECIFIC PROBLEMS IN THE USE OF ANTIPSYCHOTICS

Few drugs have such great therapeutic margins and such a wide range of therapeutic doses as these. Twenty- to thirtyfold differences in daily doses have been recorded. Requirements of most patients fall within a narrower range, usually from 200 to 800 mg daily based on chlorpromazine doses. Occasional patients may do well with higher doses. A recent study indicates that doses of

2,000 mg daily may enhance improvement in some chronic schizophrenic patients under the age of 40 years who have been hospitalized less than 10 years. While no patient should be considered a drug failure without an intensive course of therapy, routine use of such massive doses may represent overtreatment for many. Blood levels of phenothiazines have been difficult to measure and their significance is far from clear; concentrations of chlorpromazine in plasma may ultimately provide a guide to optimal doses (Curry 1970). More studies of the differences between patients in metabolizing these drugs may elucidate problems in dosage but, for the moment, the situation is akin to that of other drugs whose plasma levels are not readily measured: The proper dose is a sufficient quantity to maximize therapeutic goals and minimize unwanted effects.

Duration of treatment is an unsettled question--at least, duration of long-term treatment. Acute responses of patients newly treated with drugs are variable, ranging from days to weeks. Most clinicians would feel that failure of acute or newly admitted schizophrenics to improve after 6 to 8 weeks of adequate treatment with a drug would be reason to try another. Newly treated chronic patients might require 12 to 24 weeks of treatment before a change of medication would be warranted. Improvement tends to be more rapid earlier than later on, when therapeutic gains creep.

Assuming that complete or partial remission is attained, how long should treatment be continued? As far as one can tell, it should probably be indefinitely for most patients. The consequence of replacing drug with placebo in stabilized hospitalized patients revealed a linear rate of clinical relapse over a four-month period, affecting 45 per cent of these patients (Caffey *et al.* 1964). Of considerable interest was the fact that a sharp reduction in maintenance doses to three-sevenths of those usually given resulted in only a 15 percent relapse rate over the same period. Apparently, many patients receive higher than necessary maintenance doses of drug. Still, it might be argued that 55 percent of patients remain in clinical remission after being off drug for a substantial period and that "drug holidays" might be in order. The difficulty is that, despite the most earnest attempts, patients who maintained improvement could not be distinguished from those who relapsed. Consequently, the most practical approach would be to consider indefinite uninterrupted treatment for most patients. The consequences of doing otherwise are quite evident; lapses in maintenance therapy with antipsychotic drugs are presently the most frequent cause of readmission to a mental hospital following discharge. On the other side of the coin, the value of phenothiazines in preventing psychiatric hospitalization seems to be well established (Engelhardt *et al.* 1967).

Antipsychotic drugs have been used effectively and safely in conjunction with most other psychiatric therapies. The lack of improvement of patients treated with ineffective drugs or placebos casts doubt upon the efficacy of the other therapies, although the evidence was inferential. A direct test in the case of group psychotherapy has been made, with little evidence to suggest that group psychotherapy is of much value in the total management of schizophrenics, or that it interacts with drug therapy to produce a greater effect than the latter alone (Gorham and Pokorny 1964). More recently, individual psychotherapy of chronic schizophrenics and its interaction with drug therapy has also been studied. Although both in combination reduced the florid symptoms of these patients, psychotherapy alone did little or nothing for the same patients (Grinspoon, Ewalt, and Shader 1967). The hoariest therapies of all, occupational and industrial therapy, were also found to offer little or nothing not afforded by other therapies. It should be emphasized that these are mere beginnings in the evaluation of the various approaches to treating schizophrenics and one should not overgeneralize. Yet, one thing seems clear: Drugs do not prevent any benefits from other therapies, and vice versa.

Although there was some initial hesitance in using electroconvulsive therapy (ECT) in conjunction with reserpine, due to hypotensive and apneic episodes, the danger with phenothiazines is not as great. Generally, one can combine these treatments quite safely if one recognizes the lowered convulsive threshold and is prepared in advance to handle complications. ECT may still be indicated for agitated schizophrenics who do not respond to antipsychotic drugs alone.

Until comparatively recently, not much attention was given to the biopharmaceutical preparation of these drugs. A recent study indicates that the biological availability of drug may be far greater in some dosage forms than in others (Hollister *et al*. 1970). Chlorpromazine was most reliably given by intramuscular injection, by which plasma levels were uniformly and promptly attained; the intramuscular dose was about four times as potent as the same dose given orally. Oral preparations were by no means totally reliable, liquid concentrates being somewhat better than coated tablets. Delayed-action preparations were the least reliable, and of dubious need in the case of drugs that are highly cumulative. We still have very little knowledge about how other factors, such as the presence of food or other drugs in the stomach, may affect absorption of orally administered drug. Failure of a patient to respond adequately may be less the fault of the drug than its dosage form; a brief trial of parenteral administration followed by maintenance with liquid concentrate might be tried in such patients before switching to another drug.

SUMMARY

Antipsychotics are the most strongly established of all pharmacotherapies for emotional disorders. Increasing evidence indicates that, in the case of schizophrenic patients, these drugs contribute most therapeutic benefits, with little direct evidence that many traditional therapies add more. The great number available requires that clinicians limit the number of drugs they attempt to master. By selecting from three chemical subclasses of phenothiazine derivatives and from representatives of the thioxanthene and butyrophenone derivatives, it should be possible to exploit the full range of pharmacological differences with an array of five drugs. The dose required by individual patients is highly variable so that it is imperative that dosage be individualized. No drug should be considered a failure unless it has been pushed to relatively high dosage. On the other hand, maintenance therapy should be based on the lowest dosage adequate to maintain therapeutic gains. Although many patients may go on for several months without drug and remain stable, they cannot be clearly identified from those who may relapse. Consequently, maintenance therapy should be considered for an indefinite period.

REFERENCES

Adelson, D., and Epstein, L. J. 1962. A study of phenothiazines with male and female chronically ill schizophrenic patients. *J. Nerv. Ment. Dis.* 134:543.

Caffey, E. M., Jr.; Diamond, L. S.; Frank, T. V.; Grasberger, J. C.; Herman, L.; Klett, C. J.; and Rothstein, C. 1964. Discontinuation or reduction of chemotherapy in chronic schizophrenics. *J. Chronic Dis.* 17:347.

Casey, J. F.; Bennett, I. F.; Lindley, C. J.; Hollister, L. E.; Gordon, M. H.; and Springer, N. N. 1960a. Drug therapy in schizophrenia: a controlled study of the relative effectiveness of chlorpromazine, promazine, phenobarbital, and placebo. *Arch. Gen. Psychiat.* 2:210.

Casey, J. F.; Lasky, J. J.; Klett, C. J.; and Hollister, L. E. 1960b. Treatment of schizophrenic reactions with phenothiazine derivatives: a comparative study of chlorpromazine, triflupromazine, mepazine, prochlorperazine, perphenazine, and phenobarbital. *Amer. J. Psychiat.* 117:97.

Casey, J. F.; Hollister, L. E.; Lasky, J. J.; Klett, C. J.; and Caffey, E. M. 1961. Combined drug therapy of chronic schizophrenics: a controlled evaluation of placebo, dextroamphetamine, imipramine, isocarboxazid, and trifluoperazine added to maintenance doses of chlorpromazine. *Amer. J. Psychiat.* 117:997.

Curry, S. H. 1970. Chlorpromazine: concentrations in plasma, excretion in urine and duration of effect. *Proc. Roy. Soc. Med.* in press.

Engelhardt, D. M.; Rosen, B.; Freedman, N.; and Margolis, R. 1967. Phenothiazines in prevention of psychiatric hospitalization. IV. Delay or prevention of hospitalization - a re-evaluation. *Arch. Gen. Psychiat.* 16:98.

Galbrecht, C. R., and Klett, C. J. 1968. Predicting response to phenothiazines: the right drug for the right patient. *J. Nerv. Ment. Dis.* 147:173.

Goldberg, S. C. 1968. Prediction of response to anti-psychotic drugs. In *Psychopharmacology. A Review of Progress 1957-1967.* D. Efron (ed.). Washington, D. C.: U. S. Govt. Printing Office, p. 1101.

Gorham, D. R., and Pokorny, A. D. 1964. Effects of a phenothiazine and/or group psychotherapy with schizophrenics. *Dis. Nerv. Syst.* 25:77.

Green, D. E., and Forrest, I. S. 1966. In vivo metabolism of chlorpromazine. *Canad. Psychiat. Assoc. J.* 11:299.

Grinspoon, L.; Ewalt, J. R.; and Shader, R. 1967. Long-term treatment of chronic schizophrenia. *Int. J. Psychiat.* 4:116.

Hollister, L. E.; Overall, J. E.; Bennett, J. L.; Kimbell, I., Jr.; and Shelton, J. 1967. Specific therapeutic actions of acetophenazine, perphenazine and benzquinamide in newly admitted schizophrenic patients. *Clin. Pharmacol. Ther.* 8:249.

Hollister, L. E.; Curry, S. H.; Derr, J. E.; and Kanter, S. L. 1970. Studies of delayed-action medication. V.-Plasma levels and urinary excretion of four different forms of chlorpromazine. *Clin. Pharmacol. Ther.* 11:49.

Hordern, A. 1961. Medical Progress. Psychiatry and the tranquilizers. *New Eng. J. Med.* 265:585.

Janssen, P. A. J. 1970. Chemical and pharmacological classification of neuroleptics. In *Modern Problems of Pharmacopsychiatry*, vol. 5. *The Neuroleptics.* D. P. Bobon, P. A. J. Janssen, and J. Bobon (eds.). Basel: S. Karger, p. 33.

Kinross-Wright, J. 1967. The current status of phenothiazines. *J.A.M.A.* 200:461.

Klett, C. J., and Moseley, E. C. 1965. The right drug for the right patient. *J. Consult. Clin. Psychol.* 29:546.

Kurland, A. A.; Hanlon, T. E.; Tatom, M. H.; and Michaux, M. H. 1961. The comparative effectiveness of six phenothiazine compounds, phenobarbital and inert placebo in the treatment of acutely ill patients: global measures of severity of illness. *J. Nerv. Ment. Dis.* 133:1.

Lasky, J. J.; Klett, C. J.; Caffey, E. M., Jr.; Bennett, J. L.; Rosenblum, M. P.; and Hollister, L. E. 1962. Drug treatment of schizophrenic patients: a comparative evaluation of chlorpromazine, chlorprothixene, fluphenazine, reserpine, thioridazine, and triflupromazine. *Dis. Nerv. Syst.* 23:698.

Michaux, M. H.; Hanlon, T. E.; Ota, K. Y.; and Kurland, A. A. 1964. Phenothiazines in the treatment of newly admitted state hospital patients: global comparison of eight compounds in terms of an outcome index. *Curr. Ther. Res.* 6:331.

National Institute of Mental Health, Psychopharmacological Service
  Center Collaborative Study Group 1964. Phenothiazine treatment
  in acute schizophrenia. *Arch. Gen. Psychiat.* 10:246.
National Institute of Mental Health and Psychopharmacology Research
  Branch Collaborative Study Group 1967. Differences in clinical
  effects of three phenothiazines in "acute" schizophrenia. *Dis.
  Nerv. Syst.* 28:369.
Overall, J. E.; Hollister, L. E.; Honigfeld, G.; Kimbell, I. H., Jr.;
  Myer, F.; Bennett, J. L.; and Caffey, E., Jr. 1963. Comparison
  of acetophenazine with perphenazine in schizophrenics: demonstration
  of differential effects based on computer-derived diagnostic
  models. *Clin. Pharmacol. Ther.* 4:200.
Platz, A. R.; Klett, C. J.; and Caffey, E. M., Jr. 1967. Selective
  drug action related to chronic schizophrenic subtype (a comparative
  study of carphenazine, chlorpromazine and trifluoperazine).
  Dis. Nerv. Syst. 28:601.

CHEMOTHERAPY OF MANIC-DEPRESSIVE DISORDER

Baron Shopsin and Samuel Gershon

Neuropsychopharmacology Research Unit
New York University School of Medicine

New York, New York

I. INTRODUCTION

The term "affective disorders" is used for a group of mental illnesses with a primary disturbance of affect, and comprising those behavior disorders characterized principally by increased or decreased activity and thought, expressive of a predominating mood of depression or elation.

The abnormalities of activity, affect, and thought, as a periodic occurrence, were first described by the French psychiatrists, Baillarger (1853, 1854) and Falret (1854, 1864) under the name of *folie circularie*. These contrasting affective states, depression and elation, whether occurring as isolated attacks or with periodicity, were seen by Kraepelin (1913) as variations of a single morbid process based upon physiological determinants. Including depressions of later life (involutional melancholia), he designated the condition as "manic-depressive insanity." After this concept was established, the more attenuated or borderline states were described, which we now term cycloid or cyclothymic temperaments. Far commoner than the attenuated forms of manic-depressive psychoses are the neurotic depressive reactions that figure so prominently in contemporary clinical practice.

The concept of manic-depressive psychoses probably has become obscured in recent years and the unit of manic-depressive disease, as defined by Kraepelin, needs redefinition based on clinical and genetic evidence with the aid of modern statistical techniques. Evidence has now accumulated to indicate that the disease is likely to be heterogeneous and that it contains at least two discrete groups (Leonhard 1957; Perris 1966; Angst 1966). Mania occurs in one of these groups and patients exhibit both manic and depressive phases during the course of their illness. This group has been designated "bipolar" by most investigators. In the other group there are only episodes of depression, and this has been coined the "unipolar" group by some (Perris 1966). In addition to these qualitative and quantitative clinical distinctions, genetic (Penrose 1945; Winokur and Clayton 1967; Von Trostorff 1968; Cadoret, Winokur, and Clayton 1970) and prognostic criteria developed in recent years suggest other differences among manic and depressive disorders as well.

Ironically, despite their clinical polarization, the manic and depressive patient share many common features, including inherent illness cyclicity and frequent rate of relapse. Aside from their subjective anguish, patients suffering from the biopolar or unipolar manifestations of affective illness frequently present with a common history of family alienation, divorce, frequent hospitalization, an inability to consistently hold gainful employment, and a tendency toward self-destruction and destructive behavior, both involving at times civil law authorities.

The serious and almost tragic nature of manic-depressive disorder, therefore, poses important and challenging therapeutic responsibilities in dealing with these affective disease entities.

II. CHEMOTHERAPY OF MANIA

Before psychiatrists came on the scene, the violent inmate of an insane asylum was put in a padded cell or straight jacket. If that did not prove beneficial, he was likely to be beaten or immersed in cold water -- what might now be considered "aversive therapy" of an unacceptably brutal nature. Even after the specialty took form, until the 1930's, psychiatrists could only do their best to prevent the patient from destroying himself, isolate him, use warm baths or wet packs, or employ various chemical agents that were far from specific, and wait for spontaneous remissions. In all but the mildest cases, custodial care in the form of hospitalization was usually mandatory.

Although documented control studies comparing treatment modalities of this condition are rare and leave the question of unequivocal treatment superiority an open one, few would dispute the fact that modern chemotherapy presents a distinct advance over the cruder previous treatment methods. The dilemma that now confronts practicing psychiatrists and researchers is, rather, in knowing which psychoactive drug is most specific or beneficial in controlling the acute manic attack, and which psychoactive agent or agents are capable of preventing relapses.

Depending upon the severity of the manic reaction, its influence

Discarded Drugs: Rauwolfia Alkaloids

Introduced in the United States by Kline in 1954, the rauwolfia-derived drugs have virtually disappeared from the shelves of most American mental hospitals. Jarvik (1965) writes that "there seems to be no question at this time that the phenothiazine drugs are far superior to the rauwolfia alkaloids in the treatment of psychotic disorders." This viewpoint is maintained in most standard textbooks (e.g., Clark and del Giudice 1970).

The major effects of rauwolfia drugs apparently are in moderating pathologic motor behavior. In general, reserpinized patients can become more manageable in a hospital setting, although a small number have ever benefited sufficiently to be discharged (Luby 1967). Aggressive, assaultive, and hyperactive patients are said to be calmed to a point where seclusion, restraints, and the use and maintenance of electroconvulsive therapy (ECT) can be avoided. Ban (1969) indicates that some clinicians still consider this substance one of the most effective psychopharmacological preparations for the control of manic patients. For this purpose he suggests a combination of intramuscular and oral medication complemented, if needed, with barbital. A review of the literature, however, offers no support for this; the available reports suggest, rather, that the rauwolfias may induce deleterious effects (Jarvik 1965; Luby 1968; Lehmann and Ban 1970) in manic individuals.

The observations by Barsa and Kline (1955) on the course of reserpine therapy are classic. According to these authors, the drug action can be divided into three phases: (1) an initial sedative phase followed, toward the end of the first week, by (2) excitation, behavioral and motor hyperactivity, as well as a dramatic exacerbation of florid psychotic symptoms usually lasting for two to three weeks, succeeded by (3) an integrative phase during which the patient becomes more cooperative and responsive to milieu programs. This treatment response would in itself preclude the use of rauwolfia drugs in the treatment for mania. The additional facts of (1) the proved treatment superiority of chlorpromazine (Wirt and Simon 1959; Lasky et al. 1962; Simon et al. 1965; Goldman 1966), (2) the rauwolfia-induced side effect of depression (Ban 1969; Lehmann and Ban 1970), and (3) the inability to use rauwolfia drugs in combination with ECT, further limit their clinical attractiveness.

Since one of the undesirable side effects of rauwolfia treatment in mania is said to be a swing toward depression, it is interesting to note that the use of combined imipramine-reserpine therapy has been proposed for intractable depression (Poldinger 1963), in which improvement follows the induction of a transient mania. This conspicuous stimulating effect resembles the sudden mood reversals that occur occasionally in cyclic manic-depressive disease (Haskovec and Rysanek 1967).

Convulsive Therapy: Flurothyl

Convulsive treatment is still used in treating manic patients, and it is usually believed to combine speed of action with a specific removal of manic symptoms. The main disadvantages of such treatment, apart from the inconvenience of administration, are that it may induce organic sequelae including clouding, confusion, and memory impairment. It does not prevent episodic recurrences of mania and the duration of symptom-free intervals is not shortened.

Flurothyl (hexafluorodiethyl ether) is a CNS stimulant that is used as a convulsive agent in the therapy for mental disorders, including mania (Esplin and Zablocka 1965). Comparison trials between ECT and flurothyl (Kurland, Cuervo, and Krantz 1960; Fink *et al.* 1961) indicate that the two procedures are similar in safety and efficacy. The advantage claimed for flurothyl is that many patients prefer the drug to electroshock, the basis for this preference presumably being the anesthetic-like state that precedes the convulsion. Electroshock therapy is currently administered after induction of sleep with barbiturates, and contractions are minimized by the concomitant use of succinylcholine so that the anesthetic-like state accompanying the use of flurothyl presents no obvious advantage. Fink *et al.* (1961) reported that flurothyl convulsions are less predictable and less easily induced than are electroshock seizures. Commercially available under the name Indoklon, this agent, given by inhalation or parenterally, fails to demonstrate any clear advantages over ECT. It seems the only clear-cut advantage of any convulsive therapy in mania, since this treatment is of little fundamental help in such conditions, is its effective sedation. It is almost always supplemented by pharmacotherapy.

Adjunctive Psychoactive Drugs

Belladonna Alkaloids

The belladonna alkaloids, by virtue of their CNS effects of sedation and tranquilization, are useful in manic illness. The action of scopolamine (hyoscine) is rapid and effective in harnessing the behavioral and motor disturbances accompanying mania. Atropine in massive doses (more than 200 mg parenterally) has been suggested as most effective in the treatment of agitated, anxious patients (Innes and Nickerson 1965), although the number treated by this method is inadequate to establish the importance of these characteristics in the selection of cases or to assess the results in comparison with responses to other, more common, types of therapy.

Hypnotics and Sedatives

Though the popularity and usefulness of barbiturates as sedatives has waned somewhat with the increased use of "major" and "minor" tranquilizers, these drugs are nevertheless excellent for producing sedation and tranquility. Such barbiturates as sodium amytal certainly have a place as adjunctive treatment for acute manic episodes. The CNS depression following ingestion of chloral hydrate, although less marked than that produced by the barbiturates, also makes this hypnotic useful as a treatment supplement for managing manic individuals. Paraldehyde may also be considered useful, especially in hospitalized patients refusing oral chloral hydrate. Paraldehyde has the disadvantage, however, of inebriating the patient; this condition may cloud the clinical picture and contribute to diagnostic confusion.

The barbiturates, chloral hydrate, and paraldehyde may, in the presence of pain or severe anxiety, produce excitement or delirium (Sharpless 1965). These effects may be more academic than actual, since they have not been observed in any of our studies in which these drugs have been used routinely.

Effective Antimanic Drugs

Phenothiazine Derivatives

Chlorpromazine. Since Lehmann and Hanrahan (1954) recognized chlorpromazine's beneficial effects in controlling manic excitement and agitation, this drug has become a standard treatment for this condition. Chlorpromazine is, in fact, one of the most frequently used substances in treating manic patients.

Inasmuch as vigorous intervention is usually necessary in controlling the manic episode, intramuscular medication is often considered preferable for treatment initiation in hospital. This route of administration offers the quickest effect and eliminates the possibility of "cheeking" and eventual disposal of medication by the patient. In less severe cases, oral liquid chlorpromazine is preferable to tablets or capsules for similar reasons. Concomitant use of oral and intramuscular chlorpromazine is recommended for commencing treatment. When the patient's behavior and comportment is improved, intramuscular medication may be discontinued and capsules or tablets substituted for oral liquid chlorpromazine. Since underdosage is probably the most frequent mistake in treating this condition, care must be taken to insure adequate dose administration.

Klein and Davis (1969) suggest that procyclidine be started immediately with initiation of chlorpromazine treatment. In our experience, most patients do not require antiparkinsonian medication. The routine administration of such agents is therefore not recommended unless or until such side effects as extrapyramidal symptoms become apparent.

Thioproperazine and thioridazine. Many other phenothiazine preparations are used in the therapy of manic patients, including various compounds containing amino alkyl and piperazinylalkyl side chains. Ban, Papathomopulos, and Schwartz (1962) have reported favorable therapeutic results with discontinuous thioproperazine treatment. These authors indicate that the dosage of thioproperazine is swiftly raised to produce marked extrapyramidal manifestations. This is followed by a drug-free interval providing for remission of neurological signs. At least three such courses are required for therapeutic outcome.

Thioridazine, which bears an ethylpiperidyl group, has good neuroleptic potency and efficacy (Domino 1968; Cole and Davis 1968); its pharmacological activity makes it a reasonable choice in the treatment for mania. Klein and Davis (1969) suggest that the need for heavier sedation makes chlorpromazine the phenothiazine drug of choice. Then, too, since toxic retinitis may occur when thioridazine is used in large doses, and regular, high doses are necessary to treat manic episodes, it is wiser to start with chlorpromazine or haloperidol. Thioridazine can be substituted for these latter neuroleptics during the resolution of the manic phase.

A computer search (Sandoz 1970) indicates that there have been at least fifty publications dealing with the use of thioridazine in manic-depressive patients. Of these, forty-one reports make no distinction as to the nature of the illness, that is, whether the subject was suffering from a manic or depressive episode. In all these cases, the manic-depressive patients were included with other patients having different psychiatric diagnoses, and the results in manic-depressives (whatever the mood) cannot be isolated. Nine other publications mention specifically that manic patients were treated with thioridazine. However, in six of these reports (Bercel 1961; Sherman 1961; Bauer 1962; D'Elia and Rocco 1963; Colombi and Ferrio 1965; Kloos 1967) the manic patients were included in a larger group of psychiatric patients given this drug, and treatment outcome in the manics was either not reported or was impossible to determine.

The three remaining reports in which treatment outcome in manics is discussed were based on uncontrolled trials. Couleon *et al.* (1964) reported on nine patients in the acute manic phase who were treated with ECT, followed by thioridazine and Nembutal. The favorable results reported (amelioration within ten days to two weeks) are therefore impossible to evaluate in terms of thioridazine's contribution. Gomez-Reino and Fernandez-Vincente (1962) reported that, in their open trial, seven patients suffering an "endogenous mania" were treated with thioridazine alone, and that five patients had an excellent response, two showing good improvement. Given in doses of 50 mg three times a day initially, medication was gradually increased to an optimum level of 200 to 400 mg daily, held at this level for two weeks, and then reduced to a maintenance level of 150 mg per day. The onset of response is not indicated. Herrera and Vilaprino (1964) reported an obvious improvement (within three to ten days) in all of their sixteen manic patients. Initial dosage was 300 to 500 mg daily, and duration of treatment lasted from 30 to 176 days.

All three studies are open, differ in given dosages, and they lack elegance in experimental design; collectively they contribute little, if anything, to defining the treatment efficacy of thioridazine in manic illness.

Butyrophenones. The butyrophenone, haloperidol, is available for oral use in the United States as an antipsychotic agent, and clinical trials with this drug indicate treatment efficacy for control or relief of psychomotor agitation, aggressiveness, assaultiveness, hostility, and other symptom parameters associated with acute or chronic psychoses (Goldstein, Clyde, and Caldwell 1968). Several reports underline its particular efficacy in the treatment of manic disorder.

Angyal (1967) reported in Budapest that, in all diagnostic categories investigated, the most striking impact of haloperidol was seen in cases of mania, complete cure being obtained in twelve and considerable improvement in three of the seventeen patients. Daily dosage varied from 1.5 to 17 mg, depending on symptom severity, and was divided into three aliquots. Oral administration was supplemented with intramuscular injection where necessary, the daily dose being 2 to 3 ampules (1 ampule = 1 ml = 5 mg) for one or two days, which was always sufficient to make the patient cooperative enough for oral ingestion.

In the same study of twenty-two cases of manic excitement, haloperidol was used as a single intravenous injection of 2.5 to 5 mg. Full control of these states was achieved by a single intravenous injection within five to fifteen minutes without any apparent risk to the patient. Haloperidol was considered (personal observation) superior to all other types of drugs in any kind of psychomotor excitement, agitation, outbursts of aggressiveness, or violence.

After several years' experience with haloperidol, Rees and

Davies (1965) reported in Australia that haloperidol is a most useful drug in the management of acute mania. In a study of fifty manic patients treated with haloperidol, forty-two showed improvement, thirty-five demonstrating treatment response without the use of other drugs. Thirteen were discharged, using maintenance haloperidol dosage. Haloperidol was considered invaluable in effectively controlling the behavioral and mental disturbances of these acutely manic patients, and in managing them on a hospital ward. Rees and Davies reported that the improvement of manic patients is usually striking, and that comparable improvement is not achieved by phenothiazine drugs in the same period of time. This comparison represents a personal observation, however; the study did not compare the use of chlorpromazine in a similar patient population. The speed of onset of action for haloperidol was not given, nor did the study report the dosages issued.

Because haloperidol is related chemically to gamma-aminobutyric acid (GABA), an inhibitory neurohormone, the manic state provides an interesting condition on which to test the effects of this drug. Entwistle, Taylor, and MacDonald (1962), reported on ten British patients with severe mania who were treated with intramuscular, followed by oral, administration of haloperidol. Rapid control and tranquilization of the manic state were achieved in the most overactive and noisy manic patients. The effect was more rapid (2 to 6 days; mean = 4 days) with haloperidol than with chlorpromazine and greater tranquilization was effected. The haloperidol treatment response was compared to treatment responses with Largactil (chlorpromazine) and ECT in the same manic patients on previous hospitalization. The results suggested to these authors that haloperidol is a powerful neuroleptic drug, particularly useful in cases of mania; they concluded that 5 to 10 mg of intramuscularly injected haloperidol, three times daily, shortens manic episodes.

The British textbook *Clinical Psychiatry* (Mayer-Gross, Slater, and Roth 1969) describes haloperidol as particularly advantageous in manic patients with extreme degrees of psychomotor activity. This text indicates that haloperidol, administered intravenously, can reduce manic excitement in a dramatic manner and recommends repeated intravenous administration until the patient is sufficiently calmed to be maintained on oral medication thereafter.

Such pioneers and advocates of lithium as Schou (1967) and Baastrup (1968) both indicate in separate communications that an acute manic state is treated more effectively and more quickly with haloperidol and ECT than with lithium. Haloperidol is, in fact, considered by some (Ban 1969) to be one of the most effective drugs in the therapy for mania. From the available open studies, it appears that behavioral and psychomotor activity is brought under control within three days after initiating drug treatment and, in a high percentage of these cases, all symptoms are abolished in four or five days (Sargent and Slater 1963).

Open studies offering dosage information collectively indicate that the dose of haloperidol in milligrams per day has averaged 9.8 for maximum dosage, ranging from 1.0 to 42.8 mg per day during the study periods (Goldstein, Clyde, and Caldwell 1968). Investigators generally give relatively low doses at the beginning of a study, increase the dosage to achieve therapeutic effect, then lower it to the minimum consistent with therapeutic effect. A review of average daily doses of haloperidol in relation to diagnosis indicates that "other psychotic reactions," aside from the schizophrenias, require a mean dose of 6.66 mg. This represents the daily dosage consistent with a 62 percent marked or moderate improvement (Goldstein, Clyde, and Caldwell 1968). The effective doses of haloperidol, as shown by these figures, tend to be small, considerably smaller than comparable doses of chlorpromazine or other potent phenothiazines. Table 1 shows doses of some common antipsychotic agents equivalent to one milligram of haloperidol; Table 2 represents the recommended dosage schedule to initiate haloperidol therapy as suggested by McNeil Laboratories (McNeil 1970).

Klein and Davis (1969), on the other hand, indicate that they do not recommend haloperidol as specifically useful in the treatment for mania. Since there are no controlled studies that would lend themselves to a clarification of this issue, the point cannot be formally disputed. Of the five studies available of lithium carbonate treatment in manic patients, three compare lithium with chlorpromazine. In light of the available information claiming efficacy for haloperidol in manic disorder, this compound *may* represent a more adequate reference drug than chlorpromazine. Ideally, three drug groups should be used, including a chlorpromazine, a haloperidol, and a placebo group.

Lithium Salts

Since the introduction of neuroleptic compounds in psychiatric practice some twenty years ago, lithium carbonate has had great chemotherapeutic impact because its use seems to constitute the most specific pharmacological approach to the treatment for mania. The use of lithium in psychiatry, since its "serendipitous" (Gershon 1970) introduction by Cade in 1949 to its present-day "Cinderella" (Kline 1968) status, presents, however, a clear example of a hapless lag between discovery and application. As late as 1956, Goodman and Gilman stated, "the lithium ion has no therapeutic applications and, so far as is known, no biological function" (see also Drill 1958 and Wingard 1961). Such a recent and reputable text as the *Theory and Practice of Psychiatry* (Redlich and Freedman 1966) makes no mention of this drug in the treatment for manic-depressive

TABLE 1

Haloperidol 1 mg is approximately equivalent to:

Chlorpromazine	50–75 mg
Thioridazine	50–75 mg
Trifluoperazine	1– 5 mg
Perphenazine	4.0 mg
Fluphenazine	0.5 mg

TABLE 2

Haloperidol: Recommended Adult Dose Range and Frequency of Administration**

(Based on severity of symptomatology)

Moderate	0.5–1.5 mg	2 or 3 times daily
Moderate-Severe	1.5–3.0 mg	2 or 3 times daily
Very Severe	3.0–5.0 mg	2 or 3 times daily

Daily doses higher than those recommended are seldom required.

**Prepared by McNeil Laboratories, Inc.

disorders. *Clinical Psychiatry*, the British psychiatric reference text by Mayer-Gross *et al*. (1969), devotes three and a half pages to convulsive therapy and leucotomy under the treatment of manic disorders, while allocating only one page to all existing pharmacological approaches, one-quarter page of which deals with lithium carbonate treatment.

Studies of acute mania. Although it is difficult to assess the specific therapeutic activity of lithium in mania because of the differences in research design and methodology of the available reports, these reservations notwithstanding, a composite of all recorded studies yields an improvement rate of 60 to 100 percent in mania under lithium treatment. Only one report (Guistino 1953) states that lithium administration was ineffective in manic disorder (two cases). The 70 to 80 percent mean showing distinct improvement indicates that the lithium effect is independent of age, sex, and duration of illness. Only five studies were carried out with a control group; two used placebo (Schou et al. 1954; Maggs 1963) and three employed chlorpromazine (Johnson, Gershon, and Hekimian 1968; Spring et al. 1970; Platman 1970).

A more detailed assessment of these controlled studies is a matter of considerable importance for two reasons. First, there are no other controlled studies of mania with any other therapeutic agents; second, it is difficult to obtain an exact quantitative measure of lithium's efficacy because factors other than pharmacological, such as spontaneous remission, may have played a role in most of the trials. The first controlled study, in which 38 manic patients were treated, was reported in 1954 by Schou and associates. The patients were subdivided into "typical" and "atypical" cases. Clinical assessment of mania level was made on a three-point global impression of severity. "In some cases the lithium was given in an 'open' treatment for a certain period. In other cases a 'blind' scheme was adopted: the patients receiving lithium salts or placebo for a short period, usually two weeks. Every two weeks the medication was shifted in a random manner from lithium to placebo and vice versa, and changes from lithium to lithium and placebo to placebo were also used." Three lithium salts were used, the chloride, carbonate, and citrate. Dosage was 24 to 48 milliequivalents per liter (mEq/l) of lithium per day. The overall assessment was that, of 30 "typical" cases, there was a positive effect in 12, a possible effect in 15, and a negative effect in 3; of 8 "atypical" cases, a positive effect in 2, possible effect in 3, and a negative effect in 3. The possible effect was defined as distinct improvement, where spontaneous remission could not be excluded or where improvement was not as clear-cut as that classified as positive effect. The placebo data were presented in a somewhat different form that did not allow the same type of comparisons.

The next attempt at a controlled evaluation of lithium against placebo was made by Maggs in 1963 in a double-blind study with a random assignment of medication. Each of two groups had three fourteen-day trial periods, either of lithium, rest, placebo, or placebo, rest, lithium. A fixed dose of lithium carbonate, 1.5 gm per day, was used, and psychiatric assessments were made with the use of the Wittenborn scale. Because of toxicity, uncooperativeness, or unmanageability, only 18 of 28 patients completed the entire study. The statistical assessment of the findings on cluster III (manic states) and cluster V (schizophrenic excitement) of the Wittenborn scale showed that the degree of mania diminished significantly more during the second week of treatment with lithium than after similar treatment with placebo.

The third controlled study compared lithium with an active compound, chlorpromazine (Johnson, Gershon, and Hekimian 1968). In this study, a control group of schizophrenic patients with psychomotor excitation and elation were included to assess activity in nonmanic excitation. A total of 42 patients, 28 manic and 14 schizoaffective, were examined. The results of this study indicated a superior therapeutic effect for lithium carbonate in manic states. The remission rates obtained with lithium were 78 percent, as compared with 36 percent of patients treated with chlorpromazine. If only the manic patients who completed a trial of treatment were included, however, the data would show a 100 percent response obtained with lithium. It was observed that both drugs produced a decrease in motor activity and improved manageability, and that these effects occurred earlier with chlorpromazine. Normalization of affect and ideation with lithium occurred within eight days, but with chlorpromazine this effect was less clear, less consistent, and slower in onset. In the nonmanic states, a striking dissimilarity of action was seen. The chlorpromazine-treated schizo-affective patients all showed various degrees of improvement, whereas only one of seven patients treated with lithium showed moderate improvement. The remainder manifested a worsening of their condition, which may be attributed to the experimental design in which dosage was increased until clinical improvement or toxicity appeared (maximum lithium dosage was 3.0 gm/day). This conceivably might not have occurred if lower doses of lithium were used.

In a recent study by Platman (1970), thirteen manic patients were treated with lithium carbonate and ten manic patients with chlorpromazine in a double-blind randomly selected drug trial. Lithium carbonate proved superior to chlorpromazine on all six parameters of an objective rating scale (Psychiatric Evaluation Form [PEF]) (Spitzer, Endicott, and Fleiss 1967).

Initial dose of lithium carbonate was 1200 mg daily while that of chlorpromazine was 400 mg. The mean maximum dose reached in the lithium population was 1832 mg, and 870 mg for the chlorpromazine treatment group during the three-week drug administration period. All patients on lithium carbonate showed an 8 A.M. serum level of at least 0.8 mEq/l.

Although Spring *et al*. (1970) found lithium to be effective in the treatment for acute manic states, no significant differences were elicited when results were compared with chlorpromazine by means of a double-blind technique. Patients were randomly assigned to either drug by the flip of a coin; the group treated with lithium were given 1800 mg a day for the first week and, if there was no response, the dose was increased to a maximum of 3 grams daily; in the chlorpromazine group the drug dosage was rapidly increased depending on severity of symptoms; 1600 mg was the fixed maximum dose. In all patients showing satisfactory response to lithium, the response occurred on doses not exceeding 1800 mg of lithium carbonate daily and blood levels not exceeding 1.3 mEq/l.

If, after the initial three-week period, the therapist felt that a complete or nearly complete remission of symptoms had not been achieved, the patients were crossed over to the other drug for an additional three weeks. Under this procedure, of the twelve patients completing the first three weeks of this study, six of the seven patients on lithium responded. Three of five patients on chlorpromazine also responded. The two chlorpromazine failures were crossed over to lithium carbonate and had a complete remission. The lithium carbonate failure was crossed over to chlorpromazine and failed to respond. Although these data would seem to favor lithium, statistical analysis failed to reveal any significant difference between the two groups at the 5 percent level after the first three weeks of treatment.

The assessment of these five control studies does not permit any direct comparisons since the experimental design of each was different. In Magg's (1963) report, the fixed-dosage schedule may have resulted in inadequate lithium levels. This may be important since the drug trial ran for only two weeks, with one lithium-free day per week. In the study by Spring *et al.* (1970), we are told that a satisfactory response to lithium occurred in all cases, on doses not exceeding 1800 mg lithium carbonate daily, although the protocol did allow for a maximum lithium issuance of 3 gm daily. The reason for not increasing lithium medication is not offered. If, indeed, all patients responded to lithium with complete remission, the statistical outcome showing chlorpromazine superiority must be questioned. The possibility of too high a dosage in the schizo-affective group reported by Johnson, Gershon, and Hekimian (1968) may account for the worsening of scores in this group. Perhaps the single most important issue making comparison of these studies difficult is the lack of homogeneity of the various groups, even when more descriptive material is offered regarding clinical diagnosis. For example, in Schou's (1954) report, the "atypical" subgroup is apparently diagnostically different by clinical description from the "typical" group; the distinction is reflected in the differences in treatment outcome between the two groups. Schou (1967, 1970) has since then commented upon the unfavorable outcome with lithium in such atypical patients, and in the study by Johnson, Gershon, and Hekimian (1968) two groups, schizo-affective and manic, showed a sharply contrasting treatment response to lithium.

Characteristic patterns of lithium response. The lithium ion occupies a unique position in the chemical treatment of mania, in that it exerts diagnostically related psychopharmacological specificity which does not resemble the preclinical or clinical pharmacological profiles of the neuroleptic compounds used in manic disorder. Lithium's effect in mania differs distinctly from that of the neuroleptics (such as chlorpromazine and haloperidol) on three points. First, they have different time courses. Chlorpromazine and haloperidol usually act more rapidly than lithium, whose full effect cannot be expected for seven to ten days of treatment. This is of considerable importance when the acute and unusually violent cases of mania are treated. Second, while the sedative action of conventional neuroleptics is largely independent of the illness causing the agitation, lithium acts more specifically against mania, its best results being obtained in patients with clinical pictures dominated by mood elevation, irritability, restlessness, talkativeness, and jocularity. Third, and perhaps most important, the responses to lithium and neuroleptic treatments differ in quality. Neuroleptics, while producing an effective suppression of the manic overactivity and restlessness, are accompanied by a drugged effect of sedation and drowsiness. Thus, the phenothiazines and butyrophenones merely place a lid over the manic state; the patients usually retain, below the surface, their characteristic symptoms of mania. Lithium, on the other hand, seems to remove the manic symptoms in a more specific manner, dissolving the elevated mood, hyperactivity, restlessness, talkativeness, sleeplessness, etc. without sedation or the feeling of being drugged. The patient is "normalized," and brought into a state that cannot be distinguished subjectively or objectively (Schou 1967) from his normal, premorbid condition.

Factors affecting response: Diagnostic precision. In order to appreciate the specific therapeutic effects of lithium, it should be prescribed for patients showing a clear diagnostic indication for this drug. The manic phase of manic-depressive illness is the prime indication for lithium treatment. The ambiguities surrounding the diagnosis of manic illness, and especially that shadowy interface between manic phase, manic-depressive disorder and schizophrenia, schizo-affective type, and excited phase, present a diagnostic dilemma in that both illnesses share large components of both affective as well as behavioral disturbance. The resolution of this problem of differential diagnosis is critical, however, since several studies have indicated that patients do less well on lithium when the manic picture is clouded with "atypical" features (Schou 1954; Hartigan 1963; Fries 1969). This "atypical" group includes subjects with schizophrenic symptoms, and the significance of such differential drug responsiveness has been underlined in several recent studies (Johnson, Gershon, and Hekimian 1968; Aronoff and Epstein 1969; Shopsin, Kim, and Gershon 1970). In discussing their trial of lithium, Aronoff and Epstein noted that some of their schizo-affective cases, which they acknowledged might well have been designated "atypical manic-depressive illness" by others, showed only moderate response or symptom aggravation under lithium treatment. It is on this sort of explicitness about diagnostic ambiguities that progress in delineating lithium's therapeutic usefulness depends. The studies by Johnson, Gershon, and Hekimian (1968) and Shopsin, Kim, and Gershon (1970) underscore lithium's specificity of action; both investigations indicate strongly that lithium has no apparent sedative or neuroleptic properties and that it can, in fact, precipitate or contribute to further decompensation of schizophrenic symptomatology. The affective, psychomotor, or paranoid components of this psychiatric illness, like the core process itself, failed to show any selective symptom amelioration during treatment with lithium.

Attempts to improve the inadequate differentiating criteria in current use are being made. Hekimian *et al.* (1969) have reported on two new rating instruments designed to distinguish between manic and schizo-affective patients: the Differential Diagnostic Scale (DDS) for manic-depressive illness, and the Bellevue Differential Inventory (BDI). Satloff and Pinling (Gattozzi 1970), in their study of manic symptomatology, use films, tape recordings, drawings made by patients, as well as objective behavioral observation. They hope to devise simple and standardized methods for determining when manic phenomena occur in a manic individual. Gattozzi has reported that preliminary trends are beginning to emerge from the material studied.

Lithium specificity: Neurotoxicity. Central to the issue of lithium specificity, our group (Shopsin, Johnson, and Gershon 1970) recently reported toxic-confusional states as well as activating effects in a considerable number of schizophrenic patients (11 of 17) receiving lithium carbonate. Significant features in these cases are a general worsening of previously manifest psychoses with the appearance of bizarre affect and behavior patterns, inconsistent changes in psychomotor activity, aggravation of delusional thought, and florid hallucinatory phenomena. The frequently concomitant appearance of reduced comprehension, clouding of sensorium with confusion, memory impairment, and disorientation indicate organic brain dysfunction in these patients.

Blood lithium levels were quite modest in all instances (mean 0.750 mEq/l) and, paradoxically, the common lithium effects or toxic manifestations were not consistently present. The most consistent laboratory abnormalities consisted of EEG changes including alterations in the alpha activity, diffuse slowing, accentuation of previous focal abnormalities, and/or the appearance of previously absent focal changes. The occurrence of neurotoxicity corresponds, therefore, to the presence and severity of EEG changes (Figure 1).

Previous reports of psychotogenic effects and confusion during lithium treatment have appeared in the literature (Greenfield *et al.*

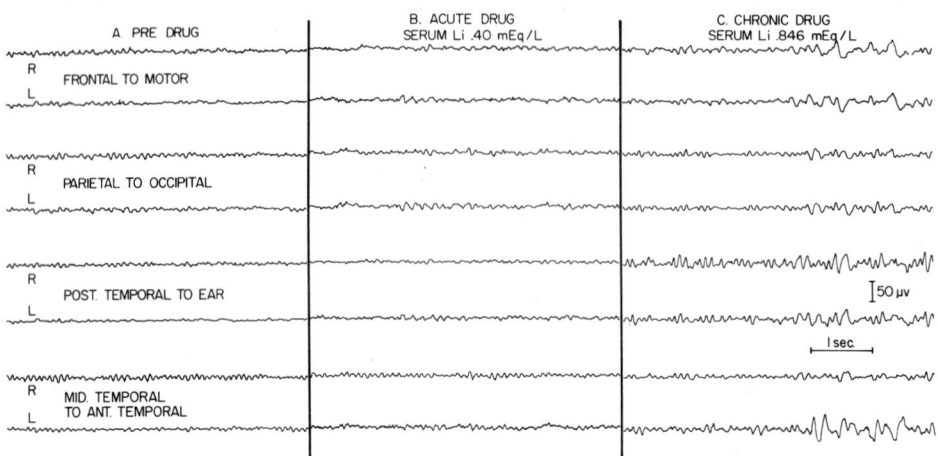

Figure 1. A. Predrug EEG (minimal asymmetry); B. EEG 2 hours after oral lithium, serum level 0.40 mEq/l (increased alpha amplitude, increased asymmetry); C. EEG during chronic lithium administration, serum level 0.846 mEq/l (moderate abnormalities -- diffuse delta activity, increased alpha amplitude, and bursts). Reprinted with permission from *J. Nerv. Ment. Dis.* 151:273, 1970.

1950; Glessinger 1954; Sivadon and Chanoit 1955; Schou 1959; Mayfield and Brown 1966; Lehmann and Ban 1970; Baldessarini and Stevens 1970; Spring *et al.* 1970).

Several studies have offered convincing evidence of changes in electrical activity of the brain during lithium treatment, relating these changes to electrolyte effects or shifts (Moracci 1931; Araki *et al.* 1965; Pfeiffer, Singh, and Goldstein 1969). Johnson, Hekimian, and Gershon (1970) noted that the most significant changes in EEG during chronic lithium administration were seen in individuals showing baseline abnormalities (Figure 2). Underlining the possible relevance of premorbid conditions to such changes, Rochford *et al.* (1970) indicated that neurologic abnormalities were found in nearly 40 percent of young adult psychiatric patients, significantly more than in controls (5 percent). The incidence of neurologic impairment did not differ significantly from one diagnostic group to another, with the exception of those patients with affective disorders. Interestingly, no neurologic abnormality was found among subjects in this latter diagnostic category. One would anticipate from such findings that neurotoxicity following lithium administration would be highest in patients with other than primary affective disorders,

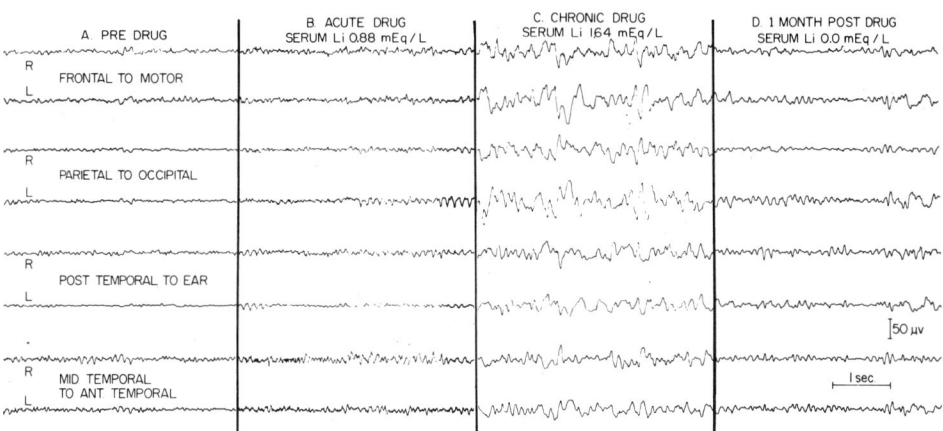

Figure 2. A. Predrug EEG (minimal asymmetry); B. EEG 2 hours after lithium ingestion, serum lithium 0.880 mEq/l (increased alpha amplitude, increased asymmetry); C. EEG during chronic lithium administration, serum lithium at 1.64 mEq/l (marked abnormalities--diffuse delta activity, increased asymmetry); D. EEG 1 month after lithium discontinued, serum level 0.00 mEq/l (persistence of left focal abnormality). Reprinted with permission from *J. Nerv. Ment. Dis.* 151:273, 1970.

that is, in subjects not diagnosed as having manic-depressive illness. This is supported by the findings in two double-blind studies using lithium or chlorpromazine in schizophrenic patients (Johnson, Gershon, and Hekimian 1968; Shopsin, Kim, and Gershon 1970). Indications are that such patients, whether by differential handling (excretion), differences in electrolyte or endocrine substrate, or "abnormal" baseline neuropathy, exhibit a decreased threshold tolerance or sensitivity for the lithium ion, which exposes them to central nervous system toxicity at moderate to low levels of serum lithium.

Therapeutic regimen: Stabilization and maintenance. Based on pharmacological studies concerning the retention and excretion of the lithium ion (Trautner *et al.* 1955), the treatment outline consists of stabilization and maintenance.

Stabilization: Once the diagnosis is established, stabilization of a patient on lithium medication is essentially a procedure similar to that of controlling a diabetic patient with insulin. Stabilization of a manic episode requires several days and is best carried out in a hospital, although this is by no means an absolute requirement. Any of the lithium salts may be used, but the most readily available and best tolerated is lithium carbonate (in capsules of 300 mg equivalent to 8.0 mEq/l of elemental lithium) (Table 3). The daily dosage during this phase is usually between 1.5 to 3.5 gm in divided doses. The size of the dose, however, is determined by such factors as the severity of clinical condition, body weight, age, and rate of renal clearance of lithium. Plasma lithium levels should be determined every three or four days during the stabilization phase by using either a flame photometer or an atomic absorption spectrometer. After commencing treatment, the plasma level of lithium will rise, and care should be taken to keep it below 2.0 mEq/l to prevent serious side effects. In addition to chemical surveillance, careful clinical observation is required. If toxic manifestations appear, or the plasma level rises above 2.0 mEq/l, the lithium dose should be reduced or the drug temporarily withdrawn. To attain a therapeutic response, the plasma lithium level usually should range between 0.6 to 1.5 mEq/l. On this regimen, the manic episode generally remits in six to ten days; more typically, in eight to ten days.

Maintenance: Continuation of high-dosage medication with lithium into the maintenance phase carries a considerable risk of toxicity.

TABLE 3

	Salt			
	LiCl	$Li_2SO_4 \cdot H_2O$	Li_2CO_3	$Li_3C_6H_5O_7 \cdot H_2O$
Molecular weight	42.4	127.96	73.89	279.96
10 milliequivalents	0.424 gram	0.37 gram	0.37 gram	0.93 gram
1 gram	23.6 milliequivalents	15.6 milliequivalents	27.0 milliequivalents	10.75 milliequivalents
10 grains (0.65 gram)	15.4 milliequivalents	10.4 milliequivalents	17.5 milliequivalents	7.0 milliequivalents

TABLE 4

Toxic Manifestations

Gastrointestinal Symptoms

1. Anorexia
2. Nausea
3. Vomiting
4. Diarrhea
5. Thirst
6. Dryness of the mouth
7. Weight loss

Neuromuscular Symptoms and Signs

1. General muscle weakness
2. Ataxia
3. Tremor
4. Muscle hyperirritability
   a. Fasciculation (increased by tapping muscle)
   b. Twitching (especially of facial muscles)
   c. Clonic movements of whole limbs
5. Choreo-athetotic movements
6. Hyperactive deep-tendon reflexes

Central Nervous System

1. Anaesthesia of skin
2. Incontinence of urine and feces
3. Slurred speech
4. Blurring of vision
5. Dizziness
6. Vertigo
7. Epileptiform seizures

Mental Symptoms

1. Mental retardation
2. Somnolence
3. Confusion
4. Restless - disturbed behavior
5. Stupor
6. Coma

Cardiovascular System

1. Pulse irregularities
2. Fall in blood pressure

3. ECG changes
4. Peripheral circulatory failure
5. Circulatory collapse

Miscellaneous

1. Polyuria
2. Glycosuria
3. General fatigue
4. Lethargy and tendency to sleep
5. Dehydration

Once the manic episode dissolves, dosage should be lowered and plasm levels continue to be measured weekly until a stable blood level is established. In this phase, the patient can be managed safely as an outpatient, providing that his plasma lithium level is checked regularly. In general, the maintenance level of plasma lithium is between 0.4 to 0.8 mEq/l, although dosage must be individualized in accordance with symptomatology, individual tolerance, and occurrence of side effects.

Toxicology. Lithium intoxications appear when more lithium is accumulated than can be excreted by the kidneys. The various toxic manifestations are summarized in Table 4, but there is no obligatory sequence of occurrence.

Acute Effects: These are of two main types. One type of undesirable effect is associated with relatively low serum lithium levels, which are more of an inconvenience than a danger. The second type is intoxication and poisoning associated with lithium serum levels of 2.0 mEq/l or more.

The first type includes anorexia, transient gastric discomfort, vomiting, diarrhea, thirst, and hand tremor. These effects often coincide with serum lithium peaks, and they may be related more to the steepness of the rise in lithium levels than to the height of the peak. These effects often disappear or diminish without reduction of dosage. Some, such as polyuria and tremor, may persist. The tremor induced by lithium does not respond to antiparkinson medication.

Toxic effects seen at blood levels between 1.5 to 2.0 mEq/l or above are more serious, and they include muscle fasciculation and twitching, hyperactive deep-tendon reflexes, ataxia, somnolence, confusion, dysarthria, and, rarely, epileptiform seizures (Gershon and Yuwiler 1960). These effects are often associated with reversible electroencephalographic alterations (Mayfield and Brown 1966; Johnson, Gershon, and Hekimian 1968). Electrocardiographic changes may occur occasionally (Schou et al. 1954; Schou 1957 and 1962). In severe cases of lithium poisoning, the central nervous system is primarily affected. Consciousness may be impaired, resulting in coma in some cases. In such severe cases, the muscles may be hypertonic or rigid with hyperactive deep-tendon reflexes, and manifest muscle tremor and fasciculations. Such toxic symptoms as tremor, ataxia, Rombergism, slurred speech, dysdiadochokinesia, and nystagmus may perhaps be considered as manifestations of cerebellar disturbance.

There is no specific antidote for lithium intoxication. Since lithium is the cause of the poisoning, the first treatment consists of eliminating this ion from the organism. Adjunctive treatment measures are aimed at averting the complications accompanying protracted states of unconsciousness, and infection. Table 5 outlines the various treatment modalities employed in the management of severe lithium poisoning. Treatment is basically the same as that used in barbiturate poisoning: (1) elimination by lavage if there is likely to be a significant amount of lithium in the stomach, (2) correction of fluid and electrolyte imbalance, and (3) regulation of kidney function. Infection prophylaxis, regular roentgenograms of the lungs, frequent determinations of blood pressure, and preservation of adequate respiration are essential. Obviously, blood and urine lithium determinations require continuous monitoring of the elimination of the ion. Forced diuresis, alkalinization of the urine, and administration of aminophylline indicate that it is possible to reduce the duration of severe lithium intoxication to two weeks or less. Lithium does not cause permanent side effects or damage.

Subacute and Chronic Effects: The possible value of lithium as a prophylactic treatment for manic-depressive disorder necessitates the careful evaluation of any side effect and complication developing during lithium ingestion. Over the years, numerous reports dealing with various endocrine and metabolic effects related to lithium carbonate maintenance have appeared in the literature; except for thyroid dysfunction, the diverse array of side effects has been met with little concern, apparently overshadowed by the greater interest paid to lithium's clinical efficacy in the affective illnesses.

The antithyroid and goitrogenic effects of lithium have been well documented (Baastrup 1967; Schou et al. 1968; Sedvall et al. 1968; Wiggers 1968; Shopsin, Blum, and Gershon 1969; Berens et al. 1969; Shopsin 1970). Alterations in carbohydrate metabolism (Van der Velde and Gordon 1969; Plenge, Mellerup, and Rafaelsen 1969; Heninger and Mueller 1970; Shopsin, Stern, and Gershon 1970), and steroid metabolism (Platman and Fieve 1968; Goodwin, Murphy, and Bunney 1968; Murphy, Goodwin, and Bunney 1969; Shopsin and Gershon 1970) related to lithium therapy have also been recorded, as have pitressin-resistant

TABLE 5

MANAGEMENT OF SEVERE LITHIUM POISONING*

Primarily via Renal Excretion:
4/5 of filtered lithium is reabsorbed in the proximal tubule (normal half-life of lithium is 24 hours)

A. Discontinue lithium
B. Stat blood lithium level - then daily or bidaily levels as required.
C. Stat serum sodium and potassium estimations (follow as required).
D. ECG stat and periodically thereafter.
E. Temperature and blood pressure every four hours.
F. Infection prophylaxis (rotate patient, etc.).
G. Optional--spinal tap and EEG.
H. If question of infection exists: blood culture and viral studies of blood and CSF are indicated.

Treatment Methods Recommended:

1. Replace water and electrolytes as needed (sodium, potassium, calcium, magnesium). Total daily fluid should be at least 5 to 6 liters per day. Do not over-salinize, and avoid abrupt changes in electrolyte intake. Monitor if changes made.
2. Forced lithium diuresis via urea - 20 gm i.v. 2 to 5 times daily (urea contraindicated if severe renal impairment antedates toxicity), or mannitol 50 to 100 gm i.v. as total daily dose.
3. Increase lithium clearance with aminophylline (which also suppresses tubular reabsorption and increases blood flow). Dosage 0.5. gm by slow i.v. administration (may cause sharp but transitory hypotension).
4. Alkalinization of urine with i.v. sodium lactate has been recommended as an adjunctive measure.
5. If poisoning is severe, the patient should be dialyzed (peritoneal dialysis or artificial kidney).

*This table is a modification of one prepared for an APA exhibit, San Francisco (1970).

diabetes insipidus-like syndromes (Angrist *et al.* 1968). Several investigators have reported a reversible lithium-related leucocytosis during administration of this drug to both man and animal (Radomski *et al.* 1950; Rissetto and Gazzano 1952; Mayfield and Brown 1966; O'Connell 1970; Shopsin, Friedman, and Gershon 1970). Some of the above data concerning endocrines, and specifically a pituitary-adrenal relationship (Samuels 1951; Fursham 1965), may account for the increases in white blood cell count during lithium therapy. The reported efficacy of lithium in countering the symptoms of premenstrual tension (Sletten and Gershon 1966) and controlling postpuerperal mania (Gershon and Yuwiler 1960) strengthens the assumption of a lithium effect on diverse metabolic and hormonal systems. Finally, the effects of lithium on adeneal cyclase (cyclic AMP) activity in different animal tissues explored may be a relevant link underlying these various endocrine and metabolic perturbations (Berens 1969; Abdulla and Hamadah 1970; Ramsden 1970; Dousa and Hechter 1970).

It would appear from current knowledge and work in this area that lithium has no consistently predictable effect on endocrine function or steroid metabolism. In some instances, the available evidence for lithium's action in this regard involves animal studies; in others, infrequent clinical syndromes and chemical evidence in psychiatric patients reveal the lithium-related effect. Throughout the literature, both diagnostic and methodological problems are apparent and contribute to the lack of consistency in both human and animal studies. It would appear that, when seen, these lithium effects in man are not related to manic-depressive illness; the various endocrine, steroid, and metabolic changes seem to represent a physiological effect of this ion. These effects are readily reversible and appear innocuous.

The different reports relating lithium to altered endocrine and metabolic function may suggest that the activity or effective concentration of a number of hormones are responsive to this drug. Despite the many observations cited here, however, clinical effects reflecting endocrine disturbance during lithium treatment remain a rare occurrence. This may indicate that lithium acts as the *agent provocateur* in revealing a previously undetected disturbance in hormone metabolism or glandular function. This is particularly true in the case of lithium-related thyroid dysfunction, where the antithyroid and goitrogenic properties of lithium become clinically apparent in patients with underlying thyroid pathology. Although much of the available information awaits replication and further evaluation, the preliminary findings of lithium's effect on endocrine function suggest the alluring possibility that a singular central action (direct or indirect) of this compound accounts for many or all of these effects. Certainly, such findings merit further control studies of pituitary, thyroid, adrenal, pancreatic, and gonadal hormone function to elucidate lithium's basic mode of action.

Distribution of lithium in biological fluids. Lithium is readily absorbed after all standard forms of administration, oral, subcutaneous, intramuscular, and intraperitoneal. The oral route is the one adopted in clinical studies in man. Lithium is not bound to plasma proteins and passes from the blood stream at different rates for different tissues. Uptake is rapid in some tissues, such as liver, kidney, and spleen, but slow in others, such as muscle, bone, and brain (Schou 1958). Equilibrium is eventually established between blood and different tissues.

Although earlier communications had reported lithium as being equally distributed in body fluids (Davenport 1950; Radomski *et al.* 1950; Schou 1958), subsequent investigations in both animal and man have indicated that, to the contrary, plasma-tissue lithium ratios at equilibrium differ depending on the tissue examined. The concentration gradients across the cell wall are generally of the order of 2 to 4: muscle, kidney, and bone contain approximately twice as much lithium as plasma (Gattozzi 1970); the thyroid gland contains 3 or 4 times the amount in plasma (Schou 1958; Shopsin, Blum, and Gershon 1969; Berens, Wolff, and Murphy 1970). Studies of cerebrospinal fluid from patients on long-term lithium administration have shown that spinal fluid levels of lithium are indefinitely maintained at 40 to 60 percent of the plasma level, even under toxic conditions (Gershon and Yuwiler 1960). Animal studies carried out in our laboratories also indicate that with 28-day lithium administration, the total brain level is also about 50 percent that of the plasma level (Ho *et al.* 1970).

Following oral administration of lithium carbonate to hospitalized psychiatric patients, lithium was found in the serum and saliva of all patients within an hour after its ingestion (Shopsin, Gershon, and Pinkney 1969). Differential patterns of distribution also appeared. Control patients tended to show elevated serum and saliva lithium concentrations more rapidly than manic or schizo-affective individuals, although there was significant scatter of the assays.

The data indicated that lithium is present in saliva at concentrations about twice its level in serum. This ratio holds for all psychiatric diagnostic types, and it remains stable over a wide range of dosages and other variables. So consistent is the concentration gradient that a constant has been obtained to derive plasma levels from saliva assays. The constant derived from the equation is: $Y = (0.46X - 0.05) \pm 0.34$, where Y is the predicted serum value and X is the obtained saliva value. Similar findings have been recorded in animals by direct tissue examination (Berens, Wolff, and Murphy 1970). Saliva, therefore, may serve as a simple means of calculating the blood level of lithium.

The plasma-tissue equilibrium is a dynamic one, proportionally changing with alterations in the plasma levels. For the clinician, such dynamics of lithium distribution are relevant inasmuch as the amount present in the body may be monitored by measuring the amount in the blood or saliva. For this purpose, it is recommended that samples be drawn when the patient is in the postabsorptive state,

6 to 9 hours after the last dose. This is most readily accomplished in the morning before the first ingested daily dose. Lithium levels in either blood or salivary secretions are reliably measured by either flame photometry or by atomic absorption photometry.

Earlier reports (Trautner *et al.* 1955; Gershon and Yuwiler 1960) and more recent ones (Greenspan *et al.* 1968; Serry 1969) suggest that manic patients metabolize lithium in a unique manner. For example, manic patients are said to retain the lithium ion and to excrete it more slowly than normothymic subjects (Trautner *et al.* 1955; Gershon and Yuwiler 1960; Greenspan, Green, and Durrell 1968). The increased retention may be due to a relative shift to an intracellular location (Greenspan, Green, and Durrell 1968; Shopsin, Gershon, and Pinkney 1969). Although the matter is far from settled, such notions are refuted by the findings of Baldessarini and Stephens (1970) who reported no differences in serum lithium concentrations in a given patient at one dosage of lithium carbonate over time, including euphoric, normothymic, and depressed moods.

Investigational Drugs in the Treatment of Mania

Several other compounds have been introduced in chemotherapy for mania, but they have contributed little to improve treatment for this disorder.

Thioxanthenes

Both chlorprothixene (Gross and Kaltenback 1961) and clopenthixol (Massaut *et al.* 1962) have been given a trial in manic patients; treatment efficacy has been suggested (Ban 1969). Thiothixene has also been reputed to produce beneficial effects in manic patients in studies by Schiele (1967) and Filotto *et al.* (1967). The general use of these drugs in the treatment for mania, however, should await investigational clarification. For example, the pharmacological activity of thiothixene reported by some investigators (Hekimian and Gershon 1967) mitigates against its use in the treatment for acute mania.

Dibenzazepines and Dibenzocycloheptenes

There have been several uncontrolled trials concerning the usefulness of both imipramine and amitriptyline in the treatment and in the prophylaxis of mania.

A therapeutic response to imipramine by a manic patient was first reported by Akimoto (1961), and in a subsequent study of twenty manic patients by this same author, thirteen patients showed complete remission or marked improvement with this drug. Andersen and Kristianson (1959) and Kristjansen (1962) have separately reported prompt, favorable therapeutic responses to imipramine by manic patients.

Akimoto (1962) also indicated that treatment with amitriptyline is effective in certain cases of mania. This suggestion was supported by Stromgren and Stromgren (1962) who indicated that amitriptyline also exhibited a prophylactic effect against manic as well as depressive relapses.

There are no confirmatory reports based on systematically conducted clinical trials or specially designed controlled investigations in this area; in the absence of better documentation, the above findings can only be considered an experimental approach.

Methysergide

Preliminary studies by Dewhurst (1968) and Haskovec and Soucek (1968) indicated a marked, rapid-acting, antimanic effect for methysergide, an antiserotonin agent. This compound is obviously of tremendous tactical and theoretical interest, since several observations suggest that the metabolism of indoles, particularly of 5-hydroxytryptamine (serotonin), is disturbed in affective illness. Dewhurst reported on ten hospitalized manic patients with a history of cyclic manic-depressive phases. Of the ten patients, seven showed very good and one good improvement; one remained stationary and one deteriorated. The effects of methysergide were evident after 24 hours and well marked at 48 hours. Symptom ratings indicated that all the characteristics of mania improved, but that the thought disturbance was less affected.

In the study by Haskovec and Soucek, manic patients were given placebo for 2 to 6 days, followed by 8 to 14 days of methysergide treatment (initially by injection), and finally placed on placebo during a subsequent period. The maximum dosage was 6 mg daily for eight patients, but two who did not improve were given 9 mg daily. In this manner, eight of the ten patients showed marked improvement. Two patients refused to cooperate in the third stage, five of the remaining six relapsed on placebo, and the remaining patient stayed well. The effects were evident within 24 hours and marked after 48 hours. As in the study by Dewhurst, there seemed to be a specific remission of the major manic symptoms, with a normalization of euphoric mood, daily activity, and sleep.

In these reports methysergide seemed to be quite specific in its effect on mood as well as the manic phenomena accompanying it. This indicated to Dewhurst that the specificity of response suggested a use for methysergide as a diagnostic test in cases of undiagnosed excitement, since results would be evident within 48 hours. However, controlled cross-validation is needed and, in fact, Coppen *et al.*

(1969) have already indicated that this compound exhibited no apparent therapeutic action in their patients with moderate to severe mania, and that compared to placebo effects it may even be detrimental. These investigators administered 6 mg of methysergide for eight days, followed by placebo for eight days, or vice versa, to ten manic patients studied in double-blind controlled fashion. Patients were rated for mood, activity, talk, and behavioral disturbance on alternate days, and the outcome indicated that methysergide was no better than placebo in treatment for mania. Analysis of variance showed further that the drug was significantly less effective than placebo for talk and behavioral disturbance.

McCabe, Reich, and Winokur (1970) also reported on an open trial of methysergide in acute mania. All patients received either 6 or 8 mg of this medication daily *per os*. Patients were observed and rated daily for changes in mental status; these were recorded on a seven-symptom check list. Of the twelve patients in the study, only one responded during the four-to five-day trial. Several who did not respond were given a considerably longer trial than the usual four days, but they showed no change. Almost all patients were subsequently treated successfully with lithium carbonate, phenothiazines, or electroconvulsive therapy.

Cinnanserin

In experimental animal studies with various species, cinnanserin exhibited antiserotonin action and, like methysergide, was considered for clinical application in the treatment for acute and chronic psychoses. In an open study design (Itil 1968), the effect of cinnanserin was studied in a group of fourteen chronic schizophrenic patients. Although thought disorder was unaffected, an obvious improvement in general management and social behavior was noted in the majority of patients. After discontinuation of the drug, all but one patient showed a reversal of symptomatology. With doses higher than 600 mg daily, patients showed an increase of restlessness and an akathesia-like syndrome, as well as a worsening of psychopathology. The results of this open trial, as well as the serotonin antagonism documented in animal studies, indicate that trials with this compound in manic patients deserve exploration.

Alpha-Methyl-Para-Tyrosine

Bunney *et al.* (1970) administered alpha-methyl-para-tyrosine (α-MPT) to four manic patients in an attempt to decrease the functional brain level of dopamine and norepinephrine (NE). A specific blocker of NE and dopamine synthesis, α-MPT exhibited a beneficial effect in two patients. Although these subjects later relapsed on placebo, these authors reported that subsequent manic episodes showed only mild improvement during treatment with this drug.

Propranolol

Another compound newly tried in the treatment for manic illness is propranolol, a beta-adrenergic-blocking agent. Reporting on the rapid, distinct improvement with this drug in certain types of psychotic patients, Atsmon indicated that four of the thirteen patients treated with propranolol were manic-depressives in the manic phase. The specific effects of propranolol in these manic patients are not known since the results were reported in Hospital Tribune (1970) as follows: "Of the thirteen, seven showed complete recovery.... four of the patients showed partial recovery; two were failures." As regards propranolol treatment, the outcome for the four manic patients cannot, therefore, be ascertained.

An outstanding impression of treatment was the "complete return to normal within hours, recovery taking place from 12 to 48 hours after initial treatment." Nearly all patients received an initial dose of 600 to 800 mg daily of propranolol. The dosage was increased in some cases, and in one instance it reached 5800 mg. There was a clear-cut parallelism between the onset of amelioration of symptoms and lowering of pulse rate, followed by a lowering of blood pressure after 12 to 24 hours.

Although none of these newer compounds have proved useful in the treatment for mania, they indicate a progression of research in this area from nonspecific pharmacological agents to more specific drugs having a defined biochemical effect. It is ironic, therefore, that despite the use of these sophisticated guidelines in applying new drugs to mania, none of the compounds have proved effective. Such agents should continue to be investigated, however, and regardless of treatment outcome in this disorder, these drugs can lead to a clearer understanding of the psychological and biological components of mood and behavior.

III. PROPHYLAXIS AGAINST MANIC AND DEPRESSIVE RELAPSES

Prophylactic Chemotherapy of Recurrent Mania

There is no clear-cut definition or agreement among clinicians of what the term "prophylactic" chemotherapy implies as used in the treatment of manic-depressive illness. We consider it to mean a drug maintenance (e.g., on lithium) that affects only the amplitude and duration of manic or depressive recurrences and does not clearly modify the endogenous cyclicity of the affective disorder. For mania, maintenance dosage of medication is increased during the incipient attack in efforts to diminish its intensity and shorten exacerbation of the illness. This course of action is taken to prevent the need for hospitalization and, if possible, to maintain the afflicted individual in a functioning capacity. Such treatment response implies a prophylactic effect for the drug; perhaps the term "stabilization" (Baastrup et al. 1970) would be preferable to others.

Lithium

In attempting to extract material regarding the effect of lithium on recurrent mania from the literature, a prophylactic claim is suggested. This assessment includes all the limitations described of the effects of lithium on acute mania, in addition to other, more serious, methodological and statistical problems that exist in long-term follow-up studies.

Noack and Trautner (1951), in their report on more than thirty cases of mania, referred to the prophylactic activity of lithium. They concluded that "lithium was found to be very beneficial in terminating and preventing the maniacal phase in cases of mania, hypomania and recurrent mania - and the treatment was useless in the depressive phase of manic-depressive psychosis."

Gershon and Yuwiler (1960), in a report based on uncontrolled observations, also claimed prophylactic activity in recurrent mania. The effect observed, however, must be more carefully defined. Large doses of lithium were required to resolve the acute manic episodes, and the patients were to be continued on a much lower maintenance dose of lithium for prophylaxis. It was noted that, at intervals corresponding approximately to those leading to manic episodes, the patients experienced some of the same features that had heralded previous episodes; these have been described as hypomanic alert by Jacobsen (1965). At such times the dosage of lithium needs to be increased to produce an abatement of symptoms. Thus, the maintenance medication produces a marked diminution in the amplitude of the symptomatology and enables the patient and his family to detect and appreciate the onset of manic symptoms.

If this assessment of lithium's action is correct, then carefully monitored prophylactic studies could readily measure the degree of prophylaxis. Thus, it is the nature of lithium's action in prophylaxis of recurrent mania to restrict the amplitude of manic episodes and to bring them to within a near-normal range of affective movement, without abolishing all manifestations of manic cycles. This degree of efficacy should enable the patient to be managed without the hospitalization that would have been previously necessary. A similar type of prophylactic activity against recurrent mania was reported in the graphic summaries presented by Schou and associates (1954). Hartigan (1963) also reported a prophylactic action of lithium against recurrent mania and added a claim for its prophylactic action against recurrent depressive cycles. It is important to note the reservation in this report, that "atypical" patients, about whom there was diagnostic doubt because of conspicuous schizophrenic or paranoid features, did not do as well as those with the pure, classical forms of the diseases.

In an "open" trial of lithium in recurrent affective disorders, Melia (1967) suggested that a beneficial effect is produced by lithium. Since the analysis of his data were pooled for both manic and depressive episodes, however, no assessment of the order of activity against recurrent mania can be obtained. Thus, he reported that the number of weeks in which patients receiving lithium were free from relapse was significantly greater at the 0.05 level than the number of weeks they were free from relapse before lithium. This conclusion was based on the t test, which is not strictly valid for this kind of study. In describing the quality of the effect, Melia stated that there was a diminution, rather than cessation, in the intensity of the mood swings, that minor mood swings were manifested, but that, on lithium, the patients did not require hospitalization.

The recent study of the prophylactic use of lithium carbonate by Spring and associates (1969) is negative. These investigators treated nine manic patients with lithium carbonate after acute manic attacks, maintained the patients on prophylactic lithium, and followed their progress for three months to one year. Of the nine patients, five relapsed within one year. All relapses occurred while the patients' serum lithium level was 0.6 mEq/l or higher. In four of the five relapsing patients, the recurrent manic attacks were as severe as any they had previously experienced. In the fifth relapsing patient, the manic attacks were less severe, but their frequency was unchanged. Of the four non-relapsing patients, the follow-up period was shorter than their average interval between attacks. This report calls for careful and critical appraisal of the claims for lithium prophylaxis in recurrent mania.

Phenothiazines

The use of phenothiazines as a prophylactic measure against recurrent manic attacks has not been measured in a control fashion. The procedure is not only warranted, but "should be employed with the patient who has already demonstrated a propensity for repeated manic episodes," according to Klein and Davis (1969), who recommend fluphenazine or its equivalent.

Butyrophenones

Rapp (1970) was one of the first to report on the potential usefulness of haloperidol in the prophylaxis of "incipient hypomania." His review of only four cases and one short follow-up of eight months make any conclusion of a prophylactic effect tentative, although the apparently incipient manic episodes were avoided.

Further clinical trials are indicated.

Prophylactic Chemotherapy of Recurrent Depression

There is no clear-cut evidence that maintenance doses of any psychoactive drug prevent the recurrence of periodic depression. Given the nature of episodic illness, it follows that gathering systematic information on this issue is difficult.

Although lithium is of doubtful usefulness in the treatment for a depressive episode, a prophylactic action of lithium in recurrent depression has been suggested in several reports since 1954 (Schou et al. 1954; Andreani, Caselli, and Martelli (1958). More systematic and detailed observations of this effect were made by Hartigan (1963), Baastrup (1964), and more recently in studies by Baastrup and Schou (1967) and Angst and associates (1969). Hartigan's 1963 report is concerned exclusively with the prophylactic action of lithium in eight patients with recurrent depression whose initial depression was treated by electroplexy, and to whom lithium was given thereafter as a prophylactic. All patients had established histories of previous depressive episodes; they were observed for at least three years; and for six patients the results were reported as entirely satisfactory.

Baastrup and Schou (1967) conducted a large and important study of the action of lithium in cases of recurrent depression. Their report deals with eighty-eight patients with manic-depressive disease who had a history of two or more manic-depressive episodes during one year, or one or more episodes per year during two years. In this study, two parameters were used for the quantitative comparison of periods with and without lithium: the relapse frequency, which was designated as the average number of episodes per year, and the psychosis rate, defined as the average number of months per year during which the patient was psychotic. The results obtained showed that, on an average, patients had relapses every eight months during the period without lithium, and every sixty months during the lithium period. A patient's average time in a psychotic state was thirteen weeks a year without lithium, and one and one-half weeks a year with lithium. It is important to stress that the best results were obtained in patients with a classical manic-depressive history, and were less satisfactory in the group of "atypical" cases. Baastrup and Schou conclude, however, that lithium exhibited the prophylactic activity in depressive episodes that had already been exhibited in cases of recurrent mania.

Fieve, Platman, and Plutchik (1968a) conducted a study aimed at exploring lithium's prophylactic effects in the depressive phase of forty-three bipolar manic-depressive patients. The group was followed up for varying periods of time, from five months to two years, and was rated with objective scoring devices (including self-rating of behavior), all on a single-blind basis. The data indicated that, among patients who had been on the drug more than seven months, as compared to patients on the drug less than seven months, lithium produced, at best, a mild decrease in depression scores, and during these two periods there were no changes in frequency of depression "failures." These authors defined failure as the existence of scores on two or more indexes showing values greater than on standard deviation above the patients' own means, in the direction indicating "increase" or aggravation of depression. These ratings were done on the basis of outpatient visits, and they are different from the definition of failure by Baastrup and Schou (1967), who required hospitalization of the patient or supervision in the home. On the basis of these single-blind data, along with the double-blind inpatient studies (Fieve, Platman, and Plutchik 1968b), which indicated lithium to have weak/nonexistent antidepressant effects compared to imipramine, Fieve (1970) concluded that the alleged prophylactic effects of lithium in so-called "recurrent acute depression" might be more apparent than real, if, in fact, it has any prophylactic effect at all.

Lithium was also judged to be without prophylactic efficacy in the depressive phase of cyclic, manic-depressive disorder by Stancer *et al.* (see Gattozzi 1970).

Prophylactic Chemotherapy Against Both Manic and Depressive Relapses

Lithium

In a study of Melia (1970), eighteen patients were assigned medication randomly by a statistician. The patients eventually comprised two drug groups: one group continued to receive medication (lithium) initiated in the acute phase, and the other was given dummy (placebo) tablets.

Four of the nine patients treated with lithium did not relapse in the follow-up period, as against two patients in the placebo group. One patient in the lithium group developed toxicity and medication was withdrawn; she was counted as having relapsed on the day lithium was stopped. The mean length of remission achieved by patients on lithium was 433 days, double that of patients on placebo, 224 days. The significance of the difference between the length of remissions achieved by the lithium and the placebo groups indicated that the superiority of lithium just failed to be significant at the 5 percent level--$0.01 > p > 0.05$.

Although efforts were made to match the groups according to characteristics of age, sex, episode frequency, length of illness, and diagnosis, the heterogeneous nature of the affective entities included in the study tends to nullify the significance of similarities between groups. The patient population consisted of cyclic manic-depressives, recurrent depressives, one recurrent manic, and two patients with recurrent schizo-affective illness. In addition, some patients who at the time of the study exhibited pure affective disorders had earlier shown schizophrenic symptoms. The fate of the subjects showing schizophrenic features during previous episodes reflects the inadequacy of Melia's group-matching criteria since they indicated no prophylaxis on lithium; the mean length of remission was ± 50 days in these two patients, as compared to over 500 days in patients without previous schizophrenic features. If one were to take the length of remission (in days) of the patients in the lithium group who had both previous and present features of schizophrenia, and compared the figures to remission length in the "typical" manics ingesting lithium, the difference would be 343 to 511, respectively. This again tends to point up lithium's specificity in the affective disorders and underlines the need for tightening methodological design for adequate interpretation of the data collected.

Bennie and Fell (1969) reported the prophylactic effects of lithium in four manic-depressive individuals and one patient suffering recurrent depression. Over the course of fifteen months, the five patients relapsed six times. In three instances of depressive relapses, these were severe enough to require ECT and large doses of tranquilizers or antidepressant drugs. The authors indicate, however, that the manic or depressive recurrences might be attributed to inadequate dosage of lithium, and that the well-being reported by the majority of patients was impressive enough to make lithium "a major contribution to the management of affective psychoses." The interpretation of findings is therefore at variance with the data presented and is ambiguous, if not spurious.

Wolpert and Mueller (1969) also reported favorable results in ten bipolar manic-depressive patients maintained on lithium for up to twenty-four months.

It was not until very recently that data were presented for large groups of patients observed and treated for prolonged periods. Van der Velde (1970) reported on seventy-five patients maintained on lithium carbonate treatment. The criteria for inclusion in this prophylactic assessment included the following: the patient had a history of at least one manic and one depressive episode prior to lithium therapy; it was possible to complete a three-year follow-up; and there was an absence of symptomatology that would make diagnosis ambiguous.

Three categories of response were noted including: I, patients who continued to show no significant change in their affective states, remaining stable for at least three years following successful treatment of an acute manic episode; II, patients who initially responded during an acute manic episode but who showed manic or depressive relapses during three years while on lithium carbonate; and III, patients who showed no marked response to lithium carbonate despite prolonged and repeated trials in which serum levels were as high as 2 mEq/l. Patients in category III were given repeated and separate trials with lithium carbonate and, in some instances, other psychotropic agents were added. Patients in category II were given additional lithium whenever there was a recurrence of either manic or depressive symptomatology. Thirty-four of the 75 patients were in category I, 21 patients in category II, and 20 patients in category III.

A clear improvement of acute manic symptoms was observed in 55 of the 75 manic-depressive patients participating in the follow-up study. Only 34 of these 55 patients, however, sustained their improvement during chronic treatment. Important differences in response to lithium appeared when the patients were grouped by age: the number of positive responses in acute manic states was highest (90 percent) in the youngest age group (17 to 40 years old), lower in the group aged 40 to 60 (75 percent), and lowest in those over age 60 (35 percent). Improvement was sustained by more of the younger patients than the older ones; only 2 of the 19 patients in the group aged 17 to 40 who responded to lithium carbonate had a manic episode during the three years of study, while the comparable figure for the group aged 40 to 60 was 11 of 42 patients.

On the basis of Van der Velde's study, the ratio of manic to depressive episodes decreases with increase of age. Response to lithium carbonate varied in some patients; a positive response at one time was no guarantee for a similar response in subsequent trials.

A controlled study by Angst, Dittrich, and Grof (1969) compared the activity of lithium with imipramine in recurrent affective psychoses. No analysis was made, however, of the type of recurrent phases (manic or depressive) that were affected. They concluded that lithium is a prophylactic agent against unipolar recurrent depressive relapses, bipolar manic-depressive recurrences, and psychotic exacerbations in schizo-affective psychosis. These authors reported that results of a prophylactic trial with imipramine showed an increase in the number of depressive episodes, compared with incidence before administration of this drug. In contrast, the controlled study by Fieve and associates (1968b) suggested that patients continuously on imipramine were less depressed than when they were continuously on lithium. In their most recent study, Angst and co-workers (1970) presented data from psychiatric clinics in

Glostrup, Prague, and Zurich for 244 patients who suffered from recurrent affective disorders and were treated prophylactically with lithium. The disease course was followed by recording the numbers of psychotic episodes and hospital admissions and the duration of cycles and episodes.

Lithium treatment led to a pronounced and statistically significant reduction in the number of both episodes and hospital admissions. This was demonstrated at all three clinics and for each of the affective disorders, manic-depressive psychosis, recurrent depressive psychosis, and schizo-affective psychosis. Duration of cycles decreased with increasing age at first episode and increasing number of previous episodes. There was a slight decrease of episode duration with increasing number of episodes.

Lithium treatment also led to a statistically significant prolongation of the cycles, considerable in manic-depressive and recurrent depressive psychosis, and moderate in schizo-affective psychosis. In manic-depressive patients, there was a statistically significant shortening of episodes during lithium treatment. Again, as reported by Angst, Dittrich, and Grof (1969), there is no explicitness regarding the type of relapse (manic or depressive) affected in the bipolar patients. The claim of a prophylactic effect on schizophrenic subjects is the widest extension of all prophylactic claims for lithium.

From among a larger group of manic-depressive patients, Baastrup et al. (1970) (see also Schou 1970) selected 88 patients who (1) had two or more manic-depressive episodes during one year, or one or more episodes per year during at least two years before being started on lithium; and (2) had been given lithium continuously for at least twelve months. The patients were observed for six and one-half years; lithium was administered prophylactically for periods of one to five years. For each patient the relapse frequency (that is, average number of episode starts per year) was evaluated for the periods without lithium and with lithium, so that the patients served as their own controls in that relapse frequencies observed during the period without lithium were used to calculate the relapse frequencies to be expected during the lithium period.

In this study, the differences in relapse frequency between periods without lithium and with lithium were statistically significant at the $p < 0.001$ level. For the group as a whole, it was found that without lithium treatment the patient spent an average of thirteen weeks a year in a psychotic state, as compared to less than two weeks with lithium treatment.

Lithium prevented relapses with equal efficacy in patients having both mania and depression, and in patients with a history of depression only. A small group of atypical cases characterized by delusions, especially of persecution, responded less well. The prophylactic action of lithium was equally good in young, middle-aged, and old patients; it was also independent of duration of the illness.

In 18 of the 88 patients, relapses occurred despite continuous lithium treatment. One-third of the patients who relapsed belonged to the group of atypical cases characterized by delusions, especially of persecution. Again, atypical clinical features are obviously unfavorable for lithium prophylaxis.

In addition to the effect against manias and depressions of psychotic intensity, the author noted that, even between psychotic phases, lithium treatment led to emotional stabilization.

Although the prophylactic studies of the use of lithium have come under serious criticism on statistical and methodological grounds, they are, nevertheless, highly suggestive. If they are substantiated by further studies, it would then appear that lithium is not only effective against manic states but also against recurrences of both manic and depressive episodes. The possibility that lithium acts against both the polar manifestations of manic-depressive psychoses places it in a unique position among the psychotropic drugs, that of actually affecting the disease entity rather than simply alleviating symptomatic manifestations. It may thus warrant a more specific labeling as a mood normalizer or "thymoleptic."

Dibenzocycloheptenes

Stromgren and Stromgren (1962) indicated that amitriptyline exhibited a prophylactic effect against manic as well as depressive relapses.

IV. BEHAVIORAL TOXICITY

The concept of drug-induced "behavioral toxicity" or "behavioral side effects" has been so recently coined that a definition of what it encompasses or excludes has yet to take form. To Cole (1960), who first described the phrase as it applied to human beings, behavioral toxicity included "adverse" subjective mood changes and "decrements in objective performance" resulting from drug ingestion. The description included both behavioral changes resulting directly from the drug and such changes in response to the perception of non-behavioral effects as the "Parkinsonian syndrome."

The chemotherapy for manic-depressive illness underscores the capacity of psychotropic agents to alter emotional or mood states in certain clinically desirable directions. Some agents alter mood in a manner or direction that may be considered adverse. Two major types of drug-induced mood changes have been reported in this regard: "paradoxical" and "pendular" effects (DiMascio and Shader 1968). Such drug-induced changes are not limited to mood; similar alterations in the pattern of gross behavior also occur.

"Paradoxical" drug effects are alterations in mood or behavior in a direction opposite to the "clinically desirable" one for which the drug has been prescribed. Antidepressant drugs have "paradoxically" induced a deepening of depressive affect (Cole, Griffith, and Kaye 1965; DiMascio, Meuer, and Stifler 1968), and the imipramines (Berthiaume 1959; Fotel-Andersen and Geert-Jorgensen 1959; Hohn et al. 1961; Pilkington 1962; Rikovsky 1964; Klein 1965), amitriptyline (Hudgens et al. 1966), as well as monoamine oxidase (MAO) inhibitors (Johnson and Eilenberg 1960; Clarke 1960; Kruse and Hoermann 1960; Barsa and Saunders 1962) have paradoxically or "atypically" induced psychotic reactions manifested by confusion, thought disorganization, disorientation, visual and auditory hallucinations, distortion of perception, depersonalization, as well as concomitant affect changes. Neuroleptic compounds have paradoxically induced acute psychotic reactions accompanied by confusion and disorientation (Malitz, Hough, and Lesse 1956; Sarwer-Foner et al. 1959; Lang and Moore 1960; Sher 1962; Chaffin 1964). Recent reports indicate also that lithium can produce a toxic-confusional state, as well as aggravation of core psychopathology in schizophrenic patients (Johnson, Gershon, and Hekimian 1968; Shopsin, Kim, and Gershon 1970; Shopsin, Johnson, and Gershon 1970).

"Pendular" drug effects are drug-induced alterations that proceed in a "desired" direction to the degree (over-reactions) that the resultant state tends towards an opposite state for which the drug was initially administered. For example, chlorpromazine is known to reduce the affective expression of excited manic patients to a level that the depressive affect becomes a predominant feature (Ayd 1958; Gradwell 1960). MAO inhibitors and imipramine relieve depression, substituting for it a state of euphoria (Cole and Weiner 1960; Brune and Himwich 1963; Klein 1965). Antidepressant agents can have a pendular effect on gross behavior patterns as well. The mood-elevating and stimulating properties of imipramine (Berthiaume 1959; Hohn et al. 1961; Brune and Himwich 1963; Klein 1965), nortryptamine (Sarwer-Foner et al. 1959; Bennett 1962), and various MAO inhibitors (Sarwer-Foner et al. 1959; Kruse and Hoermann 1960; Imlah 1960; Chu and Fogel 1962; Goldberg 1964) have resulted in retarded, depressed patients passing through the desired state and becoming euphoric, hypomanic, outwardly hostile, overly talkative with flight of ideas. Poldinger (1963) reported that depressed patients pretreated with imipramine or desmethylimipramine dramatically improved after two days of reserpine administration. Improvement followed the induction of a transient mania. Systematically studying the reserpine mood reversal phenomenon, Haskovec and Rysanek (1967) indicated that this drug combination in man was "associated with a conspicuous stimulating effect" that resembled the mood reversals occasionally occurring in manic-depressive disease.

Indications are that these drug-induced behavioral side effects are neither as rare nor as unexpected as the literature would have one believe. There are a number of reasons for this point of view (DiMascio and Shader 1968): the definition of what constitutes "behavioral toxicity" has never been clearly set down; the symptom complex of "behavioral toxicity" is so highly intertwined with the clinical status of the patient that it is difficult to recognize and isolate it as being a result of drug administration; the statistical procedures of reporting results of objective methods for quantifying drug actions as group averages often obscure bi-directional changes; in reporting extreme drug responses, extreme positive responses may be mentioned, whereas extreme negative or adverse ones are seldom included. Regardless of the frequency of such extreme effects, the therapeutic consequences of these reactions are such that they demand increased awareness of the phenomena and more extensive investigation aimed at explaining them. These problems emphasize, among other things, the need for diagnostic precision in delineating and evaluating the therapeutic specificity of a particular chemical agent in the treatment for manic-depressive disorder.

V. PSYCHOACTIVE DRUGS VERSUS OTHER FORMS OF THERAPY

Of the various forms of therapy available, what may we conclude is the appropriate antimanic treatment of choice? Lacking from the evaluation of any particular treatment modality, including psychoactive drugs, are controlled studies of mania comparing one form of therapy to another. There have been no comparisons of drug therapy versus ECT, or drug therapy combined with ECT, nor have there been any trials comparing chemotherapy with pharmacologically induced convulsive treatment for mania. There are no available reports on drugs and conditioning, combined therapy with drugs and hormones, drugs and occupation therapy, drugs and milieu therapy, or drugs and psychotherapy. Since even the classic Freudian psychotherapists acknowledge the futility of analysis for manic patients ("the free interval is obviously the period of choice for analytic efforts,"-- Fenichel 1945), and ECT presents the disadvantages of organic insult as well as other physical liabilities, chemotherapy emerges as the most advantageous form of intervention in the treatment of manic patients.

VI. PSYCHOACTIVE DRUG CHOICE

Although it would appear that lithium exerts the most specific pharmacological control in normalizing a manic episode, an acute attack is managed effectively and often more rapidly with haloperidol, chlorpromazine, or intensive ECT. In cases of more protracted mania, frequent manic relapse, or the more attenuated hypomanic states, lithium seems particularly superior to any other therapy.

The severity of illness, management, and the patient's willingness to cooperate, as well as his known previous response or intolerance to a given drug treatment can govern the choice of initial treatment. For example, a positive medication effect in the past may determine initial drug treatment; spontaneous remission may have been confused with pharmacological effect, however, and the changing biological reactivity of patients may diminish treatment response or render the drug ineffective later. On the other hand, if the drug treatment was unsuccessful in the past, it need not necessarily be excluded from consideration, since underdosage is so prevalent, and useful drugs may easily be mistaken as ineffective.

Various psychoactive drug therapies may be effectively combined. For instance, administration of chlorpromazine or haloperidol may reasonably supplement lithium treatment until the unique and normalizing effects of the latter can be realized in eight to ten days. In milder cases, barbiturates or chloral hydrate may be used for sedation or behavioral control in cases where lithium alone is used. ECT is frequently, if not usually, accompanied by concomitant use of chlorpromazine or haloperidol.

VII. GENERAL CONCLUSIONS AND PRINCIPLES OF DRUG TREATMENT

Perhaps the best way to delineate the most appropriate drug treatment or treatments for mania as well as cyclic manic-depressive relapses would be to ask, "What is, in fact, needed to treat this disorder?" Ideally, a rapid, normalizing effect without sedation, overtranquilization, or other untoward side effects would be most desirable against the acute manic phase. Preventing manic or depressive relapses should (also ideally) be accomplished with a drug that maintains a patient in this normalized condition under the same specifications, with the added qualification that it produce no harmful side effects with long-term use.

Realistically, a logical approach to treatment for an acute manic episode would include the concurrent administration of a major tranquilizer with lithium carbonate. Greater treatment efficacy may be achieved with intramuscular administration of the neuroleptic drug, if available (e.g., haloperidol is not available for intramuscular use in the United States). Both medications, that is, lithium and a neuroleptic, should be initiated simultaneously, and when behavioral and motor control is achieved, dosage of the latter can be diminished (toward the eighth to tenth day of treatment). Since only lithium has been explored for its prophylactic effects against manic-depressive recurrences, and in view of the highly suggestive data now accumulated for this drug, lithium can be considered as the maintenance treatment of choice for any patient with a history of deleterious recurrences of cyclic manic-depressive disorder. Although the evidence for its prevention of acute unipolar depressive relapses is by far less convincing, there are no other psychoactive drugs that have been explored with equal intensity or whose effects have proved more beneficial in this respect.

As with any potent drug, toxicity is inevitable, and to justify its use, the severity of the presenting condition and the likelihood of benefit must be balanced against the risk of various side effects. This same consideration holds for the late side effects or complications developing during maintenance therapy, and it is here that lithium may fall from favor and again be shelved as a potentially harmful agent. Then, too, the growth in the number of new psychoactive drugs is mind-boggling for most medical practitioners, and skill in the use of drugs requires, in addition to knowledge of their pharmacologic properties, sensitivity to their psychologic implications. The use of lithium in the treatment for mania underscores these requirements.

In reviewing the vast and bewildering array of controlled and open trials of drugs in the treatment for mania, it may be concluded that the clinical activity of lithium endows it with unique pharmacological properties, which are distinctive from the rest of the field. Thus lithium is an agent with many of the clinical properties of a major tranquilizer, but it does not exhibit a significant degree of sedative activity, and it does not produce drowsiness in manic patients while controlling marked degrees of psychomotor and behavioral overactivity. The quality of the lithium response in mania is quite different from that produced by neuroleptics; this differential quality of clinical activity tends also to support the notion of psychopharmacological specificity of this ion. Differences between lithium and the other major tranquilizers are clearly established in that preclinical psychopharmacological screening profiles do not exhibit positive activity for lithium. The most exciting aspect of lithium's use in affective disorders as well as its valuable contribution to the field of medicine may yet prove to lie in the stimulus it provides to biochemical and physiologic investigation of brain function in relation to mood changes. Both lithium and the newer compounds, such as α-MPT, methysergide, cinnanserin, and propranolol, are helping to resolve the age-old dichotomy between "dynamic" and "organic" psychiatry by expressing an account of affective illness based, as far as possible, on etiology.

VIII. PROBLEMS OF DRUG EVALUATION IN MANIA: RESEARCH DESIGN AND METHODOLOGY

All issues relevant to the evaluation of any psychoactive drug apply to those used in the study of manic disorder. However, additional difficulties arise in mania from such inherent features as differential diagnosis, the self-limiting, recurring nature of the disease, and the lack of sensitive rating devices tailored specifically to study this disorder. Secondary logistic difficulties also contribute to the problem, including the relative infrequency of the disease, management problems, the nature of behavioral disturbance and spontaneous remissions, all of which are characteristic of the disorder.

Differential diagnosis is central to the problems of evaluating drug efficacy in mania (Johnson, Gershon, and Hekimian 1968; Hekimian et al. 1969; Shopsin, Kim, and Gershon 1970). If the aim of chemotherapy is greater specificity, then diagnostic explicitness is clearly germane to methodological problems in this area. The artless criteria generally used in establishing a diagnosis of cyclic manic-depressive psychosis are reflected in the differences in treatment outcome (Zall, Therman, and Myers 1968; Lipkin, Dyrud, and Meyer 1970) and in incidence of this disorder. The latter varies radically from 0.1 percent of all psychiatric hospital admissions seen at Bellevue Hospital in New York, to 5 percent (Bratfos and Haug 1968), and 30 percent (Noyes 1954) in other centers, as well as 3 to 4 per 100,000 persons of the general population (Redlich and Freedman 1966).

Criteria of effectiveness. Of the few control studies of manic depressive illness available, most explore the comparison of the test drug against placebo (Schou et al. 1954; Maggs 1963), and only in the minority has there been a comparison against another established psychoactive drug (Johnson, Gershon, and Hekimian 1968; Spring et al. 1970; Platman 1970). Lithium and chlorpromazine have been the only drugs tested in this fashion. Even in these contemporary studies, the objective criteria most frequently employed were global clinical judgments of change. The critical seriousness of such omissions in design cannot be emphasized too strongly. At the very least, minimal standards of effectiveness need to be instituted. The use of the NIMH Personal Data Inventory (PDI), for example, would provide a minimum in the collection of background data. The Bellevue Diagnostic Inventory (BDI) (Hekimian et al. 1969), and the Differential Diagnostic Scale (DDS) (Hekimian et al. 1969), records necessary information regarding the baseline psychopathology of patients entering a study. These latter scales (that is, BDI and DDS), as well as the Wittenborn and the Lorr-IMPS scales, attempt to measure specific parameters of manic pathology. It is disappointing that more explicit instruments for manic disorder are not available.

The Structured Clinical Interview (SCI) (Burdock and Hardesty 1968), however, may provide information on other psychopathological problems missed by the other rating devices, such as various motor and behavioral components. Other manifestations of behavior may be assessed more adequately by observing ward behavior as collected by the Nurse's Observation Scale for In-Patient Evaluation (NOSIE) and the Ward Behavior Inventory (WBI). Side effects data should be collected in uniform fashion, employing such instruments as the NIMH Treatment Emergency Symptom (TES) forms. Sleep records such as 24-hour sleep charts are of considerable value in manic states, since improvement in this parameter usually proceeds *pari passu* with general clinical improvement. The onset and speed of therapeutic activity, together with possible qualitative differences between two active drugs, are also important evaluations to be made.

Design. Depending upon the availability of information about the clinical pharmacology of the agent under investigation, an open design with maximum dosage flexibility is necessary in the early phases of evaluation, before control comparison studies are launched. Even in the controlled phase, fixed dosages established over a flexible incremental dose range are necessary to realize therapeutic responses or side effects of the drug under investigation. The issue of inadequate dosage has come up frequently in studies of lithium treatment for mania. This topic was recently re-opened by Dewhurst (1968) in discussing reports that attempt to evaluate the efficacy of methysergide for mania.

The current experimental designs for mania are limited because of the restrictions of sample size and the cyclic nature of the disease. Crossover trials, therefore, are not the most desirable in this condition. The study model using parallel treatment groups with randomly assigned drugs is perhaps the best available for this purpose. The test drug needs to be compared to a standard drug that is considered effective for this disorder and that exhibits a similar profile of behavioral effects. Ideally, the design should include a third group on placebo. An initial placebo period for all groups should be included to provide for drug washout, stabilization of level of pathology in the experimental environment, and to allow discard of cases attaining natural remission during the observation period. To refrain from using adjunctive chemotherapy is a critical, but delicate, issue in the study of this population, but such supplementary drug administration introduces a potential variable that is impossible to resolve in evaluating the test drug. Another possibly valuable design has been tried with lithium salts in manic patients. It is a controlled trial of both the drug and placebo, carried out with each patient individually. The drug sequence is applied in random fashion.

Prophylactic studies. It is quite obvious that the evaluation

of drug efficacy in the treatment of a particular affective episode
of manic-depressive disorder has been a conspicuously difficult task.
It may thus be readily appreciated that the determination of prophylactic efficacy of an agent against subsequent recurrences of mania
or depression constitutes a considerably greater and more complicated
undertaking. This difficulty is all the more serious in that the
cyclic nature of manic-depressive disease requires a therapy primarily designed to prevent the bipolar recurrences of this disorder.
Some of the design considerations reviewed above for drug studies
in manic disorder are applicable here as well. Other criteria for
evaluating drug efficacy in prophylactic studies differ from those
used in direct therapeutic trials; acceptable methods, however, have
yet to be developed.

Attempts to establish criteria are immediately in question,
since even the definitions of an "episode" and a "normal interval"
are in dispute, as is the assessment of any drug-related effect on
the magnitude of the manic-depressive sweep. In efforts to clarify
these issues, cruder criteria, such as "hospitalization," have been
utilized (Baastrup and Schou 1967). Numerous variables are involved
in evaluating the need for hospitalization, so that meaningful comparisons are extremely difficult. Another parameter central to any
interpretation of drug prophylaxis is the assessment of an individual's capacity to function at work (e.g., partial debilitation,
restitutio integrum, enhanced ability to function, and degrees of
each), and his level of success in interpersonal relations as well
as other situations.

Dosage schedules for maintenance are considered to be lower
than those required to treat a manifest episode. No definitive data
are available, however, of the ratio of dosage in the maintenance
phase compared to the acute episode. Another question is whether
one, two, or three comparable groups are necessary, including a
placebo population (Laurell and Ottosson 1968; Saran 1969). Since
adequate predictive standards for the course of manic recurrences
over a given period are not available, another logistic and statistical approach to follow-up studies is to evaluate the "drop-out."
The manner of handling "drop-out" statistics may give rise to the
greatest source of observer bias (Angst *et al.* 1970) in that a non-
responder with mild side effects, for example, could conceivably be
eliminated from the study, thereby significantly affecting overall
data outcome.

Another method in assessing drug efficacy in prophylactic studies has recently been demonstrated in a report by Baastrup *et al.*
(1970). The initial population studied by these investigators consisted of responders to treatment with the investigational drug during previous manic-depressive episodes. Under a discontinuation
procedure, the population was then randomly assigned to drug and (or)

placebo, forming two groups who were followed by a sequential analysis design. The patients served as their own controls in that relapse frequencies observed during the periods without lithium were used to calculate the relapse frequencies to be expected during the lithium periods. Such quantitative predictions are possible only when the group is sufficiently large, when the relapse frequency during pretreatment periods is sufficiently high, and when the observation periods are sufficiently long. With this investigational model, Schou (1970) reports the ability to clearly differentiate drug and placebo differences within six months, using a total population of eighty-eight patients. The differences in relapse frequency between periods without lithium and with lithium were of high statistical significance ($p < 0.001$).

Although this research design has considerable merit, it obviously presents certain difficulties that Schou himself has taken into consideration. Despite all the criticism this method may generate, it is the most useful in assessing prophylactic drug efficacy employed to date.

IX. MOOD DISORDERS IN CHILDREN AND ADOLESCENTS: DIAGNOSTIC PROBLEMS AND CHEMOTHERAPY WITH LITHIUM

If there are problems in evaluating chemotherapeutic agents for mania in adults, the dilemma is magnified, if not rendered impossible, regarding children. Psychiatrists do not even agree that children suffer from manic-depressive disorder. The problem of "classification" in child psychiatry has assumed such international importance that the World Health Organization established a committee to examine the world climate of opinion on this clinical issue (Miller 1968). The subject of the justification for diagnosing cyclic manic-depressions in children highlights the constitutional, clinical, and psychodynamic bewilderment surrounding the question. Many psychiatrists believe that this disease never appears before puberty, and that emotional disturbances seen in children are reactions to specific trauma or, in a number of cases, expressions of an underlying disorder such as schizophrenic illness. Others take the view that, although the occurrence is infrequent, true manic-depressive disorder is seen in children. In 1888, Mills held that all adult psychoses existed in childhood; Dixon and Greeves (1885) claimed to have observed mania frequently in childhood; to Hamilton (1903), cyclic insanity was not uncommon in troubled children; Kassanin (1931) observed affective psychoses; Kraepelin (1913) was satisfied with the facts of early onset, believing that there may be a genetic component influencing the mentality of the child from earliest infancy, but that it does not lead to a typical manic-depressive psychosis until later. Baker in 1930 also held with some force that mania was a disorder of childhood, with hallucinations and delusions. Harms (1952) described children between four and fourteen who had attacks of mania, and Creak (1952) contended that children, however infrequently, have manic-depressive psychoses. In 1952, the journal, *The Nervous Child*, published a special issue devoted to manic and depressive illness in childhood; most of the contributing authors maintained that manic-depressive illness does not occur in childhood, and that these affective states appear, rather, at puberty when such conditions are described as "prepsychotic" states. In reviewing the vast literature on the subject, the mind boggles to find that the story and the label have little concordance with our present definitions of the disorder.

Frommer (1968) believes that, regardless of the etiological content in which a child becomes depressed, depression in childhood may often go unrecognized and untreated, because its symptoms differ from those associated with depression in adults. She believes that "suffering in childhood tends to be ignored by a society which deludes itself that childhood is a halcyon period of life and fails to take the reality experienced by the child seriously." Stella Chess (1970) also recognizes childhood depression as a clinical entity, with the qualification that it appears as a reactive or secondary symptom underlying a more fundamental problem, e.g., school phobias, interpersonal family difficulties, etc.

To further complicate the issues, manifestations of mood disturbance in children may take the form of many physical complaints, including stomach pain, headache, or dizziness.

Lithium: Children. Based on these observations, it is extremely difficult to assess the results of some recent reports on lithium treatment for childhood manic-depressive disorder. Persuaded that many children suffer the pre-maturity and adolescent equivalence of manic-depressive disorder, Annell (1969) reported very effective results against manic symptoms in young Swedish children treated with lithium carbonate. "It is so definite when it works, you can practically name the day you'll see the change....generally four days after the therapeutic concentration of the drug in blood is reached. If the child is suffering a depression, the lithium effect appears less marked in that it seems only to remove some of the somatic symptoms." Annell believes that maintenance lithium therapy is good in preventing recurrences of mania, and partially successful in averting depressions. When discomfort and irritability continue, the addition of antidepressant drugs to lithium is "often quite excellent."

This author reports the clinical impression that lithium also yields good results in children whose illnesses are not basically mood disorders. She has described five such cases in which the primary disturbance was periodic stupor; a preliminary diagnosis of schizophrenia and/or organic brain damage was made in these patients.

Others among her lithium responders were first diagnosed as severely neurotic.

An assessment of lithium's effect in these children, therefore, is complicated by many issues. The dilemma of whether a diagnosis of mania is ever applicable in children is further complicated by the fact that many of the patients described by this author would be acknowledged by many clinicians as schizophrenic. The diagnostic ambiguities applicable in the adult are also operative here. Perhaps the most critical issue in questioning the validity of overall results is that lithium would appear useful in any child, regardless of presenting symptoms; such broad applicability, even for lithium, deserves serious critical evaluation.

Frommer (1968) also found lithium useful for emotionally disturbed children. Among them were children who showed behavior that, in an adult, would suggest hypomania. Lithium was also given a trial in other children, who were described as periodically falling into moods marked by depressive features (that is, somatic complaints) and temper outbursts of serious magnitude. Lithium therapy was successful in many such cases, and in the children with depressive features, whether it was given alone or in combination with other antidepressants, successful treatment outcome was reported.

Lithium: Adolescents. Concerning the effects of lithium on mood stability in young people, Klein (Gattozzi 1970) has given lithium to adolescents and young adults who, although not suffering attacks of typical manic-depressive illness, experienced high, giddy, hedonistic, impulsive symptoms that alternated with withdrawn, morose, sullen and depressive features. Their diagnosis was emotionally unstable character disorder. Finding that these patients did not respond well to antidepressant medications, and in efforts to avoid the "zombified" feelings that phenothiazines produced (although they offer better results than the antidepressants), Klein gave lithium to a small number of such subjects. Initial results were reported as excellent, with a stabilization of emotional volatility.

At the time of writing, several studies involving the use of lithium in children and adolescents are under way. Two such studies are being carried out in New York University-Bellevue Medical Center. The results of these studies will help clarify the conclusions drawn from the statements of Annell, Frommer, and Klein.

Whether or not manic-depressive disorder exists in children remains an open question. The general psychiatric consensus in the United States does not recognize mania as a diagnostic entity in childhood, and there is no provision for such nomenclature in the American Psychiatric Association's diagnostic manual. Longitudinal studies will be required to help resolve this problem eventually and, in this regard, it may be meaningful to delineate and study certain affective, behavioral, and motor components in children showing hyperkinesis as well as other behavioral disturbances. Such descriptive categories can eventually establish common references for comparing treatment groups, even in the face of disagreement on the criteria for applying classic diagnostic terms to children. Fish and Shapiro (1965) have developed a typology of children's psychiatric disorders in which patterns and degrees of integrative disturbance may reflect the level and severity of the defect. Rating children on the basis of social, language, affect, and motor symptoms (SLAM) (Fish 1968), as well as for global severity, resulting operational definitions for both the initial state and the specific types of change may represent a better index to determine which children will respond to a given drug and in what manner.

ACKNOWLEDGMENT

This work was supported by USPHS Grants MH 04669 and MH 17436.

REFERENCES

Abdulla, Y. H., and Hámadah, K. 1970. 3,5-Cyclic adenosine monophosphate in depression and mania. *Lancet* 1:378.

Akimoto, H. 1962. In Normothymics, "mood normalizers" by M. Schou. *Brit. J. Psychiat.* 109:803 (1963).

Akimoto, H.; Nakakuki, M.; Honda, Y.; Takahashi, Y.; and Toyoda, J. 1961. Clinical evaluation of the effect of central stimulants, MAO inhibitors, and imipramine in the treatment of affective disorders. *Proceedings of Third World Congress of Psychiatry* 2:958.

Andersen, H., and Kristiansen, E. S. 1959. Tofranil treatment of endogenous depression. *Acta Psychiat. Scand.* 34:387.

Andreani, G.; Caselle, A.; and Martelli, G. 1958. Clinical and electrographic findings in the treatment of mania with lithium salts. *G. Psichiat. Neuropat.* 83:273.

Angrist, B. M.; Gershon, S.; Levitan, S. J.; and Blumberg, A. G. 1968. Lithium induced "diabetes insipidus"-like syndrome. *Compr. Psychiat.* 11(no. 2):141.

Angst, J. 1966. *Zur Aetiologie und Nosologie Endogener Depressiver Psychosen.* Berlin: Springer-Verlag, p. 197.

Angst, J.; Dittrich, A.; and Grof, P. 1969. Course of endogenous affective psychoses and its modification by prophylactic administration of imipramine and lithium. *Int. Pharmacopsychiat.* 2:1.

Angst, J.; Weis, P.; Grof, P.; Baastrup, P.; and Schou, M. 1970. Lithium prophylaxis in recurrent affective disorders. *Brit. J. Psychiat.* 116(no. 535):604.

Angyal, L. 1967. Clinical experiences with the application of halopendol to mental patients. *Ther. Hung.* 15:155.

Annell, A. I. 1969. Lithium in the treatment of children and adolescents. *Acta Psychiat. Scand.* Suppl. 207:19.

Araki, I.; Ito, M.; Kostyuk, P.; Oscarsson, O.; and Oshima, I. 1965. The effects of alkaline cations on the responses of cat spinal neurons and their removal from the cell. *Proc. Roy. Soc. (Biol.)* 162:319.

Aronoff, M. S., and Epstein, R. S. 1969. Lithium failure in mania: A clinical study. Read at annual meeting of American Psychiatric Association, Bal Harbor, Florida.

Atkinson, R. M., and Ditman, K. S. 1965. Tranylcypromine: A review. *Clin. Pharmacol. Ther.* 6:631.

Ayd, F. J. 1958. Drug-induced depression: Fact or fallacy? *New York J. Med.* 58:354.

Ayd, F. J. 1961. Psychopathic reactions to antidepressant drugs. *J. Neuropsychiat.* 2:119.

Baastrup, P. C. 1964. The use of lithium in manic-depressive psychosis. *Compr. Psychiat.* 5:396.

Baastrup, P. C. 1967. Report to symposium, Lithium and Goitre, Risskov, Denmark.

Baastrup, P. C., and Schou, M. 1967. Lithium as a prophylactic agent. Its effect against recurrent depressions and manic-depressive psychosis. *Arch. Gen. Psychiat.* 16:162.

Baastrup, P. C. 1968. Supplementary information about lithium treatment of manic-depressive disorders. *Acta Psychiat. Scand.* Suppl. 203:149.

Baastrup, P. C.; Poulson, J. C.; Schou, M.; Thomsen, K.; and Amidsen, A. 1970. Prophylactic lithium: Double blind discontinuation in manic-depressive and recurrent-depressive disorders. *Lancet* 2(no. 7668):326.

Baillarger, J. 1853-1854. Note on the type of insanity with attacks characterized by two regular periods, one of depression and one of excitation. *Bull. Acad. Nat. Med. (Paris)* 19:340.

Baker 1930. In *Foundations of Child Psychiatry*. E. Miller (ed.). 1st. Ed. New York: Pergamon Press (1968), p. 262.

Baldessarini, R. J., and Stephens, J. H. 1970. Lithium carbonate for affective disorders. *Arch. Gen. Psychiat.* 22(no. 1):72.

Ban, T. A. 1969. The rauwolfias. In *Psychopharmacology*, ch. 11. Baltimore: Williams & Wilkins, p. 222.

Ban, T. A. 1969. The buterophenones. In *Psychopharmacology*, ch. 12. Baltimore: Williams & Wilkins, p. 238.

Ban, T. A. 1969. The thioxanthenes. In *Psychopharmacology*, ch. 13. Baltimore: Williams & Wilkins, p. 256.

Ban, T. A.; Papathomopulos, E.; and Schwartz, L. 1962. Clinical studies with thioproperazine (Majeptil). *Compr. Psychiat.* 3:284.

Barsa, J. A., and Kline, N. S. 1955. Treatment of 200 disturbed psychotics with reserpine. *J.A.M.A.* vol. 158.

Barsa, J. A., and Saunders, J. C. 1962. Tranylcypromine in the treatment of chronic schizophrenics. *Amer. J. Psychiat.* 118:933.

Bauer, A. 1962. Clinical experiences with thioridazine (Mellaril) on mental syndromes. Comparison with chlorpromazine and promazine. *Canad. Med. Assoc. J.* 81:549.

Bennett, I. F. 1962. The constellations of depression: Its treatment with nortriptyline. II. Clinical evaluation of nortriptyline. *J. Nerv. Ment. Dis.* 135:59.

Bennie, R. H., and Fell, G. S. 1969. Relapses during lithium therapy. *Lancet* 2:1252.

Bercel, N. A. 1961. Clinical trial of thioridazine in private practice. *Amer. Pract. Digest Treat.* 12:44.

Berens, S. C.; Bernstein, R. S.; Robbins, J.; and Wolff, J. 1969. The antithyroid effects of lithium. Paper presented at American Thyroid Association, Chicago, Illinois.

Berens, S. C.; Wolff, J.; and Murphy, D. L. 1970. Lithium concentration by the thyroid. Submitted for publication.

Berthiaume, M. 1959. Alteration of the clinical picture during Tofranil therapy. *Canad. Psychiat. Assoc. J.* Suppl. 4:187.

Bratfos, O., and Haug, J. O. 1968. The course of manic depressive psychosis. *Acta Psychiat. Scand.* 44:89.

Brune, G. G., and Himwich, H. E. 1963. Biogenic amines and behavior in schizophrenic patients. In *Recent Advances in Biological Psychiatry*. J. Wortis (ed.). vol. 5. New York: Plenum Press, p. 144.

Bunney, W. E.; Brodie, H. K. H.; Murphy, D. L.; Goodwin, F. K. 1970. Studies of amine precursors and synthesis inhibitors in depression and mania. Presented to 123rd annual meeting of American Psychiatric Association, San Francisco.

Burdock, E. I., and Hardesty, A. S. 1968. A psychological test for psychopathology. *J. Abnorm. Psychol.* 73:62.

Cade, J. F. J. 1949. Lithium salts in the treatment of psychotic excitement. *Med. J. Aust.* 36:349.

Cadoret, R. J.; Winokur, G.; and Clayton, P. J. 1970. Family history studies: VII. Manic depressive disease versus depressive disease. *Brit. J. Psychiat.* 116(no. 535):625.

Chaffin, D. S. 1964. Phenothiazine-induced acute psychotic reaction: The "psychotoxicity" of a drug. *Amer. J. Psychiat.* 121:26.

Chess, S. 1970. Personal communication.

Chu, J., and Fogel, E. J. 1962. Clinical evaluation of the thymoleptic effect of tranylcypromine. *J. Indiana Med. Assoc.* 56:40.

Clark, W. G., and del Giudice, J. (eds.) 1970. *Principles of Psychopharmacology*. New York: Academic Press.

Clarke, J. 1960. Side-effects of phenelzine. *Brit. Med. J.* 1:1204.

Cole, J. O. 1960. Behavioral toxicity. In *Drugs and Behavior*. L. Uhr and J. G. Miller (eds.). New York: John Wiley and Sons, p. 375.

Cole, J., and Davis, J. M. 1968. Clinical efficacy of the phenothiazines as antipsychotic drugs. In *Psychopharmacology: A Review of Progress - 1957-1967*. D. H. Efron (ed.). Washington, D.C.: U.S. Govt. Printing Office, p. 1057.

Cole, L.; Griffith, C.; and Kaye, H. 1965. Anginal pain and depression. A preliminary investigation. *Dis. Chest* 48:584.

Cole, R. A., and Weiner, M. F. 1960. Clinical and theoretical observations on phenelzine (Nardil), an anti-depressant agent. *Amer. J. Psychiat.* 117:361.

Colombi, D., and Ferrio, L. 1965. Results with thioridazine administered to a group of patients with chronic psychoses. *Riv. Sper. Freniat.* 89:717.

Coppen, A. 1967. The biochemistry of affective disorders. *Brit. J. Psychiat.* 113:1237.

Coppen, A.; Prange, A. J., Jr.; Whybrow, P. C.; Noguera, R.; and Paez, J. M. 1969. Methysergide in mania, a controlled trial. *Lancet* 2:338.

Couleon, M.; Couleon, H.; Anne, L.; Blohorn, R.; Clerc, G.; and Guiraldo Trengualye, J. P. 1964. Treatment of states of psychomotor excitement, especially of acute mania by combination of thioridazine, Nembutal, and ECT. *Ann. Med. Psychol.* 122(II):752.

Creak, E. M. 1952. A letter. *Nervous Child* 9:317.

Davenport, V. D. 1950. Distribution of parenterally administered lithium in plasma, brain and muscle of rats. *Amer. J. Physiol.* 163:633.

D'Elia, G., and Rocco, P. G. 1963. Use of questionnaires in a clinico-pharmacological trial of Mellaril, *Ann. Freniatria* 76:358.

Dewhurst, W. G. 1968. Methysergide in mania. *Nature* 219(no. 5153):506.

DiMascio, A.; Meuer, R. E.; and Stifler, L. 1968. Effects of imipramine on individuals varying in level of depression. *Amer. J. Psychiat.* 124(suppl.):55.

DiMascio, A., and Shader, R. I. 1968. Behavioral toxicity. In *Psychopharmacology: A Review of Progress - 1957-1967.* D.H. Efron (ed.). Washington, D.C.: U.S. Govt. Printing Office, p. 551.

Dixon and Greeves 1885. In *Foundations of Child Psychiatry.* E. Miller (ed.). 1st Ed. New York: Pergamon Press (1968), p. 262.

Domino, E. F. 1968. Substituted phenothiazine antipsychotics. In *Psychopharmacology: A Review of Progress - 1957-1967.* D.H. Efron (ed.). Washington, D.C.: U.S. Govt. Printing Office, p. 1045.

Dousa, T., and Hechter, O. 1970. The effect of NaCl and LiCl on vasopressin-sensitive adenyl cyclase. *Life Sci.* 9(part I):765.

Drill, V. A. 1958. *Pharmacology in Medicine.* 2nd Ed. New York: McGraw-Hill.

Entwistle, C.; Taylor, R. M.; and MacDonald, I. A. 1962. The treatment of mania with haloperidol (Serenace). *Journal of Mental Science* 108:373.

Esplin, D. W., and Zablocka, B. 1965. Central nervous system stimulants. Ch. 18. In *The Pharmacological Basis of Therapeutics.* S. L. Goodman and A. Gilman (eds.). 3rd Ed. New York: MacMillan, p. 352.

Falret, J. P. 1853-1854. *Clinical Lectures on Mental Medicine. General Symptomatology.* Paris: Bailliere, p. 188.

Falret, J. P. 1864. *On Mental Diseases*. Paris: Bailliere, p. 188.
Fenichel, O. 1945. *The Psychoanalytic Theory of Neurosis*. New York: W. W. Norton, p. 413.
Fieve, R. 1970. Lithium studies and manic-depressive illness. Presented to 60th annual meeting of American Psychopathological Assn., New York City.
Fieve, R. R.; Platman, S. R.; and Plutchik, R.R. 1968a. The use of lithium in affective disorders. I. Acute endogenous depression. *Amer. J. Psychiat.* 125:487.
Fieve, R. R.; Platman, S. R.; and Plutchik, R. R. 1968b. The use of lithium in affective disorders. II. Prophylaxis of depression in chronic recurrent affective disorders. *Amer. J. Psychiat.* 125:492.
Filotto, J. *et al.* 1967. Thiothixene in the treatment of affective psychoses: A pilot study. Presented at Q.P.R.A. symposium on thioxanthenes, Montreal, Canada.
Fink, M.; Kahn, R. L.; Karp, E.; Pollack, M.; Green, M. A.; Alan, B.; and Lefkowitz, H. J. 1961. Inhalant-induced convulsions. *Arch. Gen. Psychiat.* 4:259.
Fish, B. 1968. Methodology in child psychopharmacology. In *Psychopharmacology: A Review of Progress - 1957-1967*. D. H. Efron (ed.). Washington, D.C.: U.S. Govt. Printing Office, p. 989.
Fish, B., and Shapiro, T. 1965. A typology of children's psychiatric disorders. I. Its application to a controlled evaluation of treatment. *J. Amer. Acad. Child Psychiat.* 4(no. 1):32.
Fotel-Andersen, K., and Geert-Jorgensen, E. 1959. Treatment of endogenous depression with Tofranil. *Ugeskr. Laeg.* 121:1091.
Fries, H. 1969. Experience with lithium carbonate treatment at a psychiatric department in the period 1964-1967. *Acta Psychiat. Scand.* Suppl. 207:41.
Frommer, F. A. 1968. Depressive illness in childhood. In *Recent Developments in Affective Disorders*. A. Coppen and A. Walk (eds.). *Brit. J. Psychiat.* Spec. Pub. No. 2, p. 117.
Fursham, P. H. 1965. The suprarenal glands (adrenal glands). In *The Ciba Collection of Medical Illustrations, Endocrine System and Selected Metabolic Diseases*. F. H. Netter (ed.). Vol. 4. Ciba Pharmaceutical Co., p. 84 and 105.
Gattozzi, A. A. 1970. *Lithium in the Treatment of Mood Disorders*. Washington, D.C.: National Clearing House for Mental Health Information, Publication No. 5033.
Gershon, S. 1968. Use of lithium salts in psychiatric disorders. *Dis. Nerv. Syst.* 29:51.
Gershon, S. 1970. Lithium in mania. *Clin. Pharmacol. Ther.* 11:168.
Gershon, S., and Trautner, E. M. 1956. Treatment of shock dependency by pharmacological agents. *Med. J. Aust.* 1:783.
Gershon, S., and Yuwiler, A. 1960. Lithium ion: A specific pharmacological approach to the treatment of mania. *J. Neuropsychiat.* 1:229.

Glessinger, B. 1954. Evaluation of lithium in treatment of psychotic excitement. *Med. J. Aust.* 41:277.
Goldberg, L. I. 1964. Monoamine oxidase inhibitors. *J.A.M.A.* 190:456.
Goldman, D. 1966. Drugs in treatment of psychosis. In *Psychiatric Drugs*. P. Solomon (ed.). New York: Grune and Stratton, p. 136.
Goldstein, B. J.; Clyde, D. J.; and Caldwell, J. M. 1968. Clinical efficacy of the butyrophenones as anti-psychotic drugs. In *Psychopharmacology: A Review of Progress - 1957-1967*. D.H. Efron (ed.). Washington, D.C.: U.S. Govt. Printing Office, p. 1085.
Gomez-Reino y Filgueira, J., and Fernandez-Vincente, L. 1962. Our experiences with Mellaril in endogenic manic and in chronic paranoid schizophrenia. *Actas Luso Esp. Neurol. Psiquiat.* p. 159.
Goodman, L. S., and Gilman, A. Z. 1956. *The Pharmacological Basis of Therapeutics*. 2nd Ed. New York: MacMillan.
Goodwin, F. K.; Murphy, D. L.; and Bunney, W. E., Jr. 1968. Lithium in mania and depression: A double-blind behavioral and biochemical study. Presented to annual meeting, American Psychiat. Assoc., Boston.
Gradwell, G. B. 1960. Psychotic reactions and phenelzine. *Brit. Med. J.* 2:1018.
Greenfield, I.; Zuger, M.; Bleak, R. M; and Bakal, S. F. 1950. Lithium chloride intoxication. *New York J. Med.* 50:459.
Greenspan, I.; Green, R.; and Durrell, J. 1968. Retention and distribution patterns of lithium, a pharmacological tool in studying the pathophysiology of manic-depressive psychosis. *Amer. J. Psychiat.* 125:512.
Gross, H., and Kaltenback, E. 1961. Erfahrung mit dem Thioxanthenderivat Chlorprothixen in der klinischen Psychiatrie. *Wien. Klin. Wschr.* 73:64.
Guistino, P. 1953. Il citrato di litio mel trattamento degli stati di eccitazione psicotica. *Note Psychiat.* 79:307.
Haefner, H.; Heyder, B.; and Kitscher, I. 1965. Undesirable side-effects and complications with the use of neuroleptic drugs. *Int. J. Neuropsychiat.* 1:46.
Hamilton 1903. In *Foundations of Child Psychiatry*. E. Miller (ed.) 1st Ed. New York: Pergamon Press (1968).
Harms, E. 1952. Differential pattern of manic-depressive disease in childhood. *Nervous Child* 9:326.
Hartigan, G. P. 1963. The use of lithium salts in affective disorders. *Brit. J. Psychiat.* 109:810.
Haskovec, L., and Rysanek, I. 1967. The action of reserpine in imipramine resistant depressed. *Psychopharmacologia (Berlin)* 11:18.
Haskovec, L., and Soucek, I. 1968. Trial of methysergide in mania. *Nature* 219(no. 5153):507.
Hekimian, L. J., and Gershon, S. 1967. Thioxanthenes: Some clinical and physiologic effects of a thioxanthene derivative, thiothixene, in twenty newly hospitalized male schizophrenics. *J. Clin. Pharmacol.* 7:52.

Hekimian, L. J.; Gershon, S.; Hardesty, A. S.; and Burdock, E. I. 1969. Drug efficacy and diagnostic specificity in manic-depressive illness and schizophrenia. *Dis. Nerv. Syst.* 30:747.

Heninger, G. R., and Mueller, P. S. 1970. Carbohydrate metabolism in mania. *Arch. Gen. Psychiat.* 23:310.

Herrera, J. J., and Vilaprino, J. J. 1964. Thioridazine in the treatment of manic-depressive psychosis. *Acta Psiquiat. Psicol. Amer. Lat.* 10:214.

Ho, A. K. S.; Loh, H.; Craves, F.; Hitzeman, R.; and Gershon, S. 1970. The effect of prolonged lithium treatment on the synthesis rate and turnover of monoamines in brain regions of rats. *Europ. J. Pharmacol.* 10:72.

Hohn, R.; Gross, G. M.; Gross, M; and Lasagna, L. 1961. A double-blind comparison of placebo and imipramine in the treatment of depressed patients in a state hospital. *J. Psychiat. Res.* 1:76.

Hollister, L. E. 1957. Complications from the use of tranquilizer drugs. *New Eng. J. Med.* 257:170.

Hospital Tribune. Sept. 21, 1970, p. 3.

Hudgens, R. W.; Tanna, V. L.; Harley, J. D.; and Leary, D. J., Jr. 1966. Visual hallucinations with iminodibenzyl antidepressants. *J.A.M.A.* 198:81.

Imlah, N. W. 1960. Overshooting action of phenelzine. *Lancet* 1:826.

Innes, I. R., and Nickerson, M. 1965. Anti-muscarinic or atropinic drugs. In *The Pharmacological Basis of Therapeutics*. S. L. Goodman and A. Gilman (eds.). 3rd Ed. New York: MacMillan, p. 521.

Itil, T. 1968. Early clinical and EEG drug evaluation studies. Psychiatric Research Foundation of Missouri (St. Louis) Publication No. 19. Presented at Early Clinical Drug Evaluation Units meeting, Miami, Fla.

Jacobsen, J. E. 1965. The hypomanic alert: A program designed for greater therapeutic control. *Amer. J. Psychiat.* 122:295.

Jarvik, M. E. 1965. Drugs used in treatment of psychiatric disorders. In *The Pharmacological Basis of Therapeutics*. S. L. Goodman and A. Gilman (eds.). 3rd Ed. New York: MacMillan, p. 178.

Johnson, G.; Gershon, S.; and Hekimian, L. J. 1968. Controlled evaluation of lithium and chlorpromazine in the treatment of manic states: An interim report. *Compr. Psychiat.* 9:563.

Johnson, G.; Hekimian, L.; and Gershon, S. 1970. Differential drug responsiveness in psychiatric subjects. Presented to 8th annual ACNP meeting, San Diego, California.

Johnson, G.; Maccarrio, M.; Gershon, S.; and Korein, J. 1970. The effects of lithium on EEG, behavior, and serum electrolytes. *J. Nerv. Ment. Dis.* 151:273.

Johnson, J., and Eilenberg, M. D. 1960. Psychotic reactions and phenelzine (Nardil). *Brit. Med. J.* 2:857.

Kassanin 1931. In *Foundations of Child Psychiatry*. E. Miller (ed.). 1st Ed. New York: Pergamon Press (1968), p. 262.

Klein, D. F. 1965. Behavioral effects of imipramine and phenothiazines: Implications for a psychiatric pathogenetic theory and theory of drug action. In *Recent Advances in Biological Psychiatry.* J. Wortis (ed.). New York: Plenum Press, vol. 7, p. 273.

Klein, D. F., and Davis, J. M. 1969. *Diagnosis and Drug Treatment of Psychiatric Disorders.* Baltimore: Williams & Wilkins, p. 222 and p. 313.

Kline, N. S. 1954. Use of rauwolfia serpentina benth. In *Neuropsychiatric Conditions.* Ann. N.Y. Acad. Sci. 59:107.

Kline, N. S. 1968. Lithium comes into its own (editorial). Amer. J. Psychiat. 125:150.

Kloos, H. H. 1967. Experiences with neuroleptic drugs - mainly thioridazine (Mellaril R) in clinical psychiatry. *Praxis* 56:1434.

Kolb, L. C. (ed.). 1968. *Noyes' Modern Clinical Psychiatry.* 7th Ed. Philadelphia: W. B. Saunders, p. 335.

Kraepelin, E. 1909-1913. *Thieme.* 8th Ed. Leipzig.

Kraepelin, E. 1913. *Psychiatrie. Ein Lehrbuch für Studierende und Ärzte.* Leipzig.

Kristjansen, P. 1962. In B. Gerle (ed.): Clinical observations of the side effects of haloperidol. Acta Psychiat. Scand. 40:65 (1964).

Kruse, W., and Hoermann, M. G. 1960. Clinical evaluation of four anti-depressant drugs. Curr. Ther. Res. 2:111.

Kurland, A. A.; Cuervo, R.; and Krantz, J. C., Jr. 1960. The intravenous use of hexafluorodiethyl ether as a convulsant in psychiatric treatment. J. Neuropsychiat. 1:260.

Lang, A. E., and Moore, R. A. 1961. Acute toxic psychosis concurrent with phenothiazine therapy. Amer. J. Psychiat. 117:939.

Lasky, J. J.; Klett, J. C.; Caffey, E. M.; Bennet, L. J.; Rosenblum, M. P.; and Hollister, L. E. 1962. Drug treatment of schizophrenic patients. Dis. Nerv. Syst. 23:698.

Laurell, B., and Ottosson, L. J. D. 1968. Prophylactic lithium? Letter to the editor. Lancet 2:1245.

Lehmann, H. E., and Ban, T. A. 1970. Clinical use of other antipsychotic agents. In *Principles of Psychopharmacology.* W. G. Clark and J. del Giudice (eds.). New York: Academic Press, p. 621.

Lehmann, H. E., and Hanrahan, G. E. 1954. Chlorpromazine, a new inhibiting agent for psychomotor excitement and manic states. Arch. Neurol. 71:227.

Leonhard, K. 1957. *Aufteilung der Endogenen Psychosen.* 1st Ed. Berlin.

Leonhard, K. 1966. *Aufteilung der Endogenen Psychosen.* 3rd Ed. Berlin.

Lipkin, K. M.; Dyrud, J.; and Meyer, G. G. 1970. The many faces of mania. Arch. Gen. Psychiat. (Chicago) 22:262.

Luby, E. 1968. Reserpine-like drugs - clinical efficacy. In *Psychopharmacology: A Review of Progress - 1957-1967.* D.H. Efron (ed.). Washington, D. C.: U.S. Govt. Printing Office, p. 1077.

Maggs, R. 1963. Treatment of manic illness with lithium carbonate. Brit. J. Psychiat. 109:56.

Malitz, S.; Hough, P. H.; and Lesse, S. 1956. Two year evaluation of chlorpromazine in clinical research and practice. *Amer. J. Psychiat.* 113:540.

Massaut, C.; Chantraine, J.; Meunce, E.; Pairoux, R.; Paguay, J.; Arnould, F.; Burton, P.; Tinant, M.; and Piersotte, J. 1962. Clinical study of 162 patients treated with a new neuroleptic: clopenthixol (Sordinol R). *Acta Neurol. Belg.* 62:651.

Mayer-Gross, W.; Slater, E.; and Roth, M. 1969. *Clinical Psychiatry*. 3rd Ed. London: Bailliere, Tindall & Cassell, p. 232.

Mayfield, D., and Brown, R. G. 1966. The clinical laboratory and electroencephalographic effects of lithium. *J. Psychiat. Res.* 4:207.

McCabe, M. S.; Reich, T.; and Winokur, G. 1970. Methysergide as a treatment for mania. *Amer. J. Psychiat.* 127:354.

McNeil Laboratories 1970. Personal communication, V. Slotnick.

Melia, P. I. 1967. A pilot trial of lithium carbonate in recurrent affective disorders. *J. Irish Med. Assoc.* 60:160.

Melia, P. I. 1970. Prophylactic lithium: A double-blind trial in recurrent affective disorders. *Brit. J. Psychiat.* 116:621.

Meyler, L. 1966. Side effects of drugs: Adverse reactions as reported by the medical literature of the world 1963-1965. Vol. 5. New York: Excerpta Medica Foundation, p. 16.

Miller, E. 1968. The problem of classification in child psychiatry. In *Foundations of Child Psychiatry*. 1st Ed. E. Miller (ed.). New York: Pergamon Press.

Mills 1888. In *Foundations of Child Psychiatry*. E. Miller (ed.). 1st Ed. New York: Pergamon Press, p. 262.

Moracci, E. 1931. Azione di alcuni sali applicati direttamente sui centri corticali sensitivo - motori del cane. *Arch. Fisiol.* 29:487.

Murphy, D. L.; Goodwin, F. K.; and Bunney, W. E. 1969. Aldosterone and sodium response to lithium administration in man. *Lancet* 2:458.

Noack, C. H., and Trautner, E. M. 1951. Lithium treatment of manic psychosis. *Med. J. Aust.* 2:219.

Noyes, A. P. 1954. *Modern Clinical Psychiatry*. 4th Ed. Philadelphia: W. B. Saunders.

O'Connell, R. A. 1970. Leucocytosis during lithium carbonate treatment. *Int. Pharmacopsychiat.* 4:30.

Penrose, L. 1945. Survey of cases of familial mental illness. Unpubl. manuscript, Ontario Dept. of Health.

Perris, C. 1966. A study of bipolar (manic-depressive) and unipolar recurrent depressive psychoses. *Acta Psychiat. Scand.* Suppl., p. 189.

Pfeiffer, C. Z.; Singh, M.; and Goldstein, L. 1969. Single dose-effect relationship of lithium on the electrical activity of cerebral cortex and of the heart. *J. Clin. Pharmacol.* 9:298.

Pilkington, T. L. 1962. A report on Tofranil. *Mental Deficiency* 66:729.

Platman, S. R. 1970. A comparison of lithium carbonate and chlorpromazine in mania. *Amer. J. Psychiat.* 127:351.

Platman, S. R., and Fieve, R. R. 1968. Lithium carbonate and plasma cortisol response in the affective disorders. *Arch. Gen. Psychiat.* 18:591.

Plenge, P.; Mellerup, E. T.; and Rafaelsen, O. J. 1969. Effects of lithium on carbohydrate metabolism. *Lancet* 1:1012.

Poldinger, W. 1963. Combined administration of desipramine and reserpine or tetrabenazine in depressed patients. *Psychopharmacologia (Berlin)* 4:308.

Radomski, J. L.; Fuyat, H. N.; Nelson, A. A.; and Smith, P. K. 1950. The toxic effects, excretion and distribution of lithium chloride. *J. Pharmacol. Exp. Ther.* 100:429.

Ramsden, E. N. 1970. Cyclic A.M.P. in depression and mania. *Lancet* 2:108.

Rapp, M. S. 1970. Prophylactic haloperidol in incipient hypomania. *Canad. Psychiat. Assoc. J.* 15:73.

Redlich, F. C., and Freedman, D. X. 1966. *The Theory and Practice of Psychiatry*. New York: Basic Books.

Rees, L., and Davies, B. 1965. A study of the value of haloperidol in the management and treatment of schizophrenic and manic patients. *Int. J. Neuropsychiat.* 1:263.

Rikovsky, S. 1964. Incidence of imipramine-induced psychoses. *Acta Nervosa Superior.* 6:181.

Rissetto, G., and Gazzano, G. 1952. Variazioni del sangue periferico nella intossicazione sperimentale da sali di litio. *Riv. Patol. Clin.* 7:202.

Rochford, J. M.; Detre, T.; Tucker, G. J.; and Harrow, M. 1970. Neuropsychological impairments in functional psychiatric disease. *Arch. Gen. Psychiat.* 22:114.

Samuels, A. J. 1951. Primary and secondary leucocyte changes following the intramuscular injection of epinephrine hydrochloride. *J. Clin. Invest.* 30:941.

Sandoz Pharmaceuticals 1970. Computer search - personal communication, K. Tashiro.

Saran, B. M. 1969. Lithium. Letter to the editor. *Lancet* 1:1208.

Sargent, W., and Slater, E. 1963. *An Introduction to Physical Methods of Treatment in Psychiatry*. London: Livingstone.

Sarwer-Foner, G. J.; Grauer, H.; MacKay, J.; and Koranyi, E. K. 1959. Depressive states and drugs. A study of the use of imipramine "Tofranil" in open psychiatric settings. *Med. Serv. J. Canada* 15:359.

Sarwer-Foner, G. J.; Koranyi, E. K.; Meszaros, A.; and Grauer, H. 1959. Depressive states and drugs. II. The study of phenelzine dihydrogen sulfate (Nardil) in open psychiatric settings. *Canad. Med. Assoc. J.* 81:9.

Schiele, B. C. 1967. Studies with clopenthixol and thiothixene. Presented to Symposium of the Thioxanthines, Montreal, Canada.

Schou, M. 1957. Biology and pharmacology of the lithium ion. *Pharmacological Reviews* 9:17.
Schou, M. 1958. Lithium studies. 1. Toxicity. *Acta Pharmacol.* 15:70.
Schou, M. 1958. Lithium studies. 3. Distribution between serum and tissues. *Acta Pharmacol.* 15:115.
Schou, M. 1959. Lithium in psychiatric therapy. *Psychopharmacologia (Berlin)* 1:65.
Schou, M. 1962. Electrocardiographic changes during treatment with lithium and with drugs of the imipramine-type. *Acta Psychiat. Scand.* 38:331.
Schou, M. 1968. Lithium in psychiatry - A review. *Psychopharmacology: A Review of Progress - 1957-1967*. D. H. Efron (ed.). Washington, D.C.: U.S. Govt. Printing Office, p. 701.
Schou, M. 1970. Personal communication in *Lithium in the Treatment of Mood Disorders* by A. Gattozzi. Washington, D.C.: National Clearing House for Mental Health Information, Publ. No. 5033, p. 81.
Schou, M. 1970. Use of lithium. In *Principles of Psychopharmacology*. N. G. Clark and J. del Giudice (eds.). New York: Academic Press, p. 653.
Schou, M.; Amidsen, A.; Jensen, S. E.; and Olsen, T. 1968. Occurrence of goitre during lithium treatment. *Brit. Med. J.* 3:710.
Schou, M.; Juel-Nielson, N.; Stromgren, E.; and Voldby, H. 1954. The treatment of manic psychoses by the administration of lithium salts. *J. Neurol. Neurosurg. Psychiat.* 17:250.
Sedvall, G.; Jonsson, B.; Pettersson, U.; and Levin, K. 1968. Effects of lithium salts on plasma protein bound iodine and uptake of I-131 in thyroid gland of man and rat. *Life Sci.* 7:1257.
Serry, M. 1969. Lithium retention and response. *Lancet* 1:1267.
Sharpless, S. K. 1965. Hypnotics and sedatives. In *The Pharmacological Basis of Therapeutics*. S. L. Goodman and A. Gilman (eds.). 3rd Ed. New York: MacMillan, p. 132.
Sher, N. 1962. Hallucinations after chlorpromazine in an otosclerotic. *Amer. J. Psychiat.* 118:746.
Sherman, S. 1961. A clinical evaluation of Mellaril. *Amer. J. Psychiat.* 118:452.
Shopsin, B. 1970. Effects of lithium on thyroid function. *Dis. Nerv. Syst.* 31:237.
Shopsin, B.; Blum, M.; and Gershon, S. 1969. Lithium-induced thyroid disturbance: Case report and review. *Compr. Psychiat.* 10:215.
Shopsin, B.; Friedman, R.; and Gershon, S. 1970. The lithium ion related and blood dyscrasias. Submitted for publication.
Shopsin, B., and Gershon, S. 1970. Cortisol response to dexamethasone suppression in hospitalized depressives and control patients. *Arch. Gen. Psychiat.* In press.
Shopsin, B.; Gershon, S.; and Pinckney, L. 1969. The secretion of lithium in human mixed saliva: Effects of ingested lithium on elec-

trolyte distribution in saliva and serum. *Int. Pharmacopsychiat.* 2:148.

Shopsin, B.; Johnson, G.; and Gershon, S. 1970. Neurotoxicity with lithium; differential drug responsiveness. *Int. Pharmacopsychiat.* In press.

Shopsin, B.; Kim, S. S.; and Gershon, S. 1970. A controlled study of lithium vs. chlorpromazine in acute schizophrenics. Presented at 15th Annual Conference - V.A. Cooperative Studies in Psychiatry, Houston, Texas. Accepted for publication, *Brit. J. Psychiat.*

Shopsin, B.; Stern, S.; and Gershon, S. 1970. Altered carbohydrate metabolism during lithium treatment in hospitalized psychiatric patients: Absence of diagnostic specificity. Submitted for publication.

Simon, W.; Wirt, A. L.; Wirt, R. D.; and Halloran, A. V. 1965. Long term follow-up study of schizophrenic patients. *Arch. Gen. Psychiat.* 12:510.

Sivadon, P., and Chanoit, P. 1955. Clinical experience with lithium treatment of psychomotor excitation. *Ann. Medicopsychol.* 113:790.

Sletten, I. W., and Gershon, S. 1966. The premenstrual syndrome: A discussion of its pathophysiology and treatment with the lithium ion. *Compr. Psychiat.* 7(no. 3):198.

Spitzer, R. L.; Endicott, J.; and Fleiss, J. L. 1967. Instruments and recording forms for evaluating psychiatric status and history: rationale, method of development and description. *Compr. Psychiat.* 8:321.

Spring, G. K.; Schweid, D.; Gray, C.; Steinberg, J.; and Harwitz, M. 1970. A double blind comparison of lithium and chlorpromazine in the treatment of manic states. *Amer. J. Psychiat.* 126:1306.

Spring, G. K.; Schweid, D.; Steinberg, J.; and Bond, D. 1969. Prophylactic use of lithium carbonate? *J.A.M.A.* 208:1901.

Stromgren, L. S., and Stromgren, E. 1962. In Normothymics "mood normalizers" by M. Schou *Brit. J. Psychiat.* 109:803.

Talso, P. J., and Clarke, R. W. 1951. Excretion and distribution of lithium in the dog. *Amer. J. Physiol.* 166:202.

Trautner, E. M.; Morris, R.; Noack, C. H.; and Gershon, S. 1955. The excretion and retention of ingested lithium and its effect on the ionic balance of man. *Med. J. Aust.* 2:280.

Van der Velde, C. D., and Gordon, M. W. 1969. Manic-depressive illness, diabetes mellitus and lithium carbonate. *Arch. Gen. Psychiat.* 21:478.

Van der Velde, C. D. 1970. Effectiveness of lithium carbonate in the treatment of manic-depressive illness. *Amer. J. Psychiat.* 127:345.

Von Trostorff, S. 1968. Über die hereditäre Belastung bei den bipolaren und monopolaren phasischen Psychosen. *Schweiz. Arch. Neurochir. Psychiat.* 102:235.

Wiggers, S. 1968. Lithiumpavirkning af glandula thyreoidea. *Ugeskr. Laeg.* 130/37:1523.

Wingard, C. 1961. Questions and answers. *J.A.M.A.* 175:340.
Winokur, G., and Clayton, P. 1967. Family history studies: II. Sex differences and alcoholism in primary affective illness. *Brit. J. Psychiat.* 113:973.
Wirt, R. D., and Simon, W. 1959. *Differential Treatment and Prognosis in Schizophrenia.* Springfield, Ill.: Charles C Thomas.
Wolpert, E. A., and Mueller, P. 1969. Lithium carbonate in the treatment of manic-depressive disorders. *Arch. Gen. Psychiat.* 21:155.
Zall, H.; Therman, P. O. G.; and Myers, J. M. 1968. Lithium carbonate: A clinical study. *Amer. J. Psychiat.* 125:549.

CHEMOTHERAPY OF DEPRESSION

Gerald L. Klerman

Harvard Medical School -- Massachusetts General Hospital

Boston, Massachusetts

It is now thirteen years since the simultaneous introduction in 1957 of iproniazid (Marsilid), the prototypic monoamine oxidase inhibitor, and imipramine (Tofranil), the prototypic tricyclic antidepressant. Since then, a large number of new compounds has been developed and introduced for therapeutic usage. Numerous symposiums have been held and a large number of papers have appeared about the clinical efficacy of these drugs and the biochemical bases of their actions. Nonetheless, considerable controversy continues. There are unresolved questions as to toxicity and as to therapeutic efficacy. Moreover, there is a lack of consensus as to the etiology and nosology of depressions, and whether specific patient types respond better to one or another treatment.

This uncertain status of the chemotherapy of depression is in contrast to the wide acceptance of the chemotherapy of schizophrenia and related psychotic states. In the drug treatment of schizophrenia, consensus developed rapidly as to the range of utility of the phenothiazines, butyrophenones, and thioxanthines. The similar therapeutic effects of these various antipsychotic or neuroleptic compounds contribute to a general agreement on the common areas of their clinical action (Klerman 1970). In the chemotherapy of depression, however, such consensus has not developed. A number of questions continue to perplex clinical investigators and practicing therapists.

1. Do the amphetamines have any place in the current chemotherapy of depression? Do their adverse effects override their therapeutic benefits?

2. What role do the MAO inhibitors have in general therapeutic practice? As research tools? Are there specific patient types who respond to the MAO inhibitors but not to the tricyclic antidepressants?

3. Given the agreement among experienced clinicians that the tricyclic antidepressants are the most effective drugs, what is the range of their effectiveness? How much more do the tricyclics add to general improvement due to time itself and/or to the nonspecific therapeutic actions of hospitalization, milieu, treatment expectations, and placebo effect?

4. Are there specific antidepressant drugs at all? The evidence for the efficacy of phenothiazines and of minor tranquilizers suggests that the concept of specific antidepressants is outmoded. In the chemotherapy of depression, are we not dealing with a spectrum of drugs with a wide range of action?

5. Is it possible to identify subtypes of depressed persons who will respond differentially to the available treatments? To individual drugs? To electroconvulsive treatment (ECT)? To psychotherapy?

6. What is the efficacy of long-term maintenance therapy in the prevention of relapses and recurrences? A substantial number of persons with acute depressions are likely to encounter recurrences. Clinical experience indicates that between 40 and 60 percent of the persons experiencing acute depressions will have recurrences. Is it possible to predict which persons are subject to these recurrences? What is the value of maintenance therapy? With ECT? With tricyclic derivatives? With lithium?

In this paper, I shall discuss these issues as they apply to the chemotherapy of acute depressive episodes. This paper will not discuss the chemotherapy of acute mania and of recurrent manic-depressive and other affective disorders, topics covered by Shopsin and Gershon (in this volume). I shall deal with the investigational uses of chemotherapy. I shall consider drugs such as the precursors of amines, DOPA and tryptophan, and to what extent their therapeutic actions can verify the biogenic theories of depression (Schildkraut 1970). Moreover, I will review the theoretical models and research approaches in terms of their variable efficacy in the treatment of depression.

CLINICAL EFFICACY IN THE CHEMOTHERAPY OF THE DEPRESSIONS

The clinician treating the depressed person who is acutely and symptomatically ill is currently in an advantageous position. He has available to him a moderate number of effective treatments and a reasonable assurance that between the effects of time and of treatment, the majority of his depressed patients will show remission. Problems do arise because of the tendency for recurrence, but the person experiencing an acute episode usually responds rapidly.

Most depressive episodes are self-limiting. "Time" alone plus the informal psychotherapeutic efforts of family support and medical attention often suffice to bring about improvement and even remission within a matter of months. Acute depressions have a high improvement rate even without specific chemotherapy. Most acute depressive patients will have remissions with almost complete symptomatic relief, and will return to their previous level of social, intellectual, and occupational functioning.

Various compilations have been made of the spontaneous remission rate. Alexander (1953), in an extensive compilation of clinical reports of hospitalized patients in the 1920's and 1930's, described recovery or social improvement in 44 percent of hospitalized persons within the first year, and a rise to 54 percent recovery after longer periods of treatment. These trends were observed in hospitalized patients in the era before the advent of ECT. Convulsive therapy introduced in the early 1940's subsequently raised the percentage of patients who ultimately recovered and, more significantly, shortened the duration of symptomatic distress and social disability. Outpatients, often with milder illness, have even better improvement rates. Klerman and Cole (1965) pointed out that these high "spontaneous improvement" rates approximate the improvement rates reported in uncontrolled chemotherapy trials, in which 65 to 75 percent of the patients were considered improved. Of course, there are major differences in the duration of the illness and in the speed with which patients recover, and most clinical investigators believe that the current somatic therapies do decrease the intensity of symptoms and hasten the rate of recovery. Still, the similarities between results from the natural course of the illness and uncontrolled trials necessitate the execution of further controlled studies.

It is uncertain to what extent these spontaneous improvements represent pure placebo response, the effects of various psychosocial forces, the endogenous pathophysiology of the illness, genetically determined results, or responses to the psychotherapy implicit in all treatment settings. Lasagna has summarized the relevance of the placebo response to double-blind controls and to the methodology of drug trials (Lasagna 1970). Placebo studies have identified certain types of individuals who may be placebo responders. The technique of allowing a placebo washout period before the introduction of the drug promotes the separation of placebo responders and placebo remitters. As Uhlenhuth and his associates (Uhlenhuth and Duncan 1968) have pointed out, part of this placebo response may relate to the patients' awareness of novel treatment and expectation of improvement, the phenomenon labeled "Hawthorne Effect" by social psychologists.

Given these trends, it is important to establish the goals of the chemotherapy of acute depressions. Symptom-reduction and rapid action are the current aims; no available treatment "cures" acute depression in a manner analogous to antibiotic cures of infectious disease, nor do any available treatments counter the presumed vulnerability of many persons to multiple recurrences. Long-term treatment, however, as proposed with lithium, seems to maintain remission and protect against relapse and recurrence. In these respects, the chemotherapy of depressions is more akin to the chemotherapy of chronic cardiovascular or gastrointestinal disorders than to the chemotherapy of acute infectious diseases.

There is a significant mortality associated with acute depressions. Suicide is of course the major danger, but we should not forget the complications attendant to weight loss, malnutrition, sleep deprivation, exhaustion, and the other secondary effects of the symptomatic state. In the pre-ECT era, there was a substantial mortality due to malnutrition, and to intercurrent infections such as pneumonia. These complications were especially frequent in those middle-aged and aged patients in whom severe depressions were usually diagnosed as "involutional melancholia." Moreover, there is a significant morbidity to depressions--impairment in social adjustment, family life, and occupational and economic support. Consequently, if clinicians can demonstrate that chemotherapy accelerates improvement and reduces symptoms, they have elucidated its significant advantages.

In addition to "time," the physician has available to him a range of therapeutic agents including convulsive therapies, numerous drugs, and various forms of psychotherapy, individual, group, family and couples therapies. As shown in Table 1, the large number of drugs generally considered as antidepressant can be divided into three groups:

1. The amphetamines and other psychomotor stimulants.
2. The monoamine oxidase (MAO) inhibitors.
3. The tricyclic derivatives related to imipramine.

The clinician wants to know the comparative efficacy of individual drugs and if the drugs are more efficacious than time alone. He is also interested in comparing the drug classes to each other, to ECT, and to psychotherapy. Moreover, he must question whether there are subtypes of depressions that respond differentially to one form of treatment or to another.

TABLE 1

Drugs Used in the
Chemotherapy of Depressions

Main Groups	Chemical Types	Generic Names	Trade Names
Psychomotor stimulants	Amphetamines	Amphetamine	Benzedrine
		Dextroamphetamine	Dexedrine
		Combinations with barbiturate	Dexamyl
	Others	Methylphenidate	Ritalin
Monoamine oxidase inhibitors	Hydrazines	Isocarboxazid	Marplan
		Nialamide	Niamid
		Phenelzine	Nardil
	Nonhydrazines	Pargyline	Eutonyl
		Tranylcypromine	Parnate
Tricyclic compounds	Iminodibenzyls	Desipramine	Norpramin
			Pertofrane
		Imipramine	Tofranil
		Trimipramine	Unavailable commercially in U.S.A.
	Dibenzocycloheptenes	Amitriptyline	Elavil
		Nortriptyline	Aventyl
		Protriptyline	Vivactil
	Dibenzoxepin	Doxepin	Sinequan

Amphetamines and Related Psychomotor Stimulants

There is general agreement that the psychomotor stimulants, of which the amphetamines are the prototypes, have only limited clinical effectiveness in the chemotherapy of acute depressions. For some but not all depressed persons, the amphetamines and other psychomotor stimulants may temporarily produce increased alertness, and a mild to moderate elation and euphoria. These euphoric effects, however, are quantitatively of mild magnitude and in many patients the adverse effects of the drugs (anxiety, tension, sleep disturbance, irritability, and autonomic nervous system stimulation) are discomforting.[1]

The few controlled trials available cast doubt as to whether the amphetamines are more effective than placebo (Hare, Dominian, and Sharpe 1962; General Practitioner Research Group 1964). Among Veterans Administration (V.A.) inpatients (Overall 1962), limited efficacy was found for amphetamines alone or when combined with phenothiazines in the treatment of chronic apathetic, withdrawn, hospitalized schizophrenic patients (Casey et al. 1961). Moreover, in the V.A. studies, the amphetamines were not found to be any more effective than placebo; in fact, some patients became worse on amphetamines.

As indicated, the effect on mood produced by amphetamines in patients is often short-lived. That it may be more prolonged in nondepressives is the basis for its widespread use among youth and others. Yet, since the euphoric effect is often succeeded by adverse effects such as irritability, cardiovascular stimulation, and rebound fatigue and depression, and since tolerance develops rapidly, the general effectiveness of the amphetamines is uncertain. Because of the adverse effects of the amphetamines, attempts have been made to produce a combination of amphetamines and barbiturates, and this has been noted clinically as far back as 1949 (Gottlieb 1949). A number of amphetamine-barbiturate combinations have been marketed and excellent pharmacologic studies on animals and normal human beings indicate that this combination does have unique synergistic effects. In human beings, the acute administration of the combination is associated with a greater sense of mood elevation and with less of a decrement in psychomotor performance than is produced by either drug separately (Legge and Steinberg 1962). However, in the one double-blind clinical trial available (Overall et al. 1962) the combination was found inferior to imipramine and no more effective than placebo.

---

[1] The amphetamines do have demonstrated efficacy in hyperactive children, but this clinical action is outside the scope of this paper.

The main hazards of prolonged use of the psychomotor stimulants are usually considered to be psychic. However, there is growing evidence for physical dependence. With the development of tolerance, patients often increase their doses. Consequently, a widespread illicit market traffic has developed, and physicians who have been lax in their writing and supervision of prescriptions have aggravated this illicit drug market by increasing the available supply.

There are three well-defined toxic syndromes of the amphetamines. The acute toxic reaction is dose-related and at times is fatal. The chronic psychosis may appear insidiously and may be indistinguishable clinically from chronic paranoid schizophrenic states (Connell 1958). The occurrence of this schizophrenia-like psychosis is of considerable theoretical interest; its resemblance to naturally occurring schizophrenia has given impetus to important lines of investigation on actions of the amphetamines on CNS amine metabolism. Now there is increasing belief that a true withdrawal syndrome may occur that manifests itself in fatigue, hypersomnia, and increased REM sleep (Oswald and Thacore 1963).

Attempts have been made to develop nonamphetamine psychomotor stimulants. The most widely used is methylphenidate (Ritalin) which probably has some value as a mood stimulant in mild depressions. In the one controlled study available (Robin and Wiseberg 1958), it had only slightly more apparent value than placebo in moderately depressed patients. It has many clinical features in common with the amphetamines, including utility in hyperactive children with learning disorders. Two other psychomotor stimulants merit mention—phenmetrazine (marketed as Preludin) which also produces dependence, addiction, and toxic psychoses. Pipradrol has not been found to be effective as an antidepressant.

In recent years, a number of new compounds related structurally to the amphetamines have been developed in Scandinavia and the United Kingdom. These new compounds are of considerable research interest because knowledge of structure-activity relations among the amphetamines has generated important understandings of their differential actions upon mood, alertness, and appetite. Moreover, these researches on the metabolism of the amphetamines offer interesting hypotheses for the possible mechanism for the development of tolerance and for a plausible explanation of the pathogenesis of the toxic psychoses.

Monoamine Oxidase (MAO) Inhibitors

As shown in Table 1, there are a moderate number of compounds that have demonstrated MAO inhibition. As shown in Figure 1, the MAO inhibitors used in the treatment of depression can be divided on the basis of their chemical structure into two groups, the hydra-

HYDRAZINE DERIVATIVES

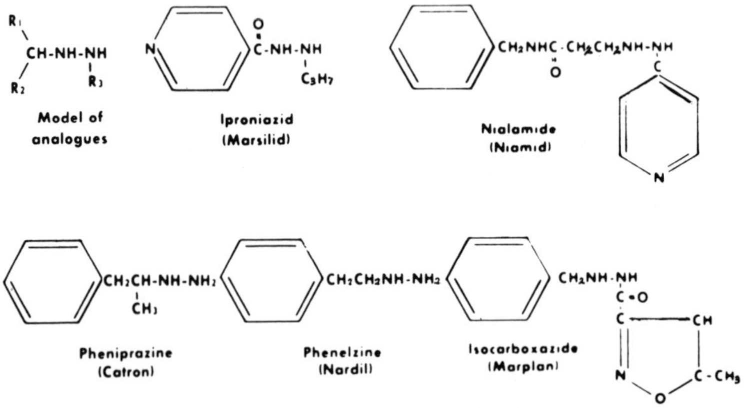

Figure 1. These agents block monoamine oxidase, an enzyme important in the catabolism of the CNS hormones serotonin and norepinephrine. Other actions may also contribute to the therapeutic effects.

zines and the nonhydrazines. Both groups share the ability to inhibit the MAO enzyme that is widely distributed in mammalian tissues and that is responsible for the oxidative deamination of the amines, including both the catecholamines and the indolealkylamines. The hydrazine compounds include isocarboxazid (Marplan), nialamide (Niamid), and phenelzine (Nardil). (The prototype MAO inhibitor, iproniazid [Marsilid], was removed from the prescription market because of liver toxicity.) Among the nonhydrazines, only one--tranylcypromine (Parnate)--is presently approved in the U.S.A. for prescription use in the chemotherapy of depression. A second nonhydrazine MAO inhibitor, pargyline (Eutonyl), is approved in the chemotherapy of hypertension. Although it is not advocated in the chemotherapy of depression, pargyline does have definite antidepressant utility. Other MAO inhibitors have been investigated for clinical efficacy but have not been approved for prescription use or, once marketed, have been removed because of toxicity.

All the compounds mentioned inhibit MAO activity *in vivo*, including in the CNS. Correlation has been demonstrated between clinical improvement and the degree of enzyme inhibition in patients, as measured by urinary excretion of peripheral metabolites. There is some question whether their antidepressant clinical effects can be attributed totally to MAO inhibition since most of these drugs have a variety of pharmacological effects (Atkinson and Ditman 1965). Moreover, Kopin has demonstrated the important role of "false" transmitters in mediating certain of the adrenergic effects of the MAO inhibitors, yet it is unclear if these are related to their antidepressant activity (Kopin 1968).

Why then are the MAO inhibitors considered less effective than the tricyclic derivatives? Part of the answer is that they are truly less effective. I have previously reviewed the evidence for the clinical efficacy of the various MAO inhibitors (Davis, Schildkraut, and Klerman 1967). In my opinion, individual MAO inhibitors do have greater than placebo efficacy. When compared with ECT and with tricyclic derivatives, however, the MAO inhibitors are demonstrably less effective. A similar situation occurred in the early days of the tranquilizers when the evidence soon accumulated that the phenothiazines, especially chlorpromazine, were more effective than reserpine. However, two additional factors must be taken into consideration when reviewing studies of the efficacy of the MAO inhibitors, the dosage employed, and the heterogeneity of depressive populations. Regarding the first factor, dosage, in clinical trials the doses are seldom pushed into the pharmacologically active dose range. Herein lies one of the serious problems with the use of the MAO inhibitors in chemotherapy, since they have a narrow dose range dictated by the frequent occurrence of adverse effects, particularly those due to their interactions with other drugs producing serious cardiovascular effects. Despite this issue of practical utility, the clinical efficacy of the MAO inhibitors has important theoretical and research implications. Adequate trials have importance in this area, even if the frequency of adverse effects limits the practical usefulness in chemotherapy.

The second problem involves the possible existence of subgroups of depressive patients specifically reactive to the MAO inhibitors. When the MAO inhibitor, tranylcypromine (Parnate), was temporarily removed from the market by the FDA in 1966, a number of experienced clinicians argued that they had treated patients whose clinical response was specific to the MAO inhibitors, that is, that they had been treated previously with other compounds, including tricyclics, and had failed to respond. Moreover, attempts to transfer these persons from MAO inhibitors to tricyclics had also failed.

A number of such striking experiences leads clinicians to believe that there are significant subgroups of patients who respond specifically to the MAO inhibitors. One possible research strategy that has not been explored fully proposes the systematic investigation of the specific amines, whether catecholamines or indolealkylamines, to which these individual patients may well respond. Within

RELATIONSHIP BETWEEN PHENOTHIAZINE DERIVATIVES AND DIBENZAZEPINE DERIVATIVES

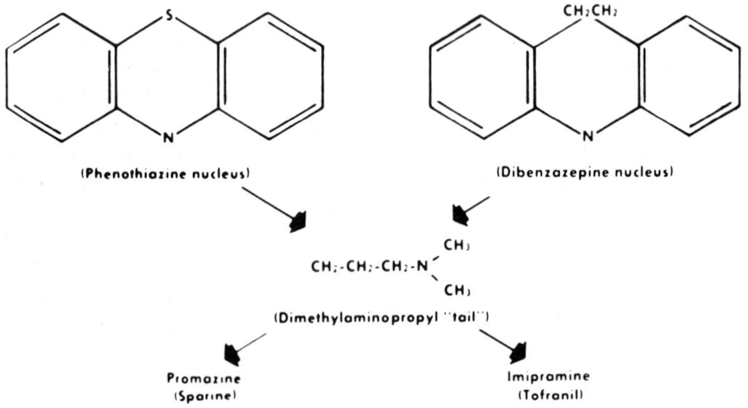

Figure 2. These drugs resemble phenothiazine derivatives chemically, but are not effective in schizophrenic reactions.

the large and heterogeneous group of depressive patients, there may be a small subtype specifically responsive to one or another MAO inhibitor. After all, phenylketonuria represents less than five percent of the total groups of mental retardation and yet it has been a most productive model for investigation and for therapy.

Because of adverse effects and the limited and contradictory evidence of their efficacy, MAO inhibitors are currently used only infrequently. Probably the pendulum has swung too far. Although it is likely that they should not be used as the drugs of first prescription, the MAO inhibitors should be administered to persons who have failed to respond to the tricyclic derivatives. They should also be used for patients who have a previous history of response to MAO inhibitors and, as has been suggested by Pare and Angst, they should be used in patients whose family members have also responded positively.

The Tricyclic Derivatives

The tricyclic derivatives are of considerable interest clinically and pharmacologically. As shown in Figure 2, their chemical structure is closely related to the phenothiazines. Review of

clinical and research experience with the tricyclic derivatives
shows clearly that they are used most widely and are the most effective drug groups. I have been involved previously in three extensive
reviews of the literature on the tricyclics--with Jonathan Cole
(Klerman and Cole 1965), with Davis and Schildkraut (Davis,
Schildkraut, and Klerman 1967), and with Paykel (Klerman and Paykel
1970). These three reviews of the literature on imipramine and related tricyclic compounds convinced me that they have selective but
important antidepressant clinical action. In view of this consensus
among clinicians, it is hard to understand why a sizeable minority
of clinical trials have failed to substantiate the view that imipramine and other tricyclic derivatives are antidepressant drugs. One
possibility, of course, is that they really are not antidepressants
and that clinicians are in error. Because of my personal clinical
experience, as well as my extensive involvement with literature reviews and the conduct of controlled therapeutic trials, I cannot
accept this judgment. Yet, Raskin, reporting on the extensive NIMH
collaborative study, comes to the conclusion that for most patients
these drugs do not offer a major source of benefit (Raskin *et al.*
1970).

How are we to understand this apparent contradiction between
the research findings of the very large NIMH study and of general
clinical and research experience? There are problems in research
methodology and mode of statistical analysis in the NIMH report.
The NIMH report does not provide a display of the percentage distributions of patients' improvement broken down by various diagnostic
types and by drugs. We are given mainly the results in terms of
their statistical significance. As clinicians, however, we are
interested also in how many patients improved and to what degree?
We need data on the frequency distributions of improvement and on
the global improvement dimensions along with statistical analyses
of individual symptom scores. The possibility also exists that the
NIMH research design contributed to negative or minor findings.
Since a large number of assessments were called for, this procedure
may have increased observer fatigue and error variance, and decreased
validity. Perhaps multihospital clinical trials would be better
served by designs incorporating fewer but more reliable and valid
outcome measures.

Looking carefully at the specific findings of the NIMH study,
rather than at the general conclusions, there is clear substantiation
of a number of major clinical trends. The tricyclic derivative
studied, imipramine, was effective in the depressive patients with
psychotic and retarded features. The schizo-affective group did
not respond well to antidepressants; they did poorly over-all, but
did respond to some degree to the phenothiazines. There was a clear
placebo response, mostly in patients under 40 with mild or neurotic
depressions, a conclusion reached previously by the New Jersey group

(Wittenborn et al. 1962), by the Massachusetts collaborative group
(Greenblatt, Grosser, and Wechsler 1962), and also by the United
Kingdom multihospital trial (Medical Research Council 1965). Thus,
the NIMH study substantiates many hypotheses of differential prediction by age, clinical type, and symptomatic state.

Differential Response to Chemotherapy

Reviewing the various clinical studies and trials, I conclude
that there is fair agreement as to the rank order of various treatments: ECT first, followed by the tricyclic derivatives, followed
by the MAO inhibitors, with placebo trailing along. One should not
discount the efficacy of placebo since a number of studies indicate
that this has a moderately high level of therapeutic benefit
(Friedman et al. 1960; Greenblatt, Grosser, and Wechsler 1964;
Klerman and Cole 1965; Lehmann 1966). The clinician, however, is
interested not only in the rank order of efficacy of treatments, but
also in the existence of specific response patterns. He also wants
to know whether this rank order of efficacy applies to all depressed
patients or if there are specific subtypes.

A number of attempts have been made to utilize therapeutic outcome as the basis for improving our understanding of the nature and
classification of depression. Largely because of the pragmatic problem of how to decide on which drug for which patient, this area has
attracted increasing attention in the past decade. Probably it is
the most important unresolved clinical research problem in the chemotherapy of depression. Can we develop a rational basis for the differential prescription of the numerous treatments of depression?
One widely held and attractive hypothesis is that certain patients
are responsive specifically to the tricyclic drugs or to MAO inhibitors. To test this hypothesis, multivariate statistical techniques,
especially factor analytic and cluster analytic techniques, have
been applied to results of clinical trials. Among the important
trends in this effort has been the revival of interest in the endogenous depressive type. This interest derives from the observation
of Kuhn and others that patients with vegetative and endogenous-like
symptoms seem to improve most with tricyclic derivatives. This
clinical observation was tested and partially substantiated by Kiloh
and Garside (1963) using advanced statistical techniques. The trend
of research does indeed suggest that patients with depressions corresponding to the endogenous pattern are likely to be responsive to
tricyclic compounds (Raskin et al. 1970; Wittenborn 1968).

In a parallel fashion, it has been hypothesized that phobic
neurotic or "atypical" depressed patients have a tendency to respond
to MAO inhibitors (Dally and Rohde 1961). Such hypotheses concerning the MAO inhibitors have not been substantiated and there is
inconsistency as to the clinical data; many patients with symptoms

similar to the descriptions of phobic anxiety states and atypical depressions have also been described as responding to imipramine (Ayd 1960; Klein 1964). Controlled clinical trials indicate the efficacy of tricyclic derivatives in depressed patients who are characterized as psychotic and/or retarded (Greenblatt, Grosser, and Wechsler 1964; Overall, Hollister, and Pennington 1966). This trend also seems confirmed by the NIMH collaborative study (Raskin 1970).

In reviewing these studies, we cannot afford to discount the importance of placebo effects in depression since, as has been mentioned previously, a substantial number of younger patients (under age 40) and those with milder illnesses respond well to time alone and to the nonspecific effects of psychotherapy. The placebo response was particularly relevant in the study by Friedman, in Philadelphia, who was not able to find a drug-imipramine difference because more than 60 percent of control patients improved in the hospital's general treatment program without benefit of specific chemotherapy.

The Heterogeneity of Clinical Depressions

These studies substantiate the hypothesis that significant patterns exist in differential responses to chemotherapy. Consequently, they draw attention again to the heterogeneity of the clinical phenomena and the continuing need for clinical research on the nature of the clinical phenomena (Klerman 1970).

As a mood, depression is part of normal human adaptation. Feelings of sadness, disappointment, and frustration are within the vicissitudes of the human condition. Currently, psychiatrists do not agree on the full range of affective phenomena to be diagnosed as clinical depression. The demarcation between normal mood and abnormal depression is unclear, so that considerably more research on the diagnostic criteria is needed. The problem is especially pressing for the many episodes of depression for which recent precipitating events are readily apparent in bereavement, adolescent developmental states, post-traumatic states, persistent social problems among minority groups, aging, and chronic illness. Clinicians tend, in their judgments, to minimize the severity of depressive states when such precipitating events are readily appparent. Drug therapy, however, is often used to modify the intensity and quality of such reactions. Results from clinical drug evaluation involving patients with such reactive states may be difficult to interpret.

As a symptom, pathologic depression often occurs secondary to other systemic or psychiatric illnesses, such as viral infections, nutritional deficiencies, or schizophrenia. Other medical conditions in which depression may be a feature include: anemia, CNS disease such as multiple sclerosis, and nutritional and vitamin deficiencies such as pellagra. Since depressions secondary to systemic or medical disease are frequent, they often pose difficult diagnostic problems, particularly in elderly people for whom the differential diagnosis between organic brain damage and depression may be difficult. In the United States, there is a tendency to overdiagnose CNS arteriosclerosis and senility, without sufficient recognition that depression may also produce slowing of general activity and reduction of intellectual activity.

In clinical practice, however, most depressions are primarily psychiatric. That is, they do not occur in the presence of demonstrable CNS or systemic disease. Pending future research, which may or may not demonstrate specific CNS pathology, most clinical depressions must be regarded as primarily psychiatric disorders, diagnosed and treated predominantly on clinical bases. In current clinical parlance, depression refers most often to a group of syndromes in which there are abnormal, persistent affect changes associated with feelings of worthlessness, guilt, helplessness, and hopelessness; anxiety, crying, suicidal tendencies, loss of interest in work and other activities; impaired capacity to perform everyday social functions, and hypochondriasis, accompanied by such physical alterations as anorexia, weight change, constipation, psychomotor retardation or agitation, headache and other bodily complaints. Even to the untrained observer, most states are clearly seen as pathological by virtue of their intensity, pervasiveness and persistence, and their interference with normal social and physiological functioning.

It is important to emphasize the existence of not one but several clinical depressive syndromes. Some psychiatrists believe that among the various depressive states there is a unique disease entity, variously called "endogenous depression," "primary affective illness," "manic-depressive illness," or "primary depression." In these patients, episodes occur without any immediate life stress and often recur, occasionally alternating with episodes of euphoria and manic excitement. Somatic therapies, including the antidepressant drugs and ECT, are most useful with these patients.

There is no agreement on the various groupings or typologies that are most applicable to the prediction of drug response. One valuable approach utilizes differential responses to drugs as possible criteria for classification--this represents a form of "pharmacological dissection." Overall and his associates have developed a phenomenological classification of depressed patients that attempts to predict response to chemotherapy of depression and that has been partially replicated (Overall, Hollister, and Pennington 1966). Pending further research, however, the existing classifications, groupings, and typologies must be considered as tentative and of heuristic value.

Age contributes a further source of heterogeneity. It is well established that the clinical course and symptomatic picture of depressions varies significantly with the person's age. Younger patients tend to be less reactive to the environment, have greater sleep disturbances, and are less likely to manifest irritability and hostility. These age trends correlate with the endogenous depressive pattern (Rosenthal and Klerman 1966). Other sources of variability are race and social class, factors that influence the clinical phenomena, and that may influence drug response (Schwab, Bialow, and Brown 1967; Tonks, Paykel, and Klerman 1970).

These heterogeneities are such that an investigator can obtain almost any chemotherapeutic result desired by altering the composition of the patient population. For example, inclusion in the study sample of high percentages of schizophrenic patients with depression or patients with schizo-affective disorders will result in over-all poor outcomes irrespective of the drug studied (Greenblatt, Grosser, and Wechsler 1964; Raskin et al. 1970). On the other hand, high percentages of younger patients with predominantly neurotic situational reactions will produce high improvement rates. In the absence of concomitant group controls, such high improvement rates may suggest an efficacious drug. Even if a control group is used, drug-placebo difference may be difficult to demonstrate, not because the drug is ineffective, but because the placebo response may be sufficiently high to obviate a drug-placebo differential (Friedman et al. 1966).

Moreover, heterogeneity of the clinical features is clearly related to differential placement in various treatment settings (Paykel, Klerman, and Prusoff 1970; Klerman et al. 1963). Changes in the definition and diagnosis of depression and in the advent of effective drugs allowing ambulatory treatment have produced significant changes in patients who are hospitalized. It is important, therefore, to recognize that the hospitalized patient represents an atypical sample of depression, usually the more severe forms of depression, or a depressed patient who has failed to respond to outpatient treatment.

CONCLUSIONS: IMPLICATIONS FOR RESEARCH ON BRAIN CHEMISTRY AND MENTAL DISEASE

Thus far, I have assessed the state of clinical practices in the chemotherapy of depression. Now it is important to consider how these clinical issues relate to problems in biochemistry of affective disorders. In part, one can give no definite answer since there are major gaps yet to be filled between the empirical evidence for the therapeutic value of these drugs and the scientific understanding of their biochemical modes of action. Relatively little can be said with certainty about the biochemical or neuropharmacologic bases for the modes of actions of these drugs although very attractive hypotheses have been formulated, particularly about the role of the biogenic amines. It may well be that the ultimate significance of the recently introduced chemotherapeutic agents will lie not so much in their therapeutic utility as in the long-term benefits from the scientific research their introduction has stimulated over the past decades, developments that offer promise of elucidating important aspects of the biology of affective states.

Throughout the brief history of modern scientific medicine, a tension has always been discernible between the laboratory and the clinic. This tension creates a potential dialogue between these two partners in medical research. At present, such a dialogue between the biochemical pharmacologist and the clinician is focused on the biology of the affective disorders. Part of this dialogue derives from the lack of adequate bridges between the laboratory and the clinic in the development of drugs in the chemotherapy of depression.

Ideally, in the evolving science of clinical pharmacology, new therapeutic agents should be developed "rationally." For this to be true, when drugs are introduced for clinical use, clinicians should make precise statements predicting clinical indications. They can derive these statements from existing knowledge of the modes of actions of the new compounds. To achieve this ideal requires at least five types of established information: (1) valid criteria to identify classes of patients with the relevant clinical syndrome, i.e., depression; (2) sufficient knowledge of etiology to allow patient groupings, i.e., criteria for etiological subclassifications; (3) animal models; (4) sufficient understanding of pathogenesis, i.e., the sequence of events leading to symptom formation of the characteristic pathophysiology to be found among depressed patients; and (5) knowledge of the specific pharmacologic actions of antidepressant drugs that allow description of the mode of treatment either to interrupt the pathogenic sequence resulting in symptom formation, or to alter the abnormal state characteristic of the disorder.

This ideal is seldom realized in most fields of medicine, least of all in psychiatry. Except for the CNS infectious diseases and certain endocrine disorders, psychiatrists do not possess such "rational" understanding. This is particularly so in the case of depression for which we have neither sufficient knowledge to allow etiologic classification of patients with depression, nor sufficient knowledge of the altered physiology to allow for predictions. Consequently, during the brief history of treating psychiatric depressed patients with drugs, therapeutic efficacy has almost always been developed from clinical experience--usually by accident.

There was little in the available animal models of iproniazid or imipramine to suggest their possible usefulness in depressed patients. The previously existing criterion for predicting clinical antidepressant action was that the compound must increase the gross psychomotor activities of animals. This criterion is derived from experience with the amphetamines and embodies the classical neuropharmacologic model of excitation versus depression as a single bipolar dimension of CNS action. By this criterion, neither imipramine nor iproniazid was predicted to be antidepressant. The unexpected demonstration of clinical efficacy of these drugs has stimulated productive lines of investigation to determine new animal models.

McKinney and Bunney have recently reviewed the evidence for animal models of depression (McKinney and Bunney 1969). Although none of the models meets the criteria for direct behavioral correlation, the theories relating amines to depression have been of considerable value in developing animal screens, particularly when testing for drugs that are MAO inhibitors or that are capable of reversing the amine-depleted state induced by either reserpine or tetrabenazine. The use of amine-depleted animals, such as those with reserpine-induced hypothermia or ptosis, is of interest because of the catecholamine mode, but it represents phenomena several steps removed from the behavioral concerns of clinical psychiatry (Litchfield 1961).

Not only have the amine models generated animal screens, but also they have direct applications in clinical trials. Enzyme inhibitors, false transmitters, amino acids and amino acid precursors have been investigated. Most of these compounds, such as L-DOPA and tryptophan, do not lend themselves to the usual processes of drug development by pharmaceutical firms, and special administrative and legal problems arise when these compounds are studied.

In the absence of clearly-defined animal models of well-understood mechanisms in the pathophysiology of affective disorders, most research in the biology of depression derives from heuristic bases. The indole and catechol hypotheses of depression stand out in this situation because they provide one type of important bridge. Before readily accepting them, one must take note of a divergence in trends in the direction of research between clinical experience and laboratory biochemical approaches. The trend of the biochemical approaches has been to find the common final pathway for the action of all antidepressant drugs through one or another of the biogenic amines. On the other hand, the clinical research, as reviewed earlier in this paper, has focused on the heterogeneity of response, strongly suggesting that there are multiple populations and subgroups, each of which may have different pathophysiological mechanisms operating. These contradictions may provide a major source of confusion and an impediment to further progress in research on the biochemistry of affective disorders.

One major source of confusion arises because "depression" has different meanings in various fields. For the neurophysiologist, depression refers to any decrease in electrophysiological activity, e.g., "cortical depression." The pharmacologist uses "depression" to refer to drug actions which decrease the activity of the target organ. Thus, the CNS depressions include drugs like the barbiturates and the anesthetics, which are unrelated either clinically or pharmacologically to antidepressant drugs. The psychologist uses the term "depression" for any decrement in optimal performance, such as slowing of psychomotor activity or reduction of intellectual functioning. For the clinical psychiatrist, however, depression covers a wide range of changes in affective state, ranging in severity from normal mood swings at one extreme, to severe melancholic psychoses at the other. Pending agreement as to terminology, confusion is likely to continue.

The use of the same term in a number of scientific fields has lent support to the view that there is a common mechanism unifying these neurophysiological, pharmacological, and clinical phenomena. As a result, many investigators have postulated that clinical depressive symptoms are the result of a depression of CNS functioning, and are best treated with a stimulant drug. This view, the "stimulant-depressant continuum," has been the classical model for neuropharmacology (Klerman 1966). It gained adherents when the amphetamines and barbiturates were the major CNS agents (Figure 3).

This model presents a single bipolar dimension to the other pole of CNS excitation. Clinical psychiatric states have been ordered on this continuum according to interruption of psychomotor activity by manic excitements presumably due to excessive CNS inhibition. Therapy based on this model, which makes use of the stimulant-depressant classification of drugs, was applied most readily when the amphetamines and barbiturates were the major CNS agents. It has also been related to Pavlovian conditioning by Eysenck and to psychoanalytic libido theory by Ostow. Recent hypotheses on catecholamines have some parallels to this older view. However, it is important to recognize that while the catecholamine hypothesis has the greatest heuristic value for current research, it has not produced sufficient results to generate objective criteria for the diagnosis of depression or for the assessment of change induced by drugs.

The complexity of actions of newer psychotropic drugs, particularly the phenothiazines and tricyclic antidepressants, makes the stimulant-depressant continuum model obsolete and overly simplistic. Moreover, since there are no firmly established neurophysiological or biochemical mechanisms in the etiology or pathophysiology of

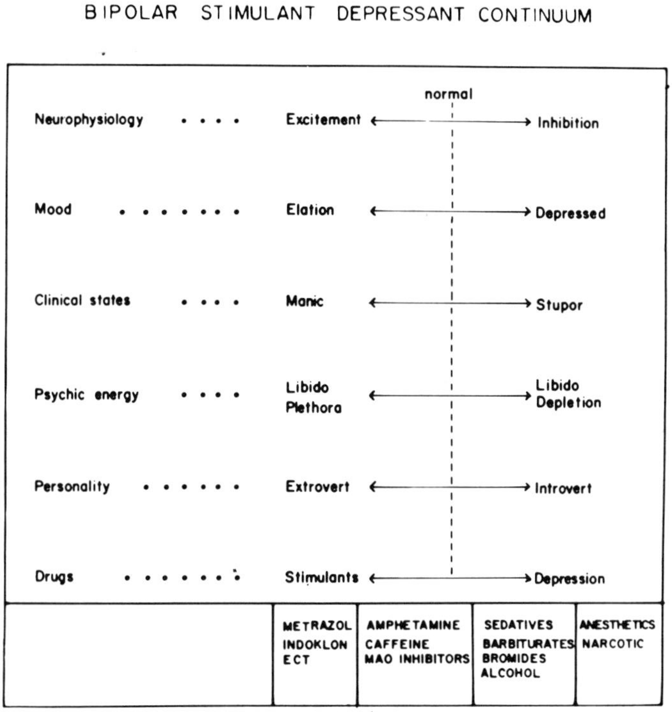

BIPOLAR STIMULANT DEPRESSANT CONTINUUM

		normal	
Neurophysiology	Excitement	← →	Inhibition
Mood	Elation	← →	Depressed
Clinical states	Manic	← →	Stupor
Psychic energy	Libido Plethora	← →	Libido Depletion
Personality	Extrovert	← →	Introvert
Drugs	Stimulants	← →	Depression
	METRAZOL INDOKLON ECT	AMPHETAMINE CAFFEINE MAO INHIBITORS	SEDATIVES BARBITURATES BROMIDES ALCOHOL / ANESTHETICS NARCOTIC

Figure 3.

depression, clinical drug evaluation must be based almost entirely on empirical therapeutic criteria rather than on knowledge of modes of action of pathological mechanisms.

The considerations about the nature of the clinical phenomena have major implications for research on brain chemistry. In addition to clinical trials with established agents, there is an important role for research on enzyme inhibitors, such as alpha-methyl-DOPA, alpha-methyl-tyrosine, and the various amino acid precursors such as DOPA and tryptophan (Bunney et al. 1968; Coppen 1967; Klerman et al. 1963; Kline and Sacks 1963; Kline, Sacks, and Simpson 1964). These investigations are important not so much because they may provide new therapeutic agents, but rather because they may offer indirect ways of testing hypotheses about the role of catecholamines and indolealkylamines in the pathogenesis of depression.

In planning these experiments, the issue of heterogeneity and possible subtypes cannot be ignored. In fact, much of the interest in developing subtypes arises out of the attempt to understand whether or not there are differential responses to imipramine. Recently, in the work on prophylactic treatment with lithium, Leonhard (1966) and the group in St. Louis (Winokur, Guze, Robins, and associates) distinguished between unipolar and bipolar affective disorders, the bipolar group including those with a history of mania (Winokur and Clayton 1967; Robins and Guze 1969). Generally, in large series (Paykel, Klerman, and Prusoff 1970), mania occurred in only about 5 percent of affective disorders within a community. Nevertheless, this 5 percent may be significant in the group specifically responsive to lithium treatment. The problem grows in magnitude when one attempts to generalize these findings to effects of lithium in the recurrent affective disorders (Angst 1961; Baastrup and Schou 1967; Schou 1968). The terminology is confusing and the diagnostic criteria have not been reliably validated. Here is where we clinicians need to bring our house in order.

The demonstration of subtypes is of considerable potential importance. Let us take as an analogous example the group of mental retardation. It is true that mongolism and phenylketonuria may represent only minorities within the group of mental retardation. Yet, research in the mongoloid group has contributed to our understanding of chromosomal anomalies, and research on phenylketonuria initiated our understanding of the aminoacidurias. A similar dissection of the large group of affective disorders into subgroups based on differential response to chemotherapy is an attractive task for the current generation of researchers. It is hoped that these patient groups can be demarcated on the basis of clinical features. This seems to be the case with responses to lithium for which the history of mania is a prime predictor. It also seems to be the case with respect to the tricyclic derivatives for which age over 40 and symptoms of the retarded, psychotic or endogenous pattern are predominant indicators. Another research strategy would be to focus on those patients who are specifically responsive to the MAO inhibitors, and selectively test one or another of the amine precursors. Here, again, the recent experience with DOPA in Parkinsonism should alert us to the need for reevaluating previous studies with precursors such as those I myself participated in, in which doses far below desirable levels may have been used.

Another major source of variability involves the patients' different abilities to metabolize the drug. Recent studies of imipramine plasma levels indicate a fantastic variability in such metabolizing. We need to develop better diagnostic techniques and to increase our knowledge of the intermediate metabolism and degradation of tricyclic derivatives.

I have attempted to review the current state of the chemotherapy of depression not only to describe the evidence for clinical efficacy but also to encourage the generating of bridges between the empirical and pragmatic treatment of patients and to create excitement about advances in the biochemistry of affective disorders. Whereas, a decade ago, research on the biochemistry of mental illness was focused on schizophrenia, in the current situation the most promising hypotheses are in the affective disorders. The earlier research on schizophrenia never realized its potential and now seems to have reached a plateau. Let us hope that ten years from now the same will not be said of the research on the biochemistry of the affective disorders.

ACKNOWLEDGMENT

Supported by Research Grant MH 13738 from the Psychopharmacology Research Branch, Division of Extramural Research Programs, National Institute of Mental Health, Health Services and Mental Health Administration, Public Health Service, Department of Health, Education and Welfare.

REFERENCES

Alexander, L. 1953. *Treatment of Mental Disorder*. Philadelphia: W. B. Saunders.

Angst, J. 1961. A clinical analysis of the effects of Tofranil in depressions. *Psychopharmacologia* 2:381.

Atkinson, R. M., and Ditman, K. S. 1965. Tranylcypromine: a review. *Clin. Pharmacol. Ther.* 6:631.

Ayd, F. J. 1960. Amitriptyline (Elavil) therapy for depressive reactions. *Psychosomatics* 1:1.

Baastrup, P. C., and Schou, M. 1967. Lithium as a prophylactic agent. Its effect against recurrent depressions and manic-depressive psychosis. *Arch. Gen. Psychiat.* 16:162.

Bunney, W. E., Jr.; Goodwin, F. K.; Davis, J. M.; and Fawcett, J. A. 1968. A behavioral-biochemical study of lithium treatment. *Amer. J. Psychiat.* 125:499.

Casey, J. F.; Hollister, L. E.; Klett, C. J.; Lasky, J. J.; and Caffey, E. M. 1961. Combined drug therapy of chronic schizophrenics. Controlled evaluation of placebo, dextroamphetamine, imipramine, isocarboxazid and trifluoperazine added to maintenance doses of chlorpromazine. *Amer. J. Psychiat.* 117:997.

Connell, P. H. 1958. *Amphetamine Psychoses*. London: Oxford University Press.

Coppen, A. J. 1967. Depressed states and indolealkylamines. In *Biological Role of Indolealkylamine Derivatives*. *Advances in Pharmacology* Vol. 6, part b. E. Costa, S. Garattini, M. Sandler, and P. Shore (eds.). New York: Academic Press, p. 283.

Dally, P. J., and Rohde, P. 1961. Comparison of antidepressant drugs in depressive illnesses. *Lancet* 1:18.

Davis, J.; Schildkraut, J. J.; and Klerman, G. L. 1967. The clinical efficacy of antidepressant drugs. Presented at annual meeting of American College of Neuropsychopharmacology, San Juan, Puerto Rico. Published 1968, Drugs used in the treatment of depression. In *Psychopharmacology, A Review of Progress 1957-1967*. Washington, D.C.: U.S. Govt. Printing Office, p. 719.

Friedman, A. S.; Granick, S.; Cohen, H. W.; and Cowitz, B. 1966. Imipramine (Tofranil) vs. placebo in hospitalized psychotic depressives (A comparison of patients' self-ratings, psychiatrists' ratings and psychological tests). *J. Psychiat. Res.* 4:13.

General Practitioner Research Group 1964. Dexamphetamine compared with inactive placebo in depression. Report of General Research Group. *Practitioner* 192:151.

Gottlieb, J. S. 1949. The use of sodium amytal and benzedrine sulfate in the symptomatic treatment of depression. *Dis. Nerv. Syst.* 10:50.

Greenblatt, M.; Grosser, G. H.; and Wechsler, H. 1962. A comparative study of selected antidepressants and EST. *Amer. J. Psychiat.* 119:144.

Greenblatt, M.; Grosser, G. H.; and Wechsler, H. 1964. Differential response of hospitalized depressed patients to somatic therapy. *Amer. J. Psychiat.* 120:935.

Hare, E. H.; Dominian, J.; and Sharpe, L. 1962. Phenelzine and dexamphetamine in depressive illness. *Brit. Med. J.* 1:9.

Kiloh, L. G., and Garside, R. F. 1963. The independence of neurotic depression and endogenous depression. *Brit. J. Psychiat.* 109:451.

Klein, D. F. 1964. Delineation of two drug-responsive anxiety syndromes. *Psychopharmacologia* 5:397.

Klerman, G. L., 1966. Modes of action of antidepressant drugs. *Pharmacotherapy of Depression*. J. Cole and J. R. Wittenborn (eds.). Springfield, Ill.: Charles C Thomas, p. 134.

Klerman, G. L. 1970. Clinical efficacy and actions of anti-psychotics. In *The Clinical Handbook of Psychopharmacology*. A. DiMascio (ed.). New York: Science House.

Klerman, G. L,, and Cole, J. O. 1965. Clinical pharmacology of imipramine and related antidepressant compounds. *Pharm. Rev.* 17:101.

Klerman, G. L., and Paykel, E. S. 1970. Depressive pattern, social background and hospitalization. *J. Nerv. Ment. Dis.* 150:466.

Klerman, G. L.; Schildkraut, J. J.; Hasenbush, L. L.; Greenblatt, M.; and Friend, D. 1963. Clinical experience with dihydroxyphenylalanine (DOPA) in depression. *J. Psychiat. Res.* 1:289.

Kline, N. S., and Sacks, W. 1963. Relief of depression within one day using an MAO inhibitor and intravenous 5-HTP. *Amer. J. Psychiat.* 120:274.

Kline, N. S.; Sacks, W.; and Simpson, G. M. 1964. Further studies on one day treatment of depression with 5-HTP. *Amer. J. Psychiat.* 121:379.

Kopin, I. J. 1968. Identification of "true" and "false" transmitters. In *Psychopharmacology, A Review of Progress 1957-1967*. Washington, D. C.: U.S. Govt. Printing Office, p. 57.

Lasagna, L. 1971. Decision processes in establishing the efficacy and safety of psychotropic drugs. *Principles and Problems in Establishing the Efficacy of Psychotropic Drugs*. Joint publication of ACNP and NIMH. Washington, D.C.: U.S. Govt. Printing Office, in press.

Legge, D., and Steinberg, H. 1962. Actions of a mixture of amphetamine and a barbiturate in man. *Brit. J. Pharmacol.* 18:490.

Lehmann, H. E. 1966. Non-MAO inhibitor antidepressants in clinical perspective. In *Antidepressant Drugs of Non-MAO Inhibitor Type*. Washington, D.C.: Public Health Service Publication, p. 122.

Leonhard, K. 1966. *Aufteilung der Endogenen Psychosen*. Third Ed. Berlin.

Litchfield, J. T. 1961. Forecasting drug effects in man from studies in laboratory animals. *J.A.M.A.* 177:34.

McKinney, W. T., and Bunney, W. E. 1969. Animal model of depression. *Arch. Gen. Psychiat.* 21:240.

Oswald, I., and Thacore, V. R. 1963. Amphetamine and phenmetrazine addiction. Physiological abnormalities in the abstinence syndrome. *Brit. Med. J.* 11:427.

Overall, J. E. 1962. Dimensions of manifest depression. *Psychiat. Res.* 1:239.

Overall, J. E.; Hollister, L. E.; and Pennington, V. 1966. Nosology of depression and differential response to drugs. *J.A.M.A.* 195:946.

Overall, J. E.; Hollister, L.; Pokorny, A.; Casey, J. F.; and Katz, G. 1962. Drug therapy in depressions. Controlled evaluation of imipramine, isocarboxazid, dextroamphetamine-amobarbital, and placebo. *Clin. Pharm. Ther.* 3:16.

Paykel, E.; Klerman, G. L.; and Prusoff, B. 1970. Treatment setting and clinical depression. *Arch. Gen. Psychiat.* 22:11.

Raskin, A.; Schulterbrandt, J. G.; Reatig, N.; and McKeon, J. J. 1970. Differential response to chlorpromazine, imipramine and placebo. *Arch. Gen. Psychiat.* 23:164.

Robin, A. A., and Wiseberg, S. 1958. A controlled trial of methylphenidate (Ritalin) in the treatment of depressive states. *J. Neurol. Neurosurg. Psychiat.* 21:55.

Robins, E., and Guze, S. B. 1971. Classification of affective disorders: the primary-secondary, the endogenous-reactive, and the neurotic-psychotic concepts. In *Recent Advances in the Psychobiology of the Depressive Illnesses*. Proceedings of a workshop sponsored by NIMH. T. A. Williams, M. M. Katz, and J. A. Shield, Jr. (eds.). Washington, D.C.: U.S. Govt. Printing Office, in press.

Rosenthal, S. H., and Klerman, G. L. 1966. Content and consistency in the endogenous depressive pattern. *Brit. J. Psychiat.* 112:471.

Schildkraut, J. J. 1970. *Neuropharmacology and the Affective Disorders*. Boston: Little, Brown.

Schou, M. 1968. Lithium in psychiatric therapy and prophylaxis. *J. Psychiat. Res.* 6:67.

Schwab, J. J.; Bialow, M.; and Brown, J. M. 1967. Sociocultural aspects of depression in medical patients II. Symptomatology and class variables. *Arch. Gen. Psychiat.* 17:539.

Tonks, C. M.; Paykel, E. S.; and Klerman, G. L. 1970. Clinical depressions among Negroes. *Amer. J. Psychiat.* 127:3.

Uhlenhuth, E. H., and Duncan, D. B. 1968. Subjective change with medical student therapists: II. Some determinants of change in psychoneurotic outpatients. *Arch. Gen. Psychiat.* 18:532.

United Kingdom Multi-Hospital Trial 1965. Medical Research Council. Clinical trial of the treatment of depressive illness. *Brit. Med. J.* 1:881.

Winokur, G., and Clayton, P. 1967. Family history studies: I. Two types of affective disorders separated according to genetic and clinical factors. In *Recent Advances in Biological Psychiatry*, vol. 9. J. Wortis (ed.). New York: Plenum Press.

Wittenborn, J. R.; Plante, M.; Burgess, F.; and Maurer, H. 1962. A comparison of imipramine, electroconvulsive therapy and placebo in the treatment of depression. *J. Nerv. Ment. Dis.* 135:131.

Wittenborn, J. R. 1968. Prediction of the individual's response to antidepressant medication. In *Psychopharmacology, A Review of Progress 1957-1967*. Washington, D.C.: U.S. Govt. Printing Office, p. 749.

INDEX

Acetylcholine
  stimulation of caudate nucleus, 113, 114
ACTH, 170, 178
Addison's disease, 172
Adrenalectomy, 168
  effect on
    ATPase activity, 187
    norepinephrine (NE) level in heart, 178
    NE brain turnover, 179, 180
    NE uptake and depletion, 179
Adrenal gland
  cofactor of tyrosine hydroxylase, 26
  cortex, 178
  pteridine-reducing enzyme, 26
  tyrosine hydroxylase, 21
Adrenocortical steroid hormones, 177
  ATPase, 187
  effect of Na^+ and K^+ in brain, 189
Affective illness, 135, 178, 237, 319
  chemotherapy, 319
  classification, 137, 163
  in children,
  unipolar and bipolar, 398
Aldosterone
  associated with ^{14}C-norepinephrine and ^{14}C-dopamine, 188
  ATPase, 187
Allopurinol, 167, 168
Aminorex
  effect on dopamine (DA) and NE conversion index, 92
  pharmacological response, 89

Amitriptyline
  effect on
    excretion of NMN:MHPG ratio, 229
    excretion of NMN:VMA ratio, 228
    NE excretion, 226
    NMN metabolism in rat brain, 230
    5-HT uptake and turnover, 216
    MHPG, 222
    NE metabolism, 217
    NE uptake and turnover, 216
    normetanephrine, 223
    VMA, 219
Amphetamine, 231, 379, 384
  as psychomotor stimulant, 383
  chick behavior, 41
  combination with barbiturate, 384
  DA, NE conversion index, 85
  depletion of NE, 83
  dopamine (DA) turnover, 83, 87
  6-hydroxydopamine, 261
  mechanism of psychosis, 53
  NE turnover, 84
  pharmacological effect, 83, 86
  rearing activity, 86
  stereotype behavior, 94
  toxic syndrome, 385
ℓ-Amphetamine
  effect on DA, NE, 87, 88
  pharmacological response, 88
Antabuse, 62, 78
Antipsychotic drugs
  chemical classes, 305
  choice of drug, 311
  clinical efficacy, 308
  pharmacological properties, 307
Arecholine, 114

ATPase
  associated with aldosterone and corticosterone, 186
  associated with catecholamine uptake, 182, 185
  ouabain action, 182
  regulation of Na^+ and K^+, 190

Barbiturates, 323
Behavior
  after α-methyl-p-tyrosine, 147, 152
  associated with low 5-HT, 173
  in rat, 38
  in White Leghorn chick, 38
  lithium toxicity, 333
  mutilation, 293
  purine metabolism, 281
  rating scale, 137
  toxicity, 354
Belladonna alkaloids, 322
Benzylamine
  as substrate of MAO isoenzyme, 9, 10, 11
Bethanechol, 114
Biogenic amines, 123
Brain
  brain stem, 32
  caudate nucleus, 113
  caudate tissue, 31, 32
  effect of adrenal steroid hormones, 179
  enzyme assays from human tissue, 39, 40
  indoleethylamine N-methyltransferase, 46, 49
  6-MeO-THBC effect on 5-HT and NE, 99, 109
  nigro-neostriatal pathway, 113
  rat, 46
  separation of MAO isoenzyme, 11
  sheep, 46
  tyrosine hydroxylase, 21, 32
  White Leghorn chick, 38
Bufotenine, 38, 53
  chick behavior, 41
  in lung, 42
  motor activity, 57
  N-methyl derivatives, 38, 53
  separation by TLC, 39
Butyrophenones, 304, 325, 332, 348
  (also see haloperidol)

Carbachol, 114
Catecholamines, 177
  associated with electrolytes, 181
  conversion index, 85, 92
  direct inhibition, 77
  drug effect on synthesis, 73, 78, 79
  feedback inhibition, 22, 27
  indirect inhibition, 79
  in plasma of depressed patient, 209
  level and biosynthesis, 29
  metabolic interaction with isoenzyme, 18
  methylation and mental illness, 37, 63
  regulation of biosynthesis, 21, 27
  synthesis, 189
  turnover, 74, 83
  turnover in hypophysectomy, adrenalectomy, thyroidectomy, and ovariectomy, 178
Catecholamine-N-methyltransferase (CNMT), 66
Catecholamine-O-methyltransferase (COMT), 66, 76
  in depressed women, 209
  L-DOPA effect, 155
Cerebrospinal fluid (CSF), 123, 124, 144, 253
Chemotherapy, 319, 379
  clinical efficacy, 380
  differential response of depression, 390
  of schizophrenia, 303-317
  prophylactic, 346, 360
p-Chloro-amphetamine, 87, 89
  effect on 5-HT depletion, 90
  effect on NE and DA, 90, 92
p-Chlorophenylalanine, 129

Chlorpromazine, 65, 80, 323, 330, 357
  dosage, 312
  lenticular deposits, 312
Chromaffin granules
  methods of homogenization, 24
  of tyrosine hydroxylase, 23, 24
Chromatography, 55, 56
  of tryptamine, 53
Cortisol, 163, 170, 172, 178, 179
  in CSF, 253
  increased NE uptake in brain slices, 179
  induced enzyme activity, 179
  in plasma in endogenous depression, 173
Cushing's disease, 172

Depression, 63, 123, 237
  associated with 5-HT and cortisol, 163
  biochemical criteria, 255
  catecholamine levels in plasma, 209
  chemotherapy, 379
  chronic, 14
  depletion of 5-HT in brain, 240
  effect of α-methyl-p-tyrosine, 152
  endogenous, 14, 164, 172, 173, 223, 243
  heterogeneity, 391
  in children, 363
  manic, 319
  MHPG excretion, 221
  neurotic, 14
  NMA levels in urine, 220
  prophylactic chemotherapy, 349
  rauwolfia alkaloid side effects, 321
  reactive, 170
  studies in patients, 137, 198
  subgroups of patients reactive to MAO inhibitors, 387
  syndrome definition, 392

Deoxyribonucleic acid (DNA), 275
Desoxycorticosterone acetate (DOCA), 178
Dexamethasone
  T3 interaction, 198
Dihydropteridine reductase, 21, 26, 29, 30
  in adrenal gland, 26
Dimethyltryptamine
  in chick, 41
  in schizophrenic patients, 61
DOM (dimethoxymethylamphetamine), 63
DOPA, 21, 27, 74, 139, 247
  effect on NE metabolism, 262
  formation, 29, 31
  in depression, 131, 135
  inhibition by epinephrine, 29
  in rat brain, 136
  in sleep, 262
DOPA decarboxylase, 77
Dopamine (DA)
  after L-DOPA administration, 136
  as false transmitter of 5-HT, 155
  depression of caudate nucleus, 117
  effect of aminorex, phenmetrazine, 90
  effect of d-amphetamine, 83
  effect on aldosterone, 188
  effect on neurons of nigro-neostriatal pathway, 113
  effect on nigral stimulation, 118
  in caudate nucleus, 113, 115
  in depression, 127
  in urine, 139, 154
  link with behavior, 63, 74
  mechanism in schizophrenia, 62, 63
  output, 31
  turnover, 80, 87, 138, 147
Dopamine-β-hydroxylase, 74, 77
Down's syndrome, 14, 17

Electric stimulation, 188
Electrolytes, Na^+, K^+, Rb^+, 177, 180

Electrolytes *(continued)*
  NE transport, 185
  NE uptake, 182, 185
  role in catecholamine disposition, 181
Electroshock, 314, 322, 356, 357
Epinephrine, 30, 198
  inhibition of DOPA formation, 29
  subcellular fraction, 23, 24

Fenfluramine, 87, 91
  depletion of 5-HT, 91
Flurothyl, 322

Gamma-amino butyric acid (GABA), 113
Gel electrophoresis, 276
Genetics, 265
  deleterious gene, 276
  frequency of polymorphism, 275
  multigenic theory in schizophrenia, 279
  study in populations, 277, 278
Gout, 281

Hallucinogens
  in chicks, 41
  in normal people, 62
Haloperidol, 325, 326, 328, 357
Hamilton rating scale, 200, 205
Histamine, 52, 62
Homocysteic acid, 116
Homovanillic acid (HVA), 67, 124
  in CSF, 144
  in urine, 139
  in urine after adrenalectomy, 178
6-Hydroxydopamine, 260
  amphetamine, 261
  REM sleep, 261
5-Hydroxyindoleacetic acid (5-HIAA), 104

  after cortisol, 165, 172
  in brain of depressed patient, 128
  in CSF, 124, 125, 138, 144
  in stressed rat, 168, 170
  in urine, 202
  in young rat, 172
  storage time for assay, 259
p-Hydroxynorephedrine, 83, 94
5-Hydroxytryptamine (5-HT), 38, 48
  associated with depression, 240
  as substrate of MAO isoenzyme, 5, 9, 10, 11
  depletion by p-chloroamphetamine, 90
  effect of fenfluramine, 91
  effect on 5-HTP, 99
  effect of 6-MeO-THBC on distribution, 97, 99
  effect of pargyline, 99
  fall after cortisol, 165
  increase in plasma, 110
  in depressed patient, 127
    in brain, 163
    turnover, 138, 147
  in Down's syndrome, 14
  in hindbrain, 127
  in sleep, 240
  in stressed rat, 168, 170
  insufficiency, 242
  in thyroid, 200
  in young rat, 172
  low levels, 173
  storage time for assay, 259
  subcellular distribution, 102
  synthesis, 164
  turnover effect by amitriptyline, 216
  uptake effect by amitriptyline, 216
  with MAOI and pretreatment, 41
5-Hydroxytryptophan (5-HTP), 38
  in rapid eye movement sleep (REM), 37
  sedation, 37
  turnover, 38
  with MAOI, 37
5-HTP decarboxylase, 98, 104
Hypomania, 139, 141

INDEX

Hypophysectomy
  effect on NE level in heart, 178
Hypoxanthine guanine phosphoribosyl transferase (HGPRT), 297
  in erythrocytes, 299
  in fibroblasts, 298

Imipramine, 130
  difference of effect in men and women, 209
  effect on catecholamine and serotonin metabolism, 203
  metabolism, 198
  thyroid interaction, 197
Indoleethylamine N-methyltransferase, 38
  assay method, 40
  in chick brain, 46, 47, 48
  in rat brain, 48
  in sheep brain, 46
  Ki of chlorpromazine and lithium, 47
  Km, 47
  pH, 52
Iontophoretic application of
  acetylcholine, 117
  dopamine, 117
  α-methyldopamine, 117
Iontophoretic dopamine, 113
Isoenzymes
  definition, 3
  gel electrophoresis for separation, 4
  MAO, 4, 5

Lactic dehydrogenase (LDH), 4
Lesch-Nyhan syndrome, 292
Lithium, 80, 327, 357
  blood levels, 333, 335, 336
  characteristic patterns of response, 331
  distribution in biological fluids, 341
  dosage, 330, 336
  effect on
    EEG, 333, 335
    endocrine function, 339, 341
    manic behavior, 330
    thyroxine, 253
    VMA excretion, 251
  excretion, 343
  for adolescents, 364
  for children, 363
  intoxication, treatment, 339, 340
  MHPG excretion, 250
  neurotoxicity, 333
  prophylactic chemotherapy, 347, 349, 350
  therapeutic regimen, 335
  thyroid dysfunction as side effect, 339
  time course, 332
  toxicology, 337, 338
  treatment of acute mania, 328, 329

Malate dehydrogenase (MDH), 277
Mania, 123, 137, 150, 151, 319
  classification, 332
  in children, 362
  research design, 359
Mescaline, 38, 63
Mestranol, 170
Metanephrine, 68
  in urine, 202
Methacholine, 114
Methionine, 61, 62
  antimetabolite, 65
  methyl group donor from, 63
Methionine sulphoximine (MSO), 65
3-Methoxy-4-hydroxymandelic acid (see vanillylmandelic acid)
3-Methoxy-4-hydroxyphenylethanol (MHPT), 67
3-Methoxy-4-hydroxyphenylglycol (MHPG), 65, 67
  excretion effect with lithium, 250
  in adrenolectomized animal urine, 178
  in CSF, 222
  in hypomanic patient, 139
  in urine, 154

3-Methoxy-4-hydroxyphenylglycol
(MHPG) *(continued)*
  in urine of depressed patients, 202, 207, 217, 221
  levels with amitryptiline, 222
6-Methoxy-1,2,3,4-tetrahydro-β-carboline (6-MeO-THBC), 97
  dose-response to 5-HT, 101
  effect on
    5-HIAA, 104
    5-HT and NE, 99, 100, 108
    5-HT subcellular distribution, 102
    5-HTP decarboxylase, 104, 107
    MAO, 102
    platelets, 106
    tryptophan hydroxylase, 104
    tryptophan pyrrolase, 104
  intracerebral, 109
3-Methoxytyramine (MTYR), 68
α-Methyldopamine, 117
α-Methyl-para-tyrosine (α-MPT), 135, 147
  behavioral effect in depression, 147
  behavioral effects in patients, 137
  in adrenalectomy, 180
  in ape, 260
  in treatment of mania, 345
  production of depressive symptoms, 241
Methysergide, 129, 344
Microiontophoresis, 115
Monoamine oxidase (MAO)
  blood separation, 14
  implication for mental disorder, 3
  in adrenalectomized animal, 178
  in developing tissue, 3, 5
  in rat brain, 5, 11
  in rat heart, 5, 9, 12
  in rat liver, 5, 13
  isoenzymes, 3
  6-MeO-THBC, 98, 102
  multiple forms, 3, 4
  pattern in adult, 5, 8, 9, 11
  in child, 5, 8, 9, 11
  in serum, 14, 15, 16, 76
  polyacrylamide gel, 5
  radioactive substrate, 11
  separation technique, 11
Monoamine oxidase inhibitor
(MAOI), 383, 385
  in subgroups of depressive patients, 387
  relation to bufotenine, 42, 62, 116
  sensitivity of isoenzyme, 5
  with tryptophan, 130
Motor activity
  decrease with lithium, 330
  effect of amphetamine, 83, 84
  effect of bufotenine, 57
  related to DA turnover, 84, 114
Muscarinic activity, 115
Mutation
  effect on gene production, 275
  neutral, 278

Neurons
  basal ganglion, 113
  caudate, 113, 115, 117
  caudate, firing rate, 118
  cholinergic, 114
  dopaminergic, 114
  firing pattern, 116
  NE in, 247
Neurotransmitter, 74
  (also see NE, 5-HT, acetylcholine, and GABA)
  neurohormonal, 247
  reuptake, 76
  uptake of drug, 81
Norepinephrine
  after L-DOPA administration, 136
  associated with rage, coping behavior, self-stimulation, appetitive behavior, 241
  associated with Rb^+, 185
  cationic regulation, 190
  compartments, 27, 84
  concentration in brain after adrenalectomy, 181

Norepinephrine *(continued)*
  -containing neurons, 247
  depletion, 84, 179
    time course, 84
  drug effect on biosynthesis, 77, 78, 79
  effect of
    aminorex, 90
    amitriptyline, 217
    5-HTP, 99
    6-MeO-THBC, 99
    pargyline, 99
    phenmetrazine, 90
    therapy, 231
    thyroidectomy and ovariectomy, 178
    tricyclic antidepressant, 215
  excretion in depressed patients, 225, 227
  in adrenalectomy and hypophysectomy, 178
  in depressed patients, 127
  inhibition of tyrosine hydroxylase, 25
  kinetics, 84
  p-Cl-amphetamine effect, 90
  synthesis and binding, 63, 74
  synthesis rate in rat brain, heart, 27
  transport, 185
  turnover, 84, 138, 147
    by amphetamine, 87
    in brain adrenalectomy, 179, 180
  uptake associated with ATPase, 182, 185, 189
    electrical stimulation, 182, 189
    K^+ and Na^+, 182, 185
    ouabain, 182
  uptake by amitriptyline and imipramine, 216
  uptake in brain slices, 179
    heart, 179
  with aldosterone, 188
Norethynodrel
  effect on 5-HT and 5-HIAA, 170

Normetanephrine, 52, 68
  amitriptyline effect, 223
  in rat brain, 215
  in urine, 202

Octopamine, 28
O-methylbufotenine, 53
Ouabain
  blocking of NE uptake, 179, 182
  inhibition of ATPase, 182
Oxotremorine, 114

Paranoid psychosis
  following amphetamine, 83
Pargyline, 38, 386
  effect of 6-hydroxydopamine after pretreatment, 260
  effect on NE and 5-HT, 42, 99
Parkinsonism, 63, 113
Phenmetrazine, 87, 89, 91, 92, 385
Phenothiazine, 62, 65, 225, 304, 323, 332, 348
  and T3 interaction, 198
Physostigmine, 114
Platelets, 100
  5-HT level, 106
Probenecid, 138, 146
Pteridine, 29
Purine
  metabolism, 281
  synthesis, 290, 291
Pyridoxal deficiency, 167
Psychosis
  manic-depressive, 319, 353
  recurrent depressive, 353
  schizo-affective, 353

Receptors
  alpha-, beta-adrenergic, 242, 245
Reserpine, 29, 32, 78, 80, 257, 258, 259
  effect on tryptophan hydroxylase activity, 58

Reserpine *(continued)*
  -produced depression, 129
  rauwolfia alkaloids, 321

Sleep, 37
  effects of DOPA, 262
  5-HT role, 46, 240
  REM, 261
Schizophrenia, 61, 265, 279
  age at admission, 272
  chemotherapy, 303, 315
  combination of drug treatment, 312
  concordance rate in twins, 266
  duration of drug treatment, 313
  environmental factors, 269, 271
  genetics, 267, 268
  relation of central adrenergic and serotonergic mechanism, 63
  response to phenothiazine, 310
  transmethylation hypothesis, 61
  types, 310
Stress, 32, 163
  immobilization, 168, 172
Sucrose density gradients
  tyrosine hydroxylase, 22
  discontinuous gradients for N-methyltransferase, 46
Sympathetic nerve
  activity in NE biosynthesis, 27

β-Tetrahydronaphthylamine, 179
Thioproperazine, 29, 31, 324
Thioridazine, 324
Thyroid
  hormone, L-triiodothyronine, (T3), 197
  hyper-, 199
  hypo-, 199
  -imipramine interaction, 197
  sex differences, 209
Thyroid-stimulating hormone
(TSH), 198, 203
Thyroxine, 178
  lithium effect, 253
Tremor
  cholinergic, 114
  dopaminergic, 114
Tricyclic antidepressants, 215, 383, 388
  (see also imipramine)
  effect on NE uptake and metabolism, 218
Tryptamine
  as substrate of MAO isoenzyme, 5, 9, 10, 11
  effect on N-methyltransferase, 47, 48, 69
  in urine, 129, 203, 207
Tryptophan, 129, 130
  in brain and plasma, 167
  metabolite, 164
  with MAOI, 130
Tryptophan hydroxylase, 59
  inhibition by p-Cl-amphetamine, 90, 98, 104
Tryptophan pyrrolase, 98, 104, 165, 170, 172
Tyrosine
  -3,5-^{3}H, 85
  -^{14}C, 136
  in sympathetic nerve activity, 27
  transaminase, 179
Tyrosine hydroxylase, 21
  activity, 28, 179
  in bovine adrenal gland, 21
  induction, 32, 179
  in rat brain, 21
  in soluble fraction, 22
  particle-bound, 21, 23
  subcellular distribution, 22

Uric acid, 282
  excretion, 290
  in serum, 284, 285, 286
Uricase, 282

Vanillylmandelic acid (VMA), 65

Vanillylmandelic acid (VMA)
(*continued*)
  chromatogram, 67
  excretion effect by lithium, 251
  in urine, 154, 202, 207, 215, 217, 220

White Leghorn chick, 38

Yohimbine, 168

Zung self-rating scale, 208